MW00396074

LIVING AHIMSA DIET

MOTHER OM MEDIA • SINKING SPRING • PENNSYLVANIA • US

LIVING
AHIMSA DIET~

NOURISHING LOVE & LIFE

BY
MAYA TIWARI

This publication provides authoritative information on diet and health, but is sold with the understanding that the author and publisher are not rendering medical advice. It is the individual reader's obligation to evaluate her or his own medical needs, to determine for herself or himself whether specific medical advice is required and where necessary, to seek the services of a qualified health care professional.

A Mother Om Media Book

Copyright © 2011 by Maya Tiwari

Illustrations & Cover Art © 2011 by Maya Tiwari

Wise Earth Ayurveda® and Living Ahimsa—The Power of Peace® are unique schools of healing principles and practices developed by Maya Tiwari and based on Vedic principles. The philosophy and practices set forth in this book are copyrighted by Maya Tiwari and the Wise Earth School of Ayurveda Ltd. All public presentation and/or use by unlicensed practitioners and teaching institutions of Wise Earth Ayurveda educational programs and their Inner Medicine® content, concepts, practices, therapies creative sadhana prototypes, tables, and graphics are copyrighted worldwide, and public use of them, or any part thereof, is strictly prohibited without formal written permission from the Wise Earth School of Ayurveda, Ltd. References to Wise Earth Ayurveda and Living Ahimsa programs may be made in other publications and other websites provided the context clearly refers to Maya Tiwari as the founder of the program with this attribution containing a link back to the respective websites: www.mypeacevow.com or www.wisearth.org.

For information about book sales please contact us at:

Mother Om Media
Sales & Marketing
P.O. Box 2094
Sinking Spring, PA 19608
E-mail: sales@motherommedia.com | Website: www.motherommedia.com

For media inquiries please contact us at:

Mother Om Media
Public Relations
P.O. Box 277
New York, NY 10014
Telephone: 646-982-7595 | E-mail: press@motherommedia.com | Website: www.motherommedia.com

All rights reserved under International and Pan-American Copyright Conventions. Published in the US by Mother Om Media.

Publisher's Cataloging-in-Publication:
Tiwari, Maya.
Living ahimsa diet : nourishing love & life / by Maya
Tiwari. -- 1st ed.
 p. cm.
 Includes index.
ISBN-13: 978-0-9793279-2-6
ISBN-10: 0-9793279-2-X
1. Nutrition. 2. Medicine, Ayurvedic. 3. Health.
4. Vegetarian cooking. I. Title.
RA784.T58 2011   613.2   QBI10-600252

Book Design by Sharon Anderson, Blue Moon Design

Printed and bound in the US

First Edition: 2011

CONTENTS

ILLUSTRATIONS

FIGURES

TABLES

DEDICATION

I dedicate this work to all who strive to cultivate ahimsa—
peace, harmony, and love—within ourselves, with others,
with all species, and to be at one with Mother Nature!

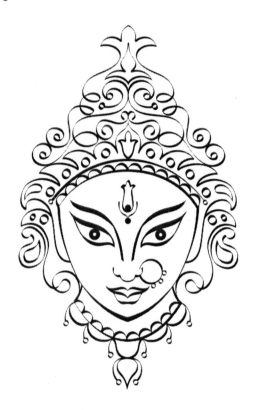

May the universe never abuse food,
Breath is food;
The body eats food,
This body rests on breath.
Breath rests on the body;
Food is resting on food.
The one who knows this
Becomes rich in food and great in fame.

— Taittiriya Upanishad 11.7

PREFACE

Years after my self-healing process, and having since helped so many others to heal themselves, I believe the most important steps for self-healing are: To stop in our tracks, be still, take pause, and allow time to breathe and reflect. The first cosmic law of *ahimsa*, practicing non-harm, informs that to fulfill our humanity as a whole person, we must strengthen our capacity to gain awareness. Awareness informs the mind of reason, logic, critical thinking, and understanding. It helps us to reconcile the habituations of daily life and to create the necessary time and space to imbibe regular pause. Once we foster this space (which is both internal and eternal), we discover the freedom to be at ease with ourselves, to reclaim our vast inner resources of love and light, and ultimately, to conquer fear, hurt, and despair.

In modern culture, disease is the only condition that gives a person the irrefutable license to immediately take leave from daily haggles to create the necessary space for retreating into the self. To take advantage of this opportunity, we need to address a common misperception that thwarts our healing process and converts it into an uphill battle. We must discard erroneous notions such as, "I can't take time for myself right now," or "I have too many other commitments to take care of," or "there is no way I can create time to do this." It is critical that we take a long, deep pause when we are facing a major challenge. The first rule of healing is that nothing else is as important as our well-being, and for this the art of pause is our greatest medicine! Once we recognize that this pause is not only essential, but also an imperative part of the rhythm of maintaining a sentient mind and healthful body, we have no choice but to take pause. We can emulate the seasons by bearing witness to their cyclical movements, pauses, and junctures. Recognize "pause" as the golden gift of sanity, mindfulness, health, and healing! Once we take pause, the process of settling into our serenity happens naturally.

I also whole-heartedly believe that we must trust that each healing crisis has its profound reason for being. It shows us how the path of disease is hallowed in the condition of who we are at that moment in time. When we learn to view illness as a time to rest and resolve inner conflict—a necessary break that gives us a chance to get back into our physical, emotional, and spiritual bodies—we can begin to reclaim the love and life necessary to dissolve negative karmas, and ward off hurt, injury, and despair. I emphasize: To cultivate this awareness we must take time to pause, reflect, and be at one with what appears to be broken inside of us. We must step back, hang loose, and put aside an over-packed and scheduled life and instead create a simple, sheltered space that is serene, uncluttered, and distanced from the baggage of our present living conditions.

HARVESTING AWARENESS & NOURISHMENT

Although *Living Ahimsa Diet: Nourishing Love & Life* primary focuses on food, true healing is not about the foods we eat, the medicines we consume, or how many yoga classes we attend weekly. It is about how we respond to everyday lifestyle choices that we make regarding our meals, medicines, relationships, family, work, and other activities—and our responses invariably equal the degree of awareness we cultivate in our lives. Among a complex mix of things, healing is about our karma, lost dreams, unfulfilled desires, and sometimes, just the plain reality of fatigue, disillusionment, and exhaustion. Crisis, like healing, is an organic juncture in the life of each and every person, rich and poor, great and small, sages and the not so saintly. When we recognize that these junctures invoke the overarching energy that supports all forms of healing, we are made whole again, so much brighter than before. The only way we can be broken or felled by disease or illness, or any other challenge for that matter, is when we respond to it as a punishment, an inconvenience, or as an intruder. (Mind you, disease becomes an intruder when we fail to recognize the gift it brings.)

Within these pages, we will explore how our bodies are made up of consciousness and spirit, and are connected to the greater continuum of energies through memory. In order to heal, we need to appease vital tissue memory and nourish and nurture the whole self. In essence, we need to reorder the same internal energy that went into disorder and creating a disease, and bring it back into a state of harmony. For this, we have to reclaim a wholesome diet, nourishment, and nurturance in the way we eat, think, breath and move, and in the sounds we create. This is a significant way to engender love within and without. When we feel nourished, the more commonsensical, intuitive, and aware we become.

I recognize that my readers are in many different levels of practice, from dedicated instructors to people who like yoga but have an "average" urban life (smoking or working under pressure, for example). It is important to know that self-healing is possible for everyone. We do not require an extraordinary level of practice and discipline, or faith and courage. We all can access that level of awareness that allows us to cure ourselves. Each one of us possesses innate power to heal, to love, and to be whole. We do not need a college education or intense spiritual discipline, or 24/7 holistic practices to be commonsensical, or to learn the wholesome way of nourishment. The most critical obstacles in the way of healing are a lack of honesty with ourselves about our current issues, and not being willing to face the truth of who we are and where we are on our life's journey. Before we can call upon faith, we must arrive at and cross over this critical juncture; it is the same juncture for each and every one of us, regardless of the degree of our education, or nature of ancestry, condition, or culture. As soon as we are able to voice the truth of our innermost selves and say, "Enough!", "I do not want to hurt anymore!", "I will strive to live a peaceful life", "I want to be happy, to be fulfilled!"—we attract what we need to progressively move forward. The benevolent grace of the universe immediately comes to our aid. Trusting this truth is what faith is about. On the heels of faith comes the absolute cure: Love.

HONOR THE PROCESS

In self-healing the process is all there is. We discover that healing is an organic function within us. In aligning ourselves from the onset to this truth, we reveal the hidden cavern of unresolved desire, fear, weakness, and hurt transported from generation to generation, from life to life through the cycle of rebirth. Our illness or distress is ours alone; we cannot live anyone else's karma, or their illness, their happiness, or their process. Whatever is the challenge, and however we feel about it (right or wrong), the glory and the fight is ours and the way we get through it—the process—is also specific to our individual karma—the content and context of who we are and where we are on our life's path. The goal through any challenge is to heal. However, the only way we can accomplish this goal is by accepting what is and invoking a clear intent to honor the journey however it unfolds.

We are better equipped to influence a successful outcome when we understand how critical it is to honor our process, however unexpected or challenging it may be. The process is often hard to face because it is not so pretty. It necessitates, at the heart of it, journeying to that place which is hidden, that place of "stuckness" and staleness that needs to be shaken loose and brazened out. If we are able to face it head-on, we open up to spirit and find resolve. In so doing, we develop a greater awareness of who we are, where we are going, and the nature of our purpose. In other words, we find our golden wings. This is what wellness and lightness of being is about—the growth we earn that ultimately brings harmony, love, and happiness to the fore. Healing is about mothering, accepting and loving the self; it requires courage to embrace and honor our progression. Bear in mind, this course of action is sacred, and requires a sanctum of privacy around it. To expunge negative energy, it is best you create a retreat for yourself so that you can more easily open the shroud to reveal honesty. It is equally important that the process be witnessed by one other person with whom you feel intimate in spirit—a spouse or a friend who listens and hears you, and who would never judge you or your process.

LOVE IS THE WAY

The Living Ahimsa way of love—the foundation of this book—is about cultivating inner harmony and light for all the length of our days. Love is always at the heart of healing. Ultimately, the truth of self-healing and spirituality is rooted in faith—that of love and compassion. As we move into the Golden Age, more and more of the general population is concluding that the old structures of organized religion, complicated philosophy, and hierarchical doctrines are outdated and must be reordered with awareness and light for all. Once we are aware of the power of our own awareness and ongoing interconnectedness to the universe, we can energetically change the worn out system that is bankrupting love and life instead of sustaining it. The simple fact is: The canons of cosmic reality and their impact on our memory's ability to retain wellness, love, and compassion must be understood if we are to harvest faith that is infinite and unfractured. If we do not have a basic comprehension of our indelible relationship to the cosmos, it would be extremely difficult to maintain our awareness, and thus our priority for love, happiness, harmony, and wellness, even when we are committed to doing so.

This work is delivered from the passion of grace and prayer, from the fullness of devout love that comes from unearthing the ancient soil of my soul. After thirty years of witnessing the miracles of healing in thousands of ways with thousands of people, I know that self-healing is always about love. Love is the tangible and illusive energy that we must never let go of. Whatever may be the illness, challenge, difficulty, disappointment, and crisis in your life, hold on to this implacable truth: You are loved. And you have the power to refill love from within. Even when love is betrayed, or when we lose a loved one, love can never be taken away from you, because you are love! I am Love! Every tissue, cell, and memory of my being is composed of the cosmically divine material of love. How well we know this certainty about ourselves is the degree to which we will use the wisdom in these pages to heal and transform everything else in our lives.

INNER LIGHT MEDITATION

The Inner Light Meditation that follows will prove to be immediately helpful in cultivating awareness through the simple art of pause, allowing the mind, emotions, and uncertainty to settle. Remember, it is not about finding immediate answers to a dilemma, but rather, about discovering the right questions. This clarity comes naturally from a mind that is poised in ease while processing the turbulence of thoughts, emotions, guilt, fear, and so on. Let us enjoin spirit and begin our journey through these leaves as One Light.

- Set up a candle (made from beeswax, or organic material) or a ghee lamp on your altar, or on a low table in a serene place in your home.
- Sit comfortably in front of the flame, preferably on the ground. Gently gaze at the flame for about ten minutes. Try not to blink.
- Follow the flickering flame with your eyes. Let your mind merge into the flame.
- Envision the outer light as your inner light. See the light permeating your heart chakra.

- Empty the mind of thoughts, offer them to the flame. Empty the heart of hurt, despair, anxiety, and loneliness.
- Ask the flame to inherit all negative emotions. It will purify your thoughts and calm the heart.
- Close your eyes softly. Continue to envision the flame in the space of your third eye, center of the forehead.
- Keep the following avowal in the background of your mind:

I am love, I am light. I am awareness.
Everything I see reveals this love.
Everything I touch reveals this light.
Everything I think reveals this awareness.

- Sit in your serenity and let this confirmation float lightly in the mind.

Peace be your journey!

Love and Blessings,
Maya Tiwari

ACKNOWLEDGMENTS

I have been blessed with an extraordinary journey—a continual unfolding of Divine Grace that serves to instigate a deep understanding of our nature in love and harmony. I am eternally grateful for all of the blessings showered me in this life, and especially for the trillions of unconditional gifts given to me by Mother Nature.

My devout reverence to the *Mother Consciousness*, who protects and guides my journey and whose work it is I serve. A sequel to my first book, *Ayurveda: A Life of Balance*, these pages continue to explore revelations from the Mother Consciousness, her powerful nature, her food and its impact on the nourishment of body, mind, memory, and spirit. This work came to fruition through the help and diligent care of many people. Firstly, I want to name Catherine Elliott Escobedo, editor-in-chief of Mother Om Media, for her excellent skills and intuitive approach with editing, proofreading, and the publishing process—her input to this work altogether is too numerous to list here; and Sharon Sita Anderson for her tireless efforts, devotion to my work, and her excellent creative work in designing this book. I thank Charles Sakshat Corbit for his heartful service at Mother Om Media and to my work at large. I thank Marnie Mikell for her artistic contribution to refining my illustrations used in this book.

I wish to thank Nina Usha Molin, MD and Sarita Linda Rocco for their stalwart efforts in disseminating Wise Earth Ayurveda education and instructorship training. Indeed, my thanks to all Wise Earth Ayurveda instructors at large who teach this work in communities all over the world. My profound gratitude to Mother Om Mission's coordinators, Arjuna Boodoo, Emerita Foster, and Alicia Jorwar, for their exhaustive efforts in serving at-risk communities with Mother Om Mission education and services. Let me also thank Lisa Insanally for her kindness and exhaustive efforts at Mother Om Mission, Guyana.

Infinite gratitude to my beloved spiritual teacher, His Holiness, Swami Dayananda Sarasvati, for the knowledge he has given me, and the grace, love, and beneficence to which I aspire. I acknowledge my birth mother, Kali Devi, and my elder mother, Jaya Devi, and the divinity they have imbued in me. My appreciation goes to my friends, Ian and Margaret Howard-Smith, for their immense personal support and generous contribution to Mother Om Mission work.

Finally, my profound gratitude goes to my guiding Seraph whose immense love rescued me from my recent healing odyssey, and awakened my heart to the deeper energy of love that is the foundation of the universe and this work. May we remember to serve the Mother Consciousness with grace, love, and gratitude.

INTRODUCTION

Neither peace nor health can be gained without first
cultivating inner harmony and health for all humankind.
Food for one must be health for all. Prosperity for one
must be abundance for all. Harmony cannot be achieved
at any level while any form of life suffers.

Thirty-six years following my odyssey through ovarian cancer, and twenty-seven years since seriously embarking on the spiritual path, I am continually reminded that the most important achievement any one of us can strive for is to harness personal awareness—our ability to preserve sacred spirit, a serene mind, and a healthful body. For too long we have contributed to the erroneous belief that disease and despair, like war and poverty, are inevitable occurrences in our lives. This is false. Our basic nature is rooted in ahimsa, good health, and inner harmony. Although disease, like death, is a natural occurrence in life, it does not have to be inevitable.

At the onset of this book, I want to explain why this important work of Living Ahimsa—a lifestyle committed to the practice of inner harmony and non-harm—focuses on *food.* Although there are millions of books and thousands or more disciplines about food and diet, the meaning and purpose of food still eludes us. The deep wisdom of the earth's nourishment that supports the development of awareness in body, mind, and spirit remains a mystery—that is, until now.

Food is never inert energy. Although we pluck it from the earth or its mother plant, prepare it or cook it, food holds an irreplaceable and complex set of memories that inform the vital functions of the body, mind, and spirit. Created from timeless generations on this planet, food is a living instrument of peace, health, prosperity, and consciousness. Within these pages we will explore our personal relationship to food and examine the deeper values of nature's nourishment; how the universe gives birth to her six seasons (in the Vedic Calendar); and how each food is directly related to its mother season (nature), composed of the ancient earth and her elements: earth, water, air, fire, and space.

Food's nourishment is our most imperative foundation of health, harmony, and consciousness. "Food is universal medicine. All life came into existence out of food. Food precedes all creatures in the order of creation." The *Taittiriya Upanishad* shares its perennial wisdom on the priceless healing power of plant food, *annam,* for people and the planet. All traditional systems of medicine honor the plant as the oldest form of medicine on earth. More and more, as we discover "new" herbs in the West, we find that traditional cultures all over the world have been using that same plant as medicine for hundreds or even thousands of years.

In fact, there is nothing new about the healing power of plants. What is new and revolutionary is our nonchalant attitude and careless approach to sacred nourishment. The world's food sources have been spiraling into degradation for more than a century. The perennial destruction of nature, the tireless onslaught of contaminants and poisons, and the engineered perversions and distortions are progressively contributing to the adversity of our nourishment. Indeed, it is a great wonderment that we can still eke out any form of joy, healing, and communal spirit from the present disastrous state of our food sources! But thankfully, we are equipped with an immutable human spirit and can therefore remedy this appalling situation. To heal, nourish, and nurture is the gift of our human nature. We must at once fervently call upon it.

Food is the only sentient matter that connects us to the memory of our karmas: past, present, and future; it is the only material substance that can advance our cosmic nature so we can discover who we truly are. In short, food can reveal our unique make-up of personal karma. Food is not merely the fodder we consume to satisfy our palates and senses. Through good health, which depends on wholesome food, we begin to see that our personal history is not about the past, but about *what we need to know about our past*. No one can alleviate the karmas of hurt, pain, and despair for us, but we can learn to reclaim a sense of wholeness in the spirit of ahimsa. In so doing, we can nourish our body and mind to wipe the slate of karmas clean of ancestral grief and burdens. Mother Nature's foods hold the memories of our forebears. Food is memory. Eating is remembering.

Although we will be exploring our relationship to food within these pages, this book is clearly not about "food" as we know it. It is about recognizing the principle and practice of ahimsa in our food—our first pillar of health and abundance. As you will discover, the centrifugal force that propels personal transformation can be summed up in two words: Living Ahimsa. To repair the violence done to nature, we must first heal the violence within ourselves. *We are nature*, and therefore it is only natural that we reclaim inner harmony and an immutable sense of nurturance. This is the reason why Living Ahimsa is ultimately the most important practice we can endeavor.

Within these pages, we will learn the necessity of reclaiming our spirit of ahimsa— good health, joy, inner harmony, and abundance for ourselves, our family, and our community. Once we set the *sankalpa*, sacred intention, of practicing ahimsa in our daily lives, it goes to work building a life of harmony, health, and non-hurting. As we explore food through the naked lens of ahimsa, my hope is that you will discover, as I did, that food is the heart of matter, the mind of memory, the imprint of our ancestors, the seed of our newborn, the spirit of our family, the land, river, sky, mountain, and universe.

The teachings within this book have been honed from more than a quarter-century of work in the Living Ahimsa principles and practices which inform that harmony and peace, like violence and despair, begin in the mind before they evolve into our foods, thoughts, actions, and lifestyles. It teaches us to embrace the diverse and manifold realities of life regardless of the differences in our cultures, traditions, and belief systems. To be whole, we must heal our culture of hurt by cultivating the work of ahimsa within ourselves. To cultivate awareness, we must first learn how to mitigate violence in a peaceful way to create harmony in ourselves, nature, and in our nourishment. Neither peace nor health can be gained without first cultivating inner harmony and health for all humankind. Food for one must be health for all. Prosperity for one must be abundance for all. Harmony cannot be achieved at any level while any form of life suffers.

I have discovered in the course of this lifetime that the more challenging the juncture, the more illumined my awareness becomes. Before this realization, I recognized that painful stages were caused by a lack of nourishment at some level of my being. A rich sense of nourishment is essential for maintaining a state of balance and harmony within. Good nourishment helps us to comfortably negotiate arduous or painful junctures in our lives. It helps us to mitigate these junctions in such a way that pain does not foster hurt, despair, disappointment, or hopelessness. In fact, in Living Ahimsa, we discover that each juncture of hurt, pain, and disease can prove to be a definitive conduit through which we become wholly renewed. Such renewal brings growth and maturity that progresses the mind, body, and spirit into a higher plane of love and awareness.

When we lose control of our wellness through illness or adversity, we need to recognize that we are being given an even greater chance to reclaim the spirit of nurturance and healing—to experience rebirth. We should accept the divine reality that body and mind will—and should—unravel and become undone from time to time. As such, we must surrender to this holy undoing. This elusive act is a necessary and progressive movement of the human psychic anatomy. In order to grow, we must not obstruct the creation and formatting of new life. Once we understand how important nourishment is to the vital human system, and how to harvest the awareness necessary to catapult us from juncture to juncture in the ever-growing process of awareness, we can embrace the broken pieces of ourselves, and recognize this phenomenon as an act of surrender to the divine will. Awareness serves to transform hurt, despair, and alienation into an illumined journey of self-love and self-discovery. The gems of our human spirit can never be taken away from us regardless of the multitude of violations we may endure.

You will discover throughout this book that the crossings we experience in life are the same ones nature experiences transitioning through the changing of seasons. Living, and eating, in harmony with the seasons is the fundamental act of love and nourishment, central to Living Ahimsa. According to Ayurveda, every physical thing in the universe is created by the same five elements. Thus, we are formed from the same ingredients as the trees, sky, sun, and grains of sand or drops of rain. The five elements in our foods feed the five elements in our bodies. Essentially, the elements of Mother Nature's seasonal foods are energetically and nutritionally designed to feed, nourish, and heal each and every one of the *dhatus* (vital tissues) of the body, mind, and senses in accord with their innate requirements, both divine and mundane.

In this work, we will learn to make food choices through our interaction with the rhythms, cycles, and stages of nature. Did you know that the seven stages of a fruitful plant are identical to the seven stages of a fruitful human life? The life cycle of a plant begins with a good seed, one that retains its essential nature from the well of universal memory and has not been tampered with or genetically manipulated. The seed transforms to sprout, young plant, mature plant, flowering plant, fruitful plant, and then returns back to the earth as seed. At every stage, the plant may be harvested and prepared as food. After it has been ingested, physically and spiritually nourishing a human being, the waste and roughage are restored to the earth. There, peacefully huddled in the womb of the Mother, the seed awaits its moment in time to emerge, then pierces through the earth to fulfill its cosmic destiny.

Our vital tissues are continually being honed by nature's rhythms with or without our awareness. By imbibing nature's foods in harmony with the seasons we are able to foster enormous strength within the body and develop a kinship with the seasonal rhythms. This is why the ancients remained attentive to the cyclical changes of both the inner and outer rhythms during each season and its transition into another. Food also feeds the mind as well as it nourishes the body; once the body is properly nourished, the mind is fed. Fulfilled with essential nourishment, we can easily transcend challenges to reclaiming our consciousness. Once harvested, consciousness influences how we respond to each and every circumstance and experience in our lives. Health, healing, and harmony are the ultimate result of nature's essential nourishment.

As any organic tender of the good earth will tell you, living by the sacred principles I will teach you—honoring the self and nature and her seasons—generates an abundance of individual health and communal harmony. To learn the cosmic secrets of Mother Nature, the *rishis* did not conduct scientific evaluations, fractionalization, or fragmentation of the good earth, her provisions, and her creatures. At one time, human intelligence was sufficient to analyze without fracturing, to know without dissecting, to trust without fear the simple wisdoms in the life of the living. We understood how living in tune with nature nourished our cosmic nature and did not obsess with superficial analysis of the protein-carbohydrate ratio in the digestive process or determine the caloric content of food.

Through the Wise Earth Ayurveda perspective of energy—a profound body of knowledge that I have developed and been teaching for 27 years—I have developed a supreme way of seeing and understanding the nature of the whole, and therefore, also its parts. A holistic system, Ayurveda cures by removing the source of disease and unhappiness, which can only happen after we *identify* the source of the disease—not just the symptoms. According to Ayurveda, the unique construction of each person holds vital clues to the quantity, quality, and nature of food an individual body requires. Intake must be balanced with the size, shape, and gender of the human *prakriti*, metabolic constitution, and each person has a unique metabolic constitution requiring specific treatments, foods, and fulfillments. For instance, when we cup our hands together (Anjali Mudra), we can measure the exact quantity of food that our stomach is designed to hold. And when we close our hands with palms touching, we send a signal to our digestive system that we are filled and satisfied, prompting it to wind down its operations.

Like all of my books, *Living Ahimsa Diet: Nourishing Love & Life* reveals many precious practices from my tradition that are intended to serve you as a sentient, conscious person striving for the knowledge of the Whole. These practices will help you better understand your infinite human power of awareness, inner harmony, and sentiency—the education and focus of the Vedas. Utilized in this spirit, these teachings enhance your own cultural or ancestral roots, while expanding awareness of cosmic wholeness.

Understanding why we use Vedic iconography and practices is important; these are not merely iconic beliefs or ornamental applications to be used for aesthetic purposes. Each icon is allegorical to a profound cosmological meaning and has significant impact upon the human mind and anatomy. Each *yantra*, *mantra*, or *asana* (yoga posture) for example, specifically replicates the sonic architectural patterns of the cosmos; therefore, when we imbibe these practices we enhance our flow of energy and trigger the identical response in nature.

As we develop our awareness through the practices in this book, we are better equipped to maintain the vibrational energy that protects love, compassion, healing, and happiness in our lives. These are simply emotional components of divinity transcended into material forms. In order to sustain these qualities in life, we must keep the vibratory field of cosmic intelligence alive and well, a critical reason why learning the vast allegorical weave of the universe's tapestry is vital to maintaining our absolute well-being. And we do not have to be a Hindu, a Pagan, Muslim, a Christian, or any other religious follower to do so. All we need do is become a conscious person with a commitment to strengthening awareness, and inner harmony: Living Ahimsa.

Along with firm reverence to Mother Nature, may the energy and wisdom in this work help to support you in whichever environment you live. It is in this spirit that I share this work. May it reach every person who seeks inner harmony, wholesome health, and world peace. May it manifest in beauty through the dream state of those who are not yet awakened to their magnificent purpose.

Part One

NOURISHING,
NURTURING & HEALING

Chapter One

HARMONY OF BODY, MIND & FOOD

We must stop the bleeding.
We must stop the hurting.
We must stop the killing.
We must become the light we strive for.

My intention in writing this book is to shift your overall awareness of food so you can learn to honor it as a primary resource for achieving excellent health and personal awareness. Within these pages, I hope to evoke a sense of what nourishment, healing, and harmony feels like within you. Some of us have very little experience, if any, with these states of being, but the power to heal and the ability to feel harmony and peace has always been within our grasp.

This ability, imbued within each of us, is part of the vast stock of cosmic resources we are given at birth. It is what I call our *Inner Medicine*—a concept I will discuss at length within these pages—and it holds our greatest potential for creating harmony, peace, and abundance for all. In order to gain access to our limitless reserve of Inner Medicine, we must first explore the subtle power of food and its intrinsic energy of ahimsa—the path of non-harm that leads to inner harmony.

First and foremost, in these pages, you will learn the necessity of reclaiming your spirit of ahimsa, and by extension, broadcasting good health, joy, and abundance to your family and community. When we understand the cyclical wisdom from which life is nourished, nurtured, and healed, we can fully awaken to our joy, freedom, and a life of non-hurting—we can learn how to cultivate our inner stock of harmony and heighten our personal field of awareness.

As we learn in this education, the greatest prosperity and joy is held within the self. Your stock of Inner Medicine, once accessed, spills forth to bless everyone and everything around you. We are in a time of massive transition away from the dark days of centuries-long human activities that have been injuring the Mother Consciousness—the maternal bedrock of the universe from which all life is nourished and sustained. Now, in the broken pieces of social, economic, emotional, nutritional, and spiritual security, we each have a golden chance to see the light, to garner the awareness necessary to be a torch for hope and love. We must slim down the excesses, gather our dreams closer, and own the right to fulfill our hopes.

We must stop the bleeding. We must stop the hurting. We must stop the killing. We must become the light we strive for. This is the essence of my Living Ahimsa teachings.

In this book, you will find Living Ahimsa practices that support nature and our food, and nurture the body, mind, speech, and actions of everyday life. By developing an awareness of harmony, we reject violence, transform negative karmas, and create unlimited access to consciousness. Once healing begins, personal awareness shifts into global consciousness and the Mind of Peace emerges.

Each one of us can help heal millions of lives, one at a time, by transforming our own disease, poverty, and despair into health, harmony, and prosperity. This work is centered on the cultivation of harmony in our lives. We can achieve this by focusing on the inevitable starting point—*food*, and by strengthening our most precious asset—*awareness*. Without cultivating our innate ability of awareness it would be impossible to preserve the integrity of our nourishment and health. Therefore, let's begin by exploring the meaning of "personal awareness."

MADE OF HARMONY

I discovered in my early journeys that life is not about pursuing multiple pathways, fostering ambition or an unfathomable sense of ego—pursuits destined to fracture us in one way or another. Life has designed for us one true path—a path that guarantees each of us the right to live in harmony and integrity with all things. This path is clearly laid out for us when we look through the eyes of awareness. Although it appears that we have trillions of choices thrust upon us each day, for those who seek harmony and vibrancy in our lives we truly have but one—to cultivate greater awareness. Ultimately, it is the most sublime choice we have as human beings.

Discovering how we are essentially created from harmony, by harmony, and for harmony is rewarding work for those of you who find yourselves at a pivotal junction in your journey toward the light, as I did so many decades ago. I developed the work of Living Ahimsa—The Power of Peace as a direct response to the hurt and pain I felt during my years prior to cancer. Moreover, I have seen the devastation of hurt, despair, disease, and disharmony as I walk my journey of guiding, helping, and working with thousands of individuals and hundreds of communities over the past 30 years.

As many of you know, more than 30 years ago I walked though the firestorm of ovarian cancer that raged an internal war of pain, hurt, and despair within me. My "basic necessity body" emerged from the fiery ashes, a body held together by the light of the Mother Consciousness. Though the cancer randomly ravished my physical body, it opened a multi-dimensional vista to the place where my subtle body resides. What I did not understand at that time, but have since discovered, is that if we are completely committed to spirit, we may gain entry to the phenomenal realm where spirit and body meet, and there find healing. This is precisely what happened to me. The Living Ahimsa education teaches that we do not need to walk through the fiery ashes of deep illness to find this realm of peace.

Everyone is sensitive to love and kindness, but we are instinctively more sensitive to hurt and pain. Our common challenge is that we are not always as attuned to acts of kindness as we are to the conditions that create hurt. This is largely because *himsa*, hurt, is felt by the highly impressionable psyche. Implanted within the memories of our vital tissues, the feelings of hurt and despair can play out generation after generation like a merciless windstorm.

In the present culture we are so blocked from spirit that we have progressively become more preoccupied with our ambitions, medicines, pains, and illnesses than we are of our Inner Medicine healing capacity. But this is not a book about psychology; it is a book about your well-being—the promise of a new way to achieve the ancient peace. It is about reclaiming your body of health; your Mind of Peace; and about making ahimsa your first priority. First though, we must refuse to live with the burden of hurt.

LIVING AHIMSA: THE LAW OF NON-HURTING

It is the divine drive within us to strive for peace—to feel good, to have plenty of food, and to laugh and thrive in the fullness of life. Our natural tendency is to lead a life of non-harm, what my tradition calls "ahimsa." Living Ahimsa is about cultivating personal awareness and consciously making this a primary goal in our everyday lives. It is a way of life that includes everything from the way we think, to what we eat, to how we respond to everything around us, in general and specifically. When we become accustomed to the remarkable achievement of culling awareness within our minds, it immediately transforms our thoughts, speech, and actions, and restricts us from causing injury, pain, or hurt to the self or any living being at any time. In turn, our physical health is safeguarded. We see beauty only from the untainted Mind of Ahimsa—the Mind of Peace. To experience this reality we must explore living as conscious beings.

The Vedic way of living is rooted in the system of *dharma*, or cosmic law. From the beginning, my tradition has advocated harmony among all people and all life forms, and this awareness has led to the ethical virtues that form the roots of the Hindu lifestyle of non-violence and compassion—reverence for all forms of life and the protection of nature's resources. But over time this sense of harmony has dramatically deteriorated within my own tradition, as it has across other traditions as well. Influenced as we are by the shifting and unstable landscapes of modernity—accompanied by ignorance and afflicted awareness—a majority of people have learned to live by means of their senses and desires. We have adopted the idea that compassion, harmony, and health can actually exist apart from the food we eat, the air we breathe, the water we drink, and the thoughts we think. We ignore the fact that nature's sacred food for human sustenance is a profound gift of life, nourishment, and nurturance—the axial point from which all grace propagates. Food gives us life; therefore we must bring our attention to preserving harmony and health in nature's food source. It is time we awaken to the wisdom of the human spirit and recognize that food is the primary sustenance for humanity; without food the body expires, breath desists, life ends, and the planet dies.

Living Ahimsa means living a life of non-hurting instead of a life of hurt. If the paramount karma of humanity is to manifest harmony during this transformational time, then we must first understand what it means to live healthfully and peacefully. If we are secure in this knowledge, we can easily attain health and harmony. We must shift our thinking and our beliefs. To mine the treasure trove of the heart and reap abundant health and prosperity, we must make a commitment to cultivate inner harmony our first priority. In so doing, we become aware of the great challenges endured by Mother Nature—our source of light, water, and food. This basic shift in thinking will guide us to make a difference in our personal lives. Each one of us can make a substantial difference in preserving harmony; peace, health, and harmony all begin in the awareness of self.

At the end of this chapter I have set out a most effective practice for building awareness, The Vow of Ahimsa. You can call on this incredible practice any time you experience a sense of loss, feel un-nurtured, un-done, disappointed, hurt, angry, lonely, or grief of any kind. By taking The Vow of Ahimsa, you are declaring your intention to heal and be whole. In turn, the universal energies will help you to achieve your sacred goal.

The wording of this vow is not embedded in stone. The vow itself is a simple, malleable instrument of peace, whose seed already lies within you to help you remember the path to harmony. Each time you feel hurt or despair you can recite this vow to help you remember that you are healing at every moment. In fact, as one of the thousands of advocates who are already practicing this vow puts it, "Whenever I falter with my Vow of Ahimsa by going into that space of hurt and ill-thinking, the vow gnaws at me. It calls to me and keeps on gnawing until I respond by voicing my vow."

The revolutionary Living Ahimsa practices, which we also call *sadhanas* in Wise Earth Ayurveda, awaken the senses and our ability to connect to the greater energies of the universe. You learn to experience a sense of complete fulfillment through the art of feasting the body, mind, and soul with love and harmony. In fasting, you learn to hear the sounds of your inner self, and gain access to your Inner Medicine in order to heal yourself, nature, and all things that surround you, without medicine! This work is about rejoicing nature by feeding, feasting, fasting, nourishing, and nurturing the body, mind, and spirit.

Living Ahimsa Diet: Nourishing Love & Life provides you with the ultimate spiritual guide to maintaining a life of inner harmony in your food, your thoughts, your emotions, and your actions.

VIOLENCE IN THE FOOD SOURCE

Healing is perennial. It is not about popular phrases, trendy workshops, or obsessive practices. All healing is rooted in the cultivation of personal awareness. Having served more than a quarter of a century teaching this work, it is sometimes overwhelming to witness the rapidity of our collective movement toward impending health, economic, environmental, social, familial, and individual crisis. *Now* is the time to stop the oncoming trend of hurtful diets and diseases from taking hold among yet another generation. We have got to take immediate curative measures, as our intrinsic spiritual abundance is at grave risk.

Through the practice of Living Ahimsa we can safeguard our food source—stemming from the health of our lands, rivers, skies, and atmosphere—in order to prevent the current dilemma that is insidiously poisoning the body, mind, and spirit of our population. Through the practice of Living Ahimsa we can stop the rampant violence, disease, and despair in what's left of our communities. The interpersonal wisdom set out in these pages will help us to heal by awakening our ahimsa-conscience and invoking our inimitable sense of awareness.

Presently, we are invested in endless scientific research, costing trillions of dollars, in the areas of food, diet, and health, yet the fight against disease is failing. This predicament arises in great part from the popularized "killer diet" that has replaced a diet consisting of wholesome foods, a fact that prompts a multitude of questions: Why is the population deliberately imbibing harmful and unhealthy foods? Does this malady arise from personal choice or by designed addiction? Certainly, even the least educated person would realize that consuming polluted "fast foods," commercially grown foods, or genetically engineered "cloned or mutated foods" would negatively impact one's health and well-being. But that appears *not* to be the case. Many seem to be unaware that these so-called "food" products create potentially lethal forms of addiction, habit-forming behaviors that do not nourish, nurture, and heal. One of the most significant questions we can ask is: Why is there so little education that these unhealthful foods are linked to disease, despair, and disharmony, not only in the human population but in all species and the planet itself?

THE SHAME OF IT ALL

More than 40 years ago, the Green Revolution bequeathed a plethora of misguided ideas to the agriculture of food, like the idea that mono-cropping foods like soybeans, corn, and "feed" for livestock would solve world hunger. Instead, it was the revolutionary moment in history that brought the sacred act of farming to its knees, necessitating the use of noxious pesticides and toxic chemicals. This mistaken idea compelled many farmers to mono-crop the land, which corrupted the natural stasis of millions of micro-organisms. As a result, our soil is depleted of its valuable nutrients, and therefore the symbiotic relationship among the elements—between plant and soil (Mother Earth and her offspring)—has been denigrated and damaged.

Evidenced by a multitude of scientifically proven facts, mono-cropping the earth for any reason whatsoever only serves to deplete the top soil, pollute the skies and rivers, produce greenhouse gases, which, in turn, contribute to global warming. It eradicates rain forests and ancient heritage trees, forcing species extinction. In short, these harmful agricultural methods corrupt the serene balance of the health, harmony, and purity of Mother Earth. To make matters worse, conventional farmers are forced to pummel her with an artillery of poisons to "save" her crops from infestation. Because we humans have a symbiotic relationship with Mother Earth, we hurt when she hurts, we cry when she cries, and we die when she dies. The plethora of new diseases emerging every day and the growing rate of suicides among farmers all over the world is evidence that we are intricately connected to the well-being of the good earth.

Living Ahimsa is about the power of sacred nourishment—which engenders an intrinsic sense of selfless sharing and communal unity. As extraordinary as this act may appear, the Vedic seers and yogis performed simple acts of *yajna* (peaceful sacrifice for the benefit of the greater community) such as imbibing small amounts of polluted milk while offering prayers for the cows to be healed. In this way, the cows received the magical communion of their sacred intention. This is one example of the Mind of Peace flooding the vibratory field through the process of thought. In a smaller but significant way, we too can do our part to engender communal wellness. For instance, to alleviate the fear of these gentle animals, we can take a small amount of milk in our right palm and offer a prayer for their well-being, as well as for the farmers and the good earth. In this way of Living Ahimsa, we renegotiate our states of un-wellness and create a sense of harmony within. Every act of selfless humanity cremates our fears.

For the shared love of food, each and every one of us must contribute to change the inured and hurtful practices that are progressively eroding our individual harmony and collective humanity. We must find a starting point to do so. Begin by observing and following in the Living Ahimsa footsteps of the conscious natural farmer. Living Ahimsa takes us far beyond the visible and audible knowledge of the practical applications in our lives. It is about what is beyond the physical, emotional, psychic, and spiritual clime—the perennial, immutable solution that is wrapped in the One Peace. As such, it is much more than the fear-based evaluations or stress-driven practices we employ in our lives. It is about the all embracing energy of doing what is good for the self and knowing that is innately what is good for the animals, forests, rivers, land, and skies.

OUR HEALING JOURNEY WITH FOOD

Nature's foods, as you will learn, afford us the greatest opportunity for honing and perfecting our potential for healing. Eating wholesome foods in accord with the seasons preserves nature and life—the material that nourishes our personal, everyday awareness. Protecting nature and recognizing her bounty of food is a time-tested, direct path to discovering consciousness.

Your relationship to food can also unravel the vast mystery of your timeless karma! Food takes us through the complete cycle of evolution, from the original cosmic seed to the fragile sprout, to the flourishing plant and its fruits—our sustenance. We are composed of energy, rhythms, vibrations, memories, and elements that continually transmute into one another creating atoms, molecules, minerals, foods, and life forms. Food is the carrier of these elements, and through its transformation the body of life is formed. The full cycle sustaining life begins with consciously sowing and harvesting the good earth, preparing her wholesome foods, and imbibing them with gratitude. To complete this cycle, we return our excrement (the earth's food that has been transformed through the body's digestion and vital tissue operations) as a gift back to the earth to uphold the unbroken continuum of the Mother Consciousness—the maternal divinity that nurtures all.

The plant is our most ancient ancestor; all life was born from this sacred creation. As it emerged into its manifested state, the plant absorbed the universe's first memory, that of yajna, divine sacrifice. The Vedic seers understood that the universe was founded on the act of sacrifice, and plants unflinchingly adhere to this standard. While animals roam, birds fly, fish swim, and all the rest of life moves about, plants are rooted steadfastly in the earth. Plants bend before the tides of the seasons and yield their food to all creatures. Season after season, they dazzle us with their beauty, bringing forth exquisite flowers, fruits, fragrances, colors, and joyous sustenance. In winter they retreat into the earth to replenish the cosmic memory of their seeds. In spring they push through the dense soil to reveal another tender sprout.

According to Ayurveda, the body consists of seven vital tissues: plasma, blood, muscle, fat, bone, marrow, and reproductive tissue, which are formed from the same elements, energies, and memories that make up plant life. The purpose of nature's foods—plants, fruits, and grains—is to revitalize our vital tissues by helping them "remember" how to function in perfection. Formed from the same substances, the plant seed and the human body are eternally intertwined. Neither the seed nor the body can exist without each other. Hold a good seed in your hand and know that it unfolds the entire universe from within itself. Like the good seed, our power of awareness carries the memory of the entire universe of consciousness.

We have the potential to activate this memory through the practice of ahimsa. In order to protect our nourishment and wellness we need to learn how to inculcate the state of harmony in our thoughts, speech, and actions. You can become the light you strive for by embracing the maternal life force within you, the gold that you can mine to harvest a shared sense of accountability for all life on this planet and respect for the good earth herself. At this extraordinary moment in time, I encourage us all to make a commitment to the life-honored oath of investing in personal harmony; to reject violence; to listen and hear each other; and to respect both our individual and collective ancestral traditions. In so doing, we can start to shift global consciousness into the Mind of Peace to overcome the culture of hurt and violence. We can protect the good earth's rivers and skies, and bring her forests and foods back into a pristine state of healthful abundance.

Food as defined in the Vedas is *annam*, "that which grows on the earth," and *ahara*, "that which nourishes the body, mind, and senses, creating balance within an organism." Unlike the plant that utilizes the energy of sunlight to provide sustenance for its needs, human beings depend on the earth's foods for their sustenance. The biological process of synthesis must occur within the dhatus, or vital tissues of the body, for an organism to be fed and nourished. For this reason food plays a tremendous role in human wellness and health. Nature's foods are the primary means by which the universe transmits memory, energy, and vibration to all its species. Food is the essence of healing. Nature's foods embody *rasa*, the taste of life, and contain the universe's energetic building blocks responsible for the body, mind, and spirit being fed, nourished, and celebrated.

FOOD & AWARENESS

Everything in these pages is about sadhana—the Sanskrit word that essentially means "awakening to our true self by living in ahimsa." It means living in harmony with self and nature and recognizing every speck of life to be whole and sacred. In addition to delicious wholesome recipes, the sadhanas—seasonal food practices—presented in this book are powerful tools for harnessing the mind and bringing our thoughts into harmony with nature's rhythms. Sadhanas can be practiced simply by breathing, having a peaceful presence, a compassionate thought, saying a kind word, keeping the prayerful mind strong in times of adversity, plucking a fruit from its vine, or watching the deer feast in a green field.

Sadhanas are about being aware of the integral connection that keeps us forever embracing the Mother Consciousness. Consider the wisdom of the pages that follow an extension of your contemplation—meditation in motion—rendered more

potent in effect through the practice of sadhanas, since sadhanas heighten awareness of the divine and initiate every molecule, cell, tissue, and organ in the body
into the vibrational state of resonance imperative for healing. At the Wise Earth
School, I have observed that those who adhere to Wise Earth's revolutionary Living
Ahimsa food sadhana practices are able to attain their spiritual goals rapidly and
develop a more *sattvic* lifestyle, which I will explain in the following chapter.

Our moment-to-moment awareness of our connection to nature is at the heart
of sadhana practice. Truly living in harmony requires awareness of every bite we
eat, every word we utter, and every sound we make. When our activities flow
in the spirit of peace, we invite the memory, energy, and vibration of the universe within us. Celebrating with the full moon, observing a fast on the eleventh
day of the bright or dark moon, meditating in the golden light of dawn, making an aromatic bath a blessing, pounding the husks off whole grains with a
large mortar and pestle, planting a good seed in the rich fertile earth, chewing
grains in blissful serenity, or feeding your child from your own hands—these
are the divine moments of life that create the precious gifts of health, harmony,
and wellness.

LIVING AHIMSA: THE POWER OF PEACE

Each one of us has the ultimate power of peace in our control. We can transition
from the hectic pace of these times with serenity and peace of mind by bringing
our families close to us, nurturing our inner peace, and nourishing our bodies
with nature's wholesome repasts. Let us seize this moment to invoke a powerful yet simple practice for harmony: Join the thousands of advocates around the
globe who are making this vow their first priority. Take The Vow of Ahimsa—the
imperative path to safeguarding inner harmony and health for all.

First though, let me explore the intention behind the vow as we know that
the promises, intentions, resolutions, oaths, and vows that we make are seldom
kept. We become frustrated, disappointed, and sometimes angry by the fact that
we could not maintain the promises we have made to ourselves. Indeed, a typical
intent or resolution can quickly fall by the wayside. One reason most intentions
do not work for us is that we set unrealistic expectations for ourselves. Moreover,
we depend entirely on the fallibility of mental discipline to upkeep these vows,
evidenced by the millions of vows we take which do not work! Indeed, many
resolutions end up having the adverse effect on the mind.

Let us explore the fascinating reasons why vows as we know them do not work.
In this modern era we tend to misuse the apparatus of the mind and the senses.
We keep the mind in a state of overdrive and the senses overworked. We expect
the mind to perform in a certain way, to forge ahead, break down barriers, and
conjure up great ideas, but the mind can only perform to the extent that we under-

stand its inner-workings, and respond in the manner that equals our own awareness. In short, the manner is which we respond to any situation invariably equals the degree to which our awareness is developed.

For instance, if you come across a beggar on the street who appears to be cold and ill or hurting, the manner in which you respond speaks to the nature of your own awareness: Some people will not notice the beggar; others will frown upon his disparaging appearance; many who see him would deliberately try to avoid him; some may drop a coin or two in his lap; others may seize the chance to get rid of some annoying loose change; and some may simply say a prayer for him. And then again, there are those who would stop and talk to him; or give him their coat to keep him warm or money to buy his meals; secure a meal for him themselves; or help him get to a shelter or a hospital. Each response reveals the character of our awareness (which is basically the essence of what we have learned from our individual set of experiences and karmas).

If we are taking an oath to accomplish a certain goal, it implies that we do not have the clarity we need to accomplish this goal. Therefore taking an oath will not gain us the desired results for the simple reason that the mind is not informed enough to achieve that goal. In this sense, vows are useless, although, they do express a certain desire, an intent to do better. This intent is held in your awareness and emerges from time to time.

In Vedic education, we learn about the complex and subtle operations of the mind. For instance, we are equipped with a sakshi—inner witness—the driver of our individual awareness that keeps a flawless record of our development in consciousness. The Vow of Ahimsa is much more than a vow, resolution, or promise. It is a sankalpa. Like most Sanskrit terminology, there is simply no equitable translation in other languages for this word. We could say it is a blessing or a sacred intention, an intent that is stored in the greater mind (buddhi) witnessed by the sakshi, so that we are continually prodded by memory and prana coalescing to guide, remind, cajole and comfort us as we move along in our everyday rhythm. In this way, we remember our vow, when it counts. And when we forget to remember, we are consoled by the fact that our awareness is growing. Sooner or later we remember.

When we feel we have betrayed our vow, that very awareness of the broken or betrayed oath proves that our awareness is at work. There are no recriminations. We do not feel lessened by it, nor are we guilty or angry or unfulfilled. Instead, we become aware when we engage violence of any kind—in our thoughts, speech, or actions. We capture the nature of our thoughts and actions, because we are becoming more aware of who we are. We are infinite consciousness, free and complete. The only challenge is that we are not aware of our true nature of being. Therefore, the practice of a sankalpa helps us to remain mindful of our inner emotional, mental, and psychic processes. We become more alert and focused in our thought process. Simply put, The Vow of Ahimsa is not something to be pursued or achieved;

it is a state of being. It is a flexible mode of concentration that engenders a meditative state in motion. Our lifeways do change dramatically because our mind is being continually nourished by sankalpa. We are open to the sakshi—our inner witness—and therefore we can access our awareness. The mind becomes lighter, brighter, and more awakened to the present. Compassion grows.

THE PRACTICE: THE VOW OF AHIMSA

This vow is a vrata, a powerful practice that reflects your sacred intention. You may use any 1 of the 6 vows below. Keep your practice simple, light, and pure. Preferred practice is in the early morning, after taking a bath, and while facing east.

If you break the vow, do not recriminate yourself in any way, as habits are hard to change. Simply remember that you can always redirect your thoughts and actions toward harmony and reinitiate the vow hundreds of times if necessary. You will reinvoke the vow each season as you move through the other Living Ahimsa practices set out in this work.

INSTRUCTIONS:
- Stand or sit in a comfortable posture with hands in prayer pose, Anjali Mudra.
- Take a deep breath, collect your spirit, and repeat the vow of your choice 18 times. This sets your intention so you will be reminded by the mind itself to keep the vow.

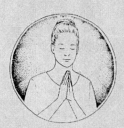

THE VOW OF AHIMSA

I take The Vow of Ahimsa
I make inner harmony my first priority

I take The Vow of Ahimsa
In my thoughts, speech, and actions

I take The Vow of Ahimsa
To protect Mother Nature and my food source

I take The Vow of Ahimsa
To preserve the heart of peace and love

I take The Vow of Ahimsa
To strengthen my power of personal awareness

I take the Vow of Ahimsa
To invest in world peace and the protection of all beings

Chapter Two

AHIMSA:
THE MIND OF PEACE

He who offers a leaf, flower, fruit or
water with devotion, that devout offering
of the pure-minded one do I accept.
— Lord Krishna
The Bhagavad Gita

A PERFECT TIME FOR HARMONY

Ahimsa means many things to many people. For the Vedic seers and Hindus, ahimsa is an everyday way of life. The vast Vedic tomes on meditation, yoga, holistic medicine, physics, astronomy, and architecture are all rooted in the universal law of ahimsa. For Mahatma Gandhi, it was the foundation for implementing civil disobedience *(satyagraha*—holding firm to the truth) in defiance of British imperial law in India. His path of ahimsa assumed courageous, yet simple forms (such as a nation harvesting salt from the sea). He demonstrated that the spirit of ahimsa can ultimately win all battles.

The forms of peaceful, non-violent action are many. From very personal— silence, fasting, prayer, charitable action, writing inspirational songs, poetry, and prose for peace—to collective campaigns, like peace marches and concerts. However, the greatest form of ahimsa is the cultivation of sacred spirit, a serene mind, and a healthful body. For this, it is of paramount importance to preserve our nutritional food source in nature.

You can practice Living Ahimsa in infinite ways, just as long as your intention is to evolve negativity and disharmony into positive vibrations of health, harmony, and hope. Keep in mind that Living Ahimsa is not about what we oppose, dislike, distrust, or have an aversion for. It is the opposite of all negative thoughts, emotions, and actions. It is the most positive act we can invoke and engender in our lives. In strengthening our collective resolve for harmony and non-hurting, we must refuse to participate in or condone violence in any form. There is only one way to accomplish this resolve and that is to create the Mind of Peace.

Each one of us is equipped with the potential for cultivating emotional, physical, and mental harmony. Did you know that our spirits are actually refined, adapted through evolution, and divinely designed to meet the demands of our time? Although we are living in a time of intense challenges, it is also an era of profound wisdom that outweighs any of its challenges. According to Hinduism, human evolution has already spanned four stages: The Age of Purity, The Age of Religion, The Age of Service, and The Age of Transformation, called *Kali Yuga*. Contrary to popular belief, Vedic astronomers believe human evolution has already completed its Kali Yuga, or cycle of transformation. The optimistic conjecture is that we are at this moment reentering *Dvapara Yuga*, the first stage of the universal cycle—an epoch of serenity and light wherein conscious behavior predominates.

This first cycle of time marks the momentous beginning of life on earth all over again. Breaking free from the darkness of Kali Yuga, we will live to see the shattering of everything that runs counter to dharma, the cosmic order. This breakdown will allow us the chance to experience a spiritual breakthrough—an opportunity to ignite the unifying spirit of ahimsa and understanding within ourselves and among all communities. We will witness the emergence of enlightened souls entering the earth, and the awakening of our soul's guiding wisdom.

At this moment, you and I are crossing the cosmic time barrier together, moving from darkness to light, from ignorance to divine knowledge. As we stand perched on the dawn of universal evolution, we are called to strive for harmony of thought, speech, and action; to consciously transform our lives by practicing non-harm, ahimsa; and to preserve and honor our sacred connection to the divine—the Mother Consciousness and the abundant foods she provides us.

While most of civilization left their imprint on history through the material medium of precious possessions—gold, silver, bronze, onyx, and granite—Hinduism as a vast wisdom-culture invested in the gold of the spirit. It has bequeathed its rich legacy of intelligence to the world through the spoken word, recited daily by an unbroken chain of generations. In Hinduism, there is no right or wrong. There is only "what is," and that "what is" is God. *Everything is God.* We seek not to believe in God, but to *know* God.

To protect the dharma of all, we can never impose our ideologies and belief systems on others. However, we can share, as I do, the gems of our traditions in order to benefit all of humanity. I feel fortunate to be born into my unique tradition; its central credo is to help humanity cultivate wisdom by sharing practices that address every aspect of living, from the mundane to the sublime, in this life and beyond. We do so without attempting to convert a person to the tradition of Hinduism, which is not in my view a religion, but a vast and meaningful way of life.

THE NATURE OF THE MIND: SATTVA, RAJAS & TAMAS

Food creates the mind: It carries the memories of our ancestors, nourishes the seed that brings forth new life, gladdens the heart, and nurtures the spirit. Not only does nature sustain human memory and energy to progress our purpose, but its perfect nourishment can reveal the entire cosmic infrastructure of the mind, body, and spirit. In order to hone the mind as an instrument of peace, we need to develop an awareness of food that connects us to the immutable rhythm of this ancient earth that nourishes our health, intelligence, and the power to be whole. Healthy foods nourish a person's mind in the same way they feed and nourish the body. When we approach our food with complete awareness, we become mindful of the most precious gift on earth we have—the state of being in Oneness with it all. First though, to harvest mental wellness and emotional harmony, we must learn the constructs and characteristics of the mind. For this, we will briefly explore the *gunas*, the three primary building blocks that create and support not only our life force but all of creation.

The Bhagavad Gita, one of the many books of the ancient Vedic scriptures, informs us that food is imbued with three gunas that are responsible for the creation, sustenance, and dissolution of the body, the mind and senses, as well as the entire universe, and essentially are the three attributes of nature. Each and every speck of life in the universe is shaped by the three gunas. Through their interaction they are responsible for the evolutionary process of manifesting subtle energies into gross objects and converting material objects back into subtler energies—the cycle of birth, death, and rebirth.

Everything in nature is influenced by the balance and interplay of these three primordial energies—the principle called *triguna.* The universe is in a state of perfect order when the three gunas are in a state of balance. Whereas the *doshas*—bodily humors—concern our physiological nature, the gunas affect our psychological condition. (If you are unfamiliar with doshas, please refer to appendix one, "Wise Earth Ayurveda Body Types.") To some degree every person has all three doshas and three gunas in their constitution. Understanding this—that we are a combination of naturally occurring elements continually striving for balance—helps us unlock the power to remain healthy in body, mind, and spirit.

Each guna bears a specific nature. In descending order of merit they are: *sattva, rajas,* and *tamas*—harmony, activity, and inertia. Understanding, purity, clarity, compassion, love, and wisdom are the predominant qualities of sattva. A person with these qualities is called sattvic. Aggressiveness, competitiveness, anger, egotism, and jealousy are the attributes of rajas. A person with these qualities is called rajasic. The inherent qualities of tamas are inertia, darkness, inactivity, ignorance, and negativity. A person bearing these attributes is called tamasic. All of the Living Ahimsa practices within these pages will shift you toward a more sattvic lifestyle—one in which you are filled with a greater feeling of peace and joy—and create further distance between you and depleting rajasic and tamasic tendencies and influences.

THE QUALITIES OF THE THREE GUNAS				
GUNA	ENERGY	NATURE	CHARACTERISTICS	QUALITIES OF BEING
Sattva	Creative Potential	Pure, harmonious, in a state of balance	Understanding, purity, clarity, compassion, love, and wisdom	Compassionate, joyous, and knowledgeable, with a vast vision of the whole
Rajas	Kinetic Potential	Active, aggressive, in a state of mobility	Aggressiveness, competitiveness, anger, egotism, and jealousy	Aggressive, progressive, and goal-oriented, with a limited vision of the whole
Tamas	Destructive Potential	Inert, destructive, in a state of concealment	Inertia, darkness, inactivity, ignorance, and negativity	Negative, lethargic, and resistant to change, with a fragmented and distorted vision of the whole

Table 2.1

Although they may seem in opposition, the functions of the gunas are entirely interdependent and cohesive. An oil lamp is a good illustration of this interdependent relationship: The oil, wick, and flame must cooperate fully with each other in order to produce light. Each guna forms an indispensable component of the balanced whole. Likewise, a healthful body, mind, and spirit perform seamlessly together as do the oil, wick, and flame. If we use the triguna principle to categorize our human components, the body can be likened to tamas—entirely inert (when stripped of its awareness); the mind to rajas—ever-generating mobility; and the spirit to the immutability of sattva. Sattva gives effulgence and light to rajas and tamas; rajas motivates and moves sattva and tamas; and tamas stabilizes sattva and rajas.

EMOTIONAL HARMONY

Although the gunas are intangible, we can observe their outward characteristics particularly in ourselves. For example, a sattva-dominated individual is generous, forgiving, understanding, and experiences things with great compassion. He has a penchant for clarity, seeing truth and objectivity, and holds firm to universal ideals.

A rajas-dominated person experiences the world subjectively, placing emphasis on personal ambitions and desires, often modifying universal truths to fit convenient goals. A tamas-dominated person experiences the world in an isolated and unaware way, with desires firmly entrenched in doubts and attachments.

By understanding the attributes the three gunas exhibit within us, we can transcend tendencies toward tamasic and rajasic responses and transform ourselves into more sattvic beings. Each guna—dynamically different in energy—serves specific and necessary purposes in the overall schema of life. However, all human beings who strive for inner harmony are well advised to cultivate a more sattvic lifestyle. Just like each guna arises from pure consciousness, we too must rise above our rajasic and tamasic tendencies to develop inner harmony and good health. We must be willing to take the occasional pause, and explore the inner terrain of the self to witness our thoughts, responses, and actions in everyday life. By being alert to our Living Ahimsa practices and our responses, we can assume responsibility for becoming healthy beings. As a result, all of our choices will be informed and clear, better serving our journey.

By keeping mindful awareness of everyday habits—breathing, eating, sleeping, and desiring—we can become attuned to our emotional and mental rhythms and the cyclical rhythms of nature. We can use our knowledge of the gunas as a guide throughout the day to bolster our power of awareness; see how every choice we make, every bite we eat, every thought we think, every word we utter, and every movement we make is influenced by the gunas at work in the mind and the senses. The lesson of applying the triguna is to strive for and witness our negotiable sense of inner balance amid the mire of challenges and confusion we encounter in modern life.

The Sattvic-Minded Person Strives For:
- The mind of ahimsa: steady, clear, and pure
- Inner harmony and health
- Self-control and balance
- Physical, mental, and spiritual stamina
- Regard for elders, ancestors, and nature
- Knowledge and wisdom
- Compassion and understanding
- Constructive and caring activities

The Rajasic-Minded Person Thrives On:
- Ambition and control
- Egoism and pride
- Popularity and success
- Militancy and activism

- Limited self-control
- Anger and jealousy
- Extreme friendship or extreme enmity
- Audibility and visibility

The Tamasic-Minded Person Thrives On:
- Ignorance and darkness
- Lethargy and inactivity
- Attachment and stubbornness
- Day sleeping and excessive sleep
- Indulging in eating, sleeping, and sex
- Restlessness and irritability
- Super-egoism
- Greediness and selfishness

Since the gunas are constantly evolving qualities—from sattva to rajas to tamas—it is difficult to categorize every food, emotion, thought, or action into one guna or the other. For instance, you may have a thought that is sattvic and well-intentioned, and then certain circumstances may occur during the day that reshape that thought into a more rajasic one.

Here is a food example of what I mean. Cow's milk is considered one of the most sattvic foods on earth. Yet, when raw cow's milk is homogenized, pasteurized, or boiled for a long time it becomes rajasic. When fermented or combined with salt to make cheese, the milk becomes tamasic. Likewise, sweet fruits are generally sattvic in nature, but when pickled they become tamasic. Sattvic green vegetables, when fried in oil, become rajasic. Root vegetables are generally considered tamasic, but carrots, beets, and turnips are sattvic in nature and are exceptions to the rule. Foods, like thoughts, that grow upward into the air are generally considered to be sattvic in quality. Foods that grow downward into the earth (and emotions that dive into the lower organs of the body) are considered tamasic in quality.

A wonderful analogy for understanding the transformational nature of the gunas is illustrated by the element of water. Ice, water, and steam are three distinct forms of the water element. In the form of ice, water is frozen and held in a congealed or static configuration. Ice is a tamasic form of the element water. In liquid form, water is free flowing, adapting to the shape of its container. In this form, water is the rajasic aspect of the element water. As steam, the element of water assumes its omnipresent and sattvic nature, transcending the boundaries of ice and liquid and the limits of gravity, shape, and form.

As with the three distinct forms of water, we too can heighten the qualities of mind, thought, and nourishment by striving for peace in our daily lives. The careful attention we bring to our everyday practice can transform our foods and thoughts into the most nurturing state of sattva. Living Ahimsa practice is a spiritual tool for body and mind; practiced again and again, it hones the spirit into its wondrous state of harmony.

The power of sattva is most prevalent in nature, and therefore can be easily harnessed by the mind. The asparagus fern, which grows within the calm shaded light of the forest, exudes the same gentle energy of sattva once it has been ingested in our bodies. The coconut tree, which grows high up into the sky, bears fruit enclosed within its husk and shell so that it remains cool, milky, and gelatinous. This sattvic food, used profusely in Vedic ceremonies, comforts the mind and vital tissues. The ripened mango knows just when to let go of the branch of its mother tree so that we may feast on its succulent, sun-blushed flesh. Like a feast of fruits, we want to keep the mind and psyche sattvic—peaceful and sweet.

The rishis, ancient Vedic seers, advised us to guide our thoughts carefully so that we can reap the fragrant fruit of the mind. As noted earlier, a simple and yet profound way to accomplish this feat is to practice The Vow of Ahimsa as often as possible to generate a continuous sense of awareness while cultivating the mind of ahimsa: harmony. *I take The Vow of Ahimsa in my thoughts, speech, and actions.*

STRENGTHENING THE FRAGILE PSYCHE

A mind poised in serenity is one of the greatest gifts of life. On the other hand, a discordant mind can lead to the erosion of our health. When you consider that we have spent centuries growing accustomed to living with violence—becoming tolerant of hurtful behaviors, or simply becoming immunized to their consequences—harvesting the fruit of the mind feels like reaching an oasis after crossing a vast expanse of desert. In short, we must mitigate the root of violence in our minds to convert discordant thoughts into wholesome actions. We can do so once we make a commitment to cultivating a peaceful mind, the mind of ahimsa, and start paying attention to the cultivation of our personal awareness.

How do we learn to use the most valuable instrument of mind that each one of us possesses—the instrument of the greater mind, called buddhi? The answer is simple: by eating wholesome nourishment from magnificent nature that allows the mind to settle into its greater realm of serenity. As you will see, the buddhi, a Sanskrit word, has an innate function—that is, to bear witness to your awareness as the body and mind unwinds and reformats itself through its ever-generating inherent intelligence. Once we learn how to use our buddhi, we start to discover the unique composition of memory and karma that makes us who we are as a person. This karma, or "formatter," shapes our habits, desires, likes, dislikes, cravings, and dreams, and ultimately, as our awareness becomes stronger, we discover our individual purpose that guides us toward the wisdom we need to hone and shape our journey.

We can support the building of awareness by taking the necessary time each and every day to allow our thoughts to settle; to remain current with our multiple activities; to digest our thoughts and foods with leisure; to acknowledge when we have an obstacle; and allow the mind to digest the nature of that obstacle and reveal to us what we need to know precisely when we need to know it. In other words, we need to take incremental pauses at various points of the day. *We should strive to do nothing during these pauses;* simply hold the intention to allow everything to settle within, then rise with ease and continue the day, however it may unfold. *We should not intrude on this process.* We should allow it be whatever it is. By so doing, we will find ourselves uncovering joy, contentment, ease, success, and a prevailing sense of lightness and freedom.

It seems that our modern society is being founded on an infrastructure of accumulated guilt—a sense of fragility that has gathered from generation to generation. In my opinion, this is the most significant impediment to reclaiming our power of awareness. In fact, the emotion of guilt is never content to exist on its own. It is a deeply imprinted, culturally acquired emotion that attracts fear, anger, isolation, and depression—not a fulfilling path for a conscious being striving to achieve the Mind of Peace and therefore a life of harmony! All obstacles, however, tend to dissolve once we allow them to get assimilated and settled within our awareness. Everything changes.

The Living Ahimsa Meditation at the end of this chapter is a powerful practice for cultivating inner strength and dissolving this feeling of fragility. This meditation, along with complementary changes you will be making in your diet, will help you to clarify and strengthen your mental and psychic planes. You will become more flexible and light, with increased energy to cleanse stuck patterns of behavior, which can lead to disease and disharmony.

Disease and despair come from a state of conflict, and conflict tends to move us rapidly away from health and happiness. When we feel we are powerless in the hands of disease or illness and unable to redirect our focus and energy, we become overwhelmed and succumb to its descending force. However, when we learn to view illness as a time to take pause and resolve inner conflict—a necessary break that gives us a chance to get back into our physical, emotional, and spiritual bodies—we can ward off hurt, injury, and negative effects. We must discard erroneous notions such as, "I can't take time for myself right now," or "I have too many other commitments to take care of," or "there is no way I can create time to do this." We must create this time to take pause especially when we are facing a major challenge. The first rule of Inner Medicine is that nothing else is as important as our well-being, and for this the art of taking pause is our greatest medicine! When we continually cross dharma—the natural rhythms of life—disease occurs, compelling us, and sometimes forcing us, into a necessary place of introspection. As the survivors of deep illness know, disease affords us a golden opportunity to reclaim our state of personal awareness and our individual sanctity.

Obstacles are there to remind us that we've forgotten something of value in our lives. It forces us to take pause and awakens us to that which is good for all. Nurturing the self must include nurturing others. Health is never for the healing of one—it is always about healing all! When you heal, your family heals. My healing and your healing is pervasive energy that instantly touches the immutable soul of the entire community, humanity, and world. The protection of all life is the greater intention of leading a life of ahimsa. Our actions cannot benefit the self at the expense of others or serve humans at the expense of the animals, forests, rivers, or nature as a whole.

FIRST PILLAR OF HEALTH & HARMONY

To experience the mind of ahimsa we must become aware of the intrinsic values that support life—the values that sustain the global family, community, and all species on earth. Whether we are Hindu, Buddhist, Christian, or Judaist; a farmer, doctor, teacher, or messenger; or of rich, poor, or middle income, becoming aware will make a profound difference in our lives.

Ayurveda teaches that the soul carries *samskaras*—cognitive imprints from rebirth to rebirth that create memory and shape personal karma from life to life. The purpose of each journey in our lives is to exfoliate karma. Healing is connected to karma, and each action we perform is influenced by the dictates of our own karma. For example, health and success are the dispensation of karma, yet interestingly, our likes and dislikes, loves and hates, prosperity and poverty, illness and wellness are not necessarily shaped by our personal karmas, but by the way we respond to them.

For instance, when we drink cow's milk (which has been largely contaminated by harmful practices in modern animal farming) it can harm our bodies. However, if a sage imbibes the same milk in the spirit of a blessing for the cows, it changes the energy of noxious and hurtful actions into wholesome food and blesses the injured cows. At each venue I go to, I witness hundreds of people who are able to shift negative patterns of behavior into self-healing. The only criterion for this transformation is your readiness and willingness to cremate a life of hurting so you can reclaim your joy and discover your greater purpose.

Living Ahimsa Meditation is a primary practice for cultivating the mind of ahimsa. This practice will help you cleanse and transcend your karma in leaps and bounds, even if you do not subscribe to the principle of rebirth or karma or understand how they work. Focused recitation of the mantra provided in the practice will help you cut through habitual behaviors so you can become aware of the judgments of the mind. When a critical thought pops up you will be able to catch it before it crescendos into an opera! A judgmental mind is a great big boulder in the way of cultivating your power of awareness. Becoming aware of your mind and its function will help you learn to hold disturbing thoughts or disruptive emotions in a kind space. Inner composure comes from creating the inner sanctum of the self. You must hone your spirit to own this space of inner harmony—the only definition of good health and good spirit. Be in the flow of peace. Living Ahimsa Meditation is a profound practice in Inner Medicine healing that empowers you to renegotiate, reconcile, and wipe out conflict.

You will discover that in doing the practices within these pages, you will be able to reclaim your memories of peace, harmony, and love; cultivate pristine vision; and experience sound, dreamless sleep. You may find through the following practice, as I did, that you will have the ability to consciously enter your dream state. In so doing, you can actually direct your dream circumstances and emotions in any direction you choose with incredible lucidity. Since we are created from the vast vibrations of the cosmos, the sounds of Sanskrit mantra inherent in this practice serve to strengthen your memory field; as a result, your physical, emotional, and spiritual vulnerabilities will dissolve. Living Ahimsa Meditation is a key practice for reconciling personal karmas and deepening your keen sense of awareness. It will help you cleanse stuck patterns of behavior that lead to disease and disharmony and recognize your life as a blessing.

LIVING AHIMSA MEDITATION

> As a weary bird flies hither and thither and comes
> to rest on its perch where it is tethered, so does the
> mind come to rest at last in its own Self.
> —The Chandogya Upanishad

Living Ahimsa Meditation is a profound practice for witnessing consciousness. In this practice we cultivate awareness, strengthen inner harmony, and discover that everything is God. Based on the most ancient form of meditation called Japa (a Sanskrit word that infers putting an end to the cycles of birth), this potent practice helps us to attain a deep state of serenity and peacefulness, whilst reconciling our karmas and dissolving those we have outgrown. Living Ahimsa Meditation is an effective means of cultivating a state of absolute awareness.

Meditation is a primary practice for easing daily stress and tension. As a dedicated practice, the Living Ahimsa Meditation enlightens the spirit whilst exploring and expanding the mind and its inner pathways of consciousness. Meditation is pure concentration; that is, it directs the mind to stillness. The Sanskrit word for meditation is *dhyanam* meaning to "discern." The Upanishads says, "meditation reveals the mind." Living Ahimsa Meditation should not be viewed as a practice that is separate from your normal daily activities. Over the last few centuries, many schools of meditation have arisen. However, we must understand that meditation in not an exercise of will. Once we start our practice, we will find that it is a continuum of harmony that flows throughout each and every moment of our days. This awareness of harmony is not confined to the times of our sittings. After some time with your practice, you will find clarity and peace of mind, and gain more ease and wisdom in your transactions. The highest goal of meditation is to bring the mind to its tether of reprieve. In so doing, it surpasses perceptions, thoughts, machinations, and even our dream state. Ultimately, to attain inner harmony, we must move beyond the state of habituation and common perceptions based in the sense organs. We move above sights and sounds, beyond the elements, beyond even the grasp of intelligence, into the realm of pure consciousness that the rishis called *anandam*, "the abiding joy and complete fullness."

In Living Ahimsa Meditation we recite mantras to evoke our sonic energies to awaken the buddhi, higher mind. This meditation brings the mind to a pivotal point within the buddhi where you can effortlessly take pause, and enter the silence. The rishis recognized that the repetition (both audible and inaudible forms) of Sanskrit mantras is a proficient way to promote unobstructed awareness. Stillness of being comes from the development of our awareness; the more aware we become of each and every moment, the more inner harmony we are likely to harvest. Our stillness heals the mind by eliminating fear, grief, anger, depression, and other negative emotions, which are based in false beliefs and habituations. Living Ahimsa Meditation clarifies our perception and validates reality and a shared sense of harmony. Practicing this meditation twice daily, once in the morning and then again in the evening, will secure a pillar of harmony in your life.

THE PRACTICE: LIVING AHIMSA MEDITATION

OPTIMUM TIMING:
- Early morning or evening for 30 minutes.
- Face east in the morning; face west in the evening.

MANTRA:
Om Namah Shivaya
(Pronounced: OOM NAH-MAH SHE-VAA-YAH)

My Reverence unto Shiva—Dissolver of Ignorance and False Perceptions

THE MUDRA: Hand Posture for Living Ahimsa Meditation
Hold the Japa Beads (Mala consisting of 108 beads) in your right hand, between your

thumb, middle, and ring fingers. The right hand enhances solar force helping to transform the mind, thoughts, and emotions into the positive energy of joy. Essentially, solar energy burns *ama*, toxic waste, from the organism. Support each bead with the middle and ring fingers while you use your thumb to move the bead by pulling the thumb toward your heart. As we learn in Living Ahimsa education, the thumb represents the element of Space, the middle finger the Fire element, and the ring finger, the Water element. As these three fingers touch upon the beads, they help to shift the mind into its state of awareness by instigating its intrinsic elements.

(Use your Japa Beads for the dedicated purpose of your meditation. Store them on your altar or in a serene space after use. Do not wear them.)

THE PROCESS:

In reciting the mantra, you are creating a continuum of sound vibration that invokes awareness that flows from the mudra to mantra and back again to the sound of the mantra. The vibrational field created by reciting the mantra keeps the mind in stillness. Your audible sound becomes connected in infinite circuitry—a circle of beads set in the numerological cosmic force of 108 to fortify energy while dispersing karma. The rishis informed that 108 repetitions of the mantra firmly plants its vibration into the brain.

THE PRACTICE:

1. Sit in a comfortable and serene space. Practice three rounds of the Mala (consisting of 108 recitations of the mantra) in each sitting. In the first round, we are looking to entrain mental faculty with the sound and vibration of the mantra. Recite the mantra audibly at a leisurely pace. Keep the Mala hand relaxed.
    (I recommend practicing this first step for about a month before progressing to the next round.)

2. In the second round, recite the mantra, but this time observe a brief and coordinated pause in between each recitation of the mantra. For example,
    Om Namah Shivaya–Pause–Om Namah Shivaya–Pause–Om Namah Shivaya–Pause. . .
    (I recommend practicing the first and second rounds together for about two months before proceeding to the final step).

3. In the final round, recite the mantra internally (quietly, or inaudibly). You may find it difficult to keep the fingers moving on the beads. In this case, continue to hold the beads lightly while resting the hands in your lap. You are now in a state of meditation. Allow thoughts to flow, do not engage them. It is natural for the mind to have thoughts, do not wrangle with them. Let them be. If you find yourself engaging thoughts, resume the active recitation and mudra with your beads. Sit in stillness for some time.

(By now your efforts in practice will have yielded ease in transitioning from one step to the next. Henceforth, you are to practice all three rounds, one after the other, in seamless effort.)

OM NAMAH SHIVAYA

What to Expect from Your Practice:

- You recognize your inner-witness self and become accountable to your purpose.
- You discover how to accommodate the inevitable.
- You cultivate a strong sense of awareness by being conscious of your thought process.
- Less-than-peaceful thoughts arise in and out of meditation—accept this as a natural occurrence, acknowledge any bothersome thoughts, and adhere to your daily affirmation: *I hold each thought in the cosmic space of ahimsa.*
- You become the witness of life, and not the engager.
- You learn that you do not have to be in control of each and every situation.
- You experience a progressive shift toward more leisure of mind.
- You cultivate an informed trust in the Divine Energy.
- You start to recognize situations for what they truly are.
- You begin to cultivate a sense of objectivity so that you can make informed responses in all situations.
- Solutions to challenges become clear.

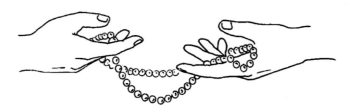

Figure 2.1 Living Ahimsa Meditation Mudra

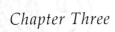

Chapter Three

VEGETARIANISM: A PATH TO PEACE

There can be no perfect peace, health,
or harmony on earth until we eradicate
the mentality of violence. For this, we must
not injure, kill, and eat animals as "food."

EATING TO NOURISH LOVE

Thousands of years ago, my Vedic ancestors understood love to be the foundation of nature. They also recognized that harmony is produced only by cooperation with all of nature and her creatures. As sentient beings, the ancients safeguarded harmony by extending reverence and gratitude to all creatures, to the forest, the mountains, and to nature as a whole. They were intelligent people who understood the remarkable set of interconnections we have with Mother Earth. They learned from nature how to sustain happy and prosperous communal living and did not involve themselves in the barbarity of today's animal annihilation in the name of food! They would not kill the very life force that supported the well-being of their families and communities, nor viciously slaughter the animals to satisfy an insatiable appetite. Instead, they worked very hard at keeping love and harmony alive.

The Vedic seers taught that what grows on the earth—plant and mineral life—is annam, the perfect and only food suitable for nourishing the human body. My ancient ancestors were expert foragers who were aware of the cadence of nature and what to harvest and reap as the seasons cycled perpetually onward. They harvested herbs, roots, fruits, and legumes without bludgeoning the forest or its animal communities. They did not view their everyday tasks as punishing or arduous work, but as necessary humanistic duties they were put on the earth to do in order to keep love and harmony thriving in their lives. They recognized the indelible cosmic qualities of love and harmony to be the bedrock of an intelligent life that sustains our humanity. Love was not about sexual affairs! Health was not about shopping in gourmet health-food stores. Harmony was not about goal-oriented successes.

We have much to learn from our ancient forebears and much more to be grateful to them for—they invested love in this planet, and their investment is eternally paying dividends. Our forebears patiently taught the animals how to serve them better. They taught the bigger animals how to harvest the land, uproot dead trees, clear pathways, and carry heavy loads in order to transport their families and goods from one place to the next. They sheared animal fur to make bedding and other items to keep the family warm. They used vegetarian animals' feces to make fuel for the fire; their urine as antiseptic for various cleansings. In return, consciously domesticated creatures provided ongoing sustenance through peaceful foods: milk and honey. Animals were considered indispensible parts of ancestral communities. Highly responsive to love and care, the animals lived up to their greatest instincts; they basked in the kindness and joy of the family by bonding with their caregivers, and especially with the children whose innocence they shared.

In my tradition, we choose vegetarian lifestyles in order to live a life of ahimsa. We choose this path out of a compelling love for life, love for Mother Earth, love for her creatures, love for her food, and love for our families, our communities, and ourselves. Truly, the practice of vegetarianism demonstrates that we are on the path to cultivating the mind of ahimsa. It is not a religion or a practice observed only by Hindus and Jains—the oldest cultures to promote vegetarianism—but a lifestyle choice with many benefits. The first pillar of health and harmony stands on the commitment to a sattvic lifestyle—in other words, Living Ahimsa, the universal principle of peace. As I see it, a personal exploration of vegetarianism is a necessary commitment in support of inner harmony and world peace.

As it stands, the most compelling reason why millions of people have converted to vegetarian diets is for better health and because they fear disease, but as human beings we have a far greater responsibility to the self and to the Mother Consciousness than to respond to fears and desires, even when these emotions are anchored in our ancestral and cultural habits. One of the divine gifts of being human in the present era is that we have a choice: we can choose to open our hearts to compassion. Health, happiness, and prosperity do not exist independently of nature; they depend entirely on the divine source within our consciousness. As our consciousness grows, our choices shift to meet our awareness. We begin to see that the personal karma and collective dharma of all must be served if we are to eradicate hurting, violence, anguish, pain, and despair. It is time that we awaken to our conscience.

The South Indian scripture *Tirukural* confirms this premise of compassionate living: "How can he practice true compassion who consumes the flesh of an animal to fatten his own flesh?" Collectively, we can find infinite strength when we make harmony our ultimate priority. Being a vegetarian is more than not killing or eating the meat of the poor, butchered creature; it is living in a state of heightened awareness and cultivating compassion for all life. It is a lifestyle that compliments human wisdom. In these pages you will learn the timeless, wholesome skills applicable to all traditions that can make the difference in the magnificent acquisition of a healthful and abundantly joyous life. For the love of life, let us make a concerted effort to safeguard all of nature's resources and Mother Nature's creatures. As noted earlier, we are fortunate to live in the most perfect universal time wherein each of us has the opportunity to awaken our sleeping memory of harmonious interdependence. Let's start this journey of understanding by applying the principle of ahimsa to the most basic yet complex need in life: *Food.*

COSMIC BUILDING BLOCKS OF HEALTH

The world is continually rediscovering that vegetarianism is a perfect path to inner harmony, health, and world peace. It is a sattvic, peace-generating lifestyle committed to imbibing nature's foods. Before we delve into vegetarianism as a powerful means to accomplishing peace, we must explore the role that the three gunas, or primordial energies, sattva, rajas, and tamas play in your choice of foods.

The ancient Ayurveda physician Sushruta tells us, "A sattvic diet gladdens the heart, nourishes the body, and revives mind and memory." The *Charaka Samhita* identifies the first foods of the earth as rice, barley, mung beans, gooseberry fruit, rainwater, rock salt, honey, cow's milk, and ghee. These foods are essential in balancing nature's primordial energies of sattva, rajas, and tamas. The balance of these three primordial energies, the triguna, is the key for creating and sustaining life. Therefore, grains, legumes, fruits, herbs, vegetables, milk, ghee, honey, raw sugar, and rock salt are the substratum for the recipes set out in this book.

Nature's foods provide a broad spectrum of provisions to put our choices for consciousness to the test. A profound way of discerning the energy of the foods we eat (and as a result, our own individual states of health) is to utilize the knowledge of the gunas. For instance, sattvic foods are those that are naturally and organically growing on the earth. They are free from pesticides and genetic manipulation, and free from the horrific corruption involved in the slaughtering of animals, fowl, and fish.

According to Ayurveda, sattvic foods should comprise the larger portion of a wholesome meal. A healthy diet should consist of a variety of seasonal foods combined in healthy proportions and eaten in an atmosphere of calm to feed and nourish the vital tissues. In turn, the tissues will support energy and strengthen the body, mind, and spirit. The cosmic formula for a long and healthy life is eating peace-generating foods in a harmonious state of mind while in a wholesome environment.

Sattvic foods are generally organic, sweet, fresh, light, unctuous, nourishing, and aromatic. While being eaten these foods produce a feeling of contentment, joy, and invigoration that lasts long after digestion occurs. The mind and senses are immediately appeased by sattvic, peace-producing foods because they transport readily digestible and nourishing sustenance to the system. Seasonal fruits (such as apples, oranges, grapes, bananas, and mangoes), grains (especially rice, wheat, and barley), and vegetables (such as leafy vegetables, broccoli, cauliflower, asparagus, and beans) that are light and fresh and easy to digest are considered the most sattvic in nature, as is the pure, organic milk of the cow. Both our food choices and their preparation play an important part in maintaining the sattva principle, as you will see. A classic Vedic dish of rice, organic cow's milk, and *gur* (raw palm sugar) is considered a quintessential sattvic meal.

Since we are created from the three gunas, each intrinsic to normal everyday living, we cannot live on sattva-producing foods alone. The body, mind, and senses need to be nourished by all three principles, with predominance in sattva (light, peaceful), secondary emphasis on rajas (bright, energizing), and least emphasis on tamas, (dark, immobile). Practically all of the 50 billion or more packaged and processed foods and medicines in the world today are of a tamasic or rajasic nature. So too is the popular "killer diet" of fast foods.

Excessively oily or spicy deep-fried foods, coffee, intoxicants—liquor, wine, beer—chocolate, candy and other processed sweets, commercially produced milk and dairy products, commercially prepared breads and crackers, are all rajasic in nature. The Bhagavad Gita informs, "… foods that are bitter, sour, pungent, salty, hot, dry, oily and burning produce pain, grief, and disease. These foods are liked by the rajasic in nature." Excessive intake of these foods, which are radically diminished in life-supporting energy, tend to disturb body chemistry, disrupt inner harmony, and dull our power of intuition.

Tamasic foods taken in excess are the most detrimental to good health. They consume a large amount of energy during digestion, weaken the digestive fire, and disturb the process of vital tissue transformation that follows digestion. People who are tamasic in nature tend to prefer foods that are dry, aged, stale, malodorous, and impure. Foods that have been processed, canned, frozen, irradiated, or tampered with in some way are tamasic in nature. Fermented foods such as soy sauce, tamari, miso, cheese, and pickles are also tamasic in nature. Animal flesh—meat, fish, fowl, and eggs—has the most tamasic qualities. Taken in excess, alcohol also becomes tamasic. Drugs such as marijuana, cocaine, hashish, opium, heroin, as well as most prescription drugs (especially painkillers, sleeping pills, and antidepressants) are extremely tamasic in their effect. Tamasic foods promote lethargy, depression, ignorance, negativity, paranoia, and general disharmony in the body and mind, and should therefore be avoided in large quantities.

There are, however, appropriate seasons to imbibe each of the three energies of sattva, rajas, and tamas in their proportionate quantities, and the recipes in this book are seasonally balanced in accord with the gunas, with each seasonal recipe influenced primarily by the peaceful tastes and tones of sattva. For instance, spring season demands more rajasic foods than in the summer when more sattvic foods are needed. The winter menu thrives on a stronger touch of tamas. Although root vegetables such as onions, potatoes, and radishes have a naturally tamasic nature since they are sheltered in the darkness of the heavy earth, they are considered good for the body when imbibed during the winter seasons, when organisms require a good degree of tamasic energy to remain stable and strong during the very cold season.

Genetically manipulated and cloned foods have the most detrimental and destructive effects on the body, mind, and senses. During these processes, the *tanmatra*—intrinsic energy quanta—of the food becomes transmuted and deranged. Since the natural memory code of the food is scrambled, the "food" no longer recognizes its own nutritional language, and therefore cannot synthesize its nutrients through the digestion process. In Vedic education, we know that several processes occur during the feeding of the vital tissues in their transformative development, and that these intrinsic processes cannot be replicated by science. Therefore, the assumption that genetically manipulated or cloned foods are identical to what nature produces is entirely erroneous and false.

For many years, I have been doing a personal practice around congested areas that sell fast foods, unhealthy foods, and unwholesome fodder. Airports and tourism spots are, indeed, ideal places to perform this rite. I offer up my prayers for the betterment of our food source, Mother Nature, and all of her creatures, and on rare occasions, imbibe a small amount of the unwholesome fodder. While digesting it, I observe certain mantras that allow the food's toxicity to be lessened. In this way, the toxicity of all foods in the vicinity is somewhat energetically mitigated. Obviously, this action is not for everyone, and I am not advocating it as a practice for the general population; I am simply providing a cultural example of small sacrifices we can make to help our fellow family on Mother Earth.

In the Hindu culture, the principle of yajna implies making a sacrifice for the welfare of the world at large. As we know, prayers have great and immediate effect. But, as we are continually experiencing the unfolding of lessons, we have to be supremely mindful each and every step of the way (especially when we take for granted how aware we already are!). We must be careful how we engage our actions and for what purpose, however well intended they may be. It is important to be especially mindful during vulnerable stages of healing or recovery. The power of an act of yajna does not yield positive results if performed while we are unclear or disoriented.

THE PEACEFUL LIFE OF A SHAKAHARI

Living Ahimsa Diet recommends the lifestyle of a *shakahari*—a vegetarian; one who nourishes their vital tissues by feasting on nature's vegetation. (I would like to interject here that it is important not to identify ourselves by the names of our food groups, not to describe ourselves as "a vegetarian, a vegan, a macrobiotic, or a meat-eater." We must let go of labels and begin to think simply in terms of being humane.) To reclaim our Inner Medicine, we must practice non-injury and non-hurting in the lifestyles we choose, which includes our diets. There can be no peace, health, or harmony on earth until we eradicate the mentality of violence. For this, we must stop the killing. We must not injure, kill, and eat animals as "food."

Mother Nature's plant foods afford us the greatest opportunity for honing the inner harmony necessary for healing. Food is life, and preserving nature protects our life force, prana. The world's present miasma of disease and violence reflects the impaired condition of our food sources caused by human tampering and corporate mischief. The path to health and harmony is eluding the world because we—as individual human beings—have either forgotten or learned to ignore the living wisdom that protects life.

We must reclaim the power of awareness in our lives before we can experience health at any level. To achieve this basic goal, we must stop propagating the pain we are causing the animals, the planet, and ourselves! We must stop the senseless slaughtering of animals. These unconscionable actions serve only to block the memory that carries our resolve of Inner Medicine healing. We may not all be able to actively participate in safeguarding nature at large, but each and every one of us has the capacity and the awareness to say "no" to violence. Ultimately, each person has a choice about what they consume and eat.

FOR THE LOVE OF OUR PLANET

According to a recent UN projection, global meat production is set to more than double from 229 million tons in 2001 to 465 million tons in 2050, with commercial milk output being projected to soar from 580 million to 1,043 million tons over the same period. Currently, 75 percent of our 260 million acres of forest have been cleared as cropland in the US to produce feed, silage to produce meat. Two hundred and twenty square feet of tropical forest is consumed to produce each pound of rain forest meat.

Hinduism Today writes, "The world's natural resources are being rapidly depleted as a result of meat-eating. Raising livestock for their meat is a very inefficient way of generating food. Pound for pound, far more resources must be expended to produce meat than to produce grains, fruits, and vegetables. For example, while 25 gallons of water are needed to produce a pound of wheat, 5,000 gallons are needed to produce a pound of California meat."

Over the past 25 years I have heard scores of stories from individuals that converted to a life of vegetarianism, meat-eaters who primarily made the change in order to cultivate personal awareness and strengthen their commitment to a life of ahimsa. Most of these individuals are students of mine who have studied at the Wise Earth School and the Mother Om Mission. For some the change was immediate, for many it took about a year to transition completely. More than 80 percent of these folks expressed concern for their well-being or the need to mitigate serious disease as the catalyst for this change. A lesser percentage were concerned about the welfare of the earth, the forests, the animals, and the environment—a concern we should all take seriously.

Writing in a recent issue of *Physics World*, British physicist Alan Calvert advised that giving up pork chops, lamb cutlets, and chicken burgers would do more for the environment than burning less oil and gas. He calculates that the animals we eat emit 21 percent of all the carbon dioxide that can be attributed to human activity. We could therefore slash man-made emissions of carbon dioxide simply by abolishing raising livestock for food.

The horrific industry of "animal farming" now contributes to 20 percent of our environment's lethal greenhouse gases as a direct result of the flatulence produced by farm animals. So alarming are these trends that the Kyoto Protocol has turned its attention to the study of this problem—a problem they recognize as a threat to the future of the entire planet. The average cow, they say, causes the same damage to the environment each year as a family car that travels 12,000 miles. In fact, although vehicles produce a far larger volume of noxious gases, methane is 21 times more harmful to the environment than carbon dioxide. To cite a report issued in 2006 from the UN Food and Farming Agency's Rome-based Food and Agriculture Organization (FAO): "The livestock industry contributes more to the greenhouse effect than cars and is also a major source of soil and water degradation."

And these animals are routinely mistreated, fed toxic and poisonous fodder, industrialized in inhumane ways, and are now about to be subjected to yet another artillery of chemicals in their feed as a quick fix to the methane problem. The reason for this measure is not to rescue the animals from their insurmountable misery, or eliminate the degrading practice of consuming the noxious meat resulting from the barbaric actions of animal farming, but to appease the human community by reducing the foul odor and polluted environment.

The answer is not to spend billions more dollars developing toxic anaerobic digestives for the poor creatures so we can comply with new regulations for handling, producing, and managing methane while enabling factory farms to further invade the community. It is to recognize that we must eradicate the practices that produce foul substances that contaminate our sense of humanity.

We are at a point in time when we can and must reevaluate our habitual and ancestral patterns of behavior. There is no more perfect time to distance ourselves from the irreverent practices of the past than right here and right now. We can no longer barter with nature and the lives of her animals for our survival because we are progressively eroding our most essential faculties: memory and intelligence; in essence, our ability to remember life as being wholesome and peaceful. Because of the impairment of our ancestral memories, we are losing our ability to recognize the sacred energy carried by other life forms.

FOR THE LOVE OF ANIMALS

Living Ahimsa is also about caring for the animals and not just about caring for family pets. I know many people who absolutely adore their dogs or cats and would even protect them with their own lives, but who do not extend this same love for animals they'd prefer to eat, animals just as intelligent, conscious, and loving. Just like the dogs and cats we welcome into our homes, chickens, turkeys, pigs, sheep, deer, and cows have their own sublime nature and personalities, likes and dislikes, and, most importantly, the ability to feel pain, suffer from depression and frustration, and experience joy. The animals have fundamental rights to life, just as humans do. In the same gleeful way that you relate to your pets, the Mother Goddess relates to all of her charges. When you participate in or contribute to the hurtfulness and injury of her animals, trees, and rivers, the Great Mother weeps like we do when our children are hurt.

According to the US Humane Society: "Each year in the United States, approximately 10 billion land animals are raised and killed for food—more than one million every hour." If each person cuts back on their animal consumption by only 10 percent, approximately one billion animals would be spared a lifetime of suffering each year. If each of us takes the sankalpa, sacred resolution, to become a vegetarian, 10 billion animals would be spared each year in the US alone. Most meat-eaters either have no idea of the devastation their diet causes worldwide, or if they do, would prefer to turn a blind eye on the pressing and catastrophic plight of the animals. No federal law truly protects animals from cruelty on the farm, and most states exempt "customary agricultural practice," regardless of the degree of abuse and violence, from the scope of their animal cruelty statutes.

Whereas the transformational fire energy in plant life replicates as nourishing digestive fire energy—*agni*—within the human body's vital tissues, organs, cells, and memory, an animal's agni is fierce and unstable, and particularly aggravates the natural balance of agni in the human system when eaten. Ultimately, this agni affects how the body responds to food and nourishment. It is impossible to separate the pain, fear, and disgrace of the slaughtered animal from its meat. When consumed by a human, it enters a living environment of plasma, blood, muscle, fat, and bone. The "injured food" leaves an indelible print in the memory of these tissues, which is reflected in the mind of the consumer. Indeed, whether or not you contribute to the principle of rebirth, killing an animal and/or eating its flesh also leads to major challenges in an individual's karma. When you realize that what enters the body will affect the mind and spirit, and that eating the slaughtered flesh of an animal cannot enhance personal consciousness, you will make a significant transition toward the sacred in your life.

Would it not be a wondrous feat of our humanity if we made decisions based primarily out of respect for the well-being of all creatures rather than from the oppressive sense of desire, fear, greed, and insatiable appetite that appear to propel our current state of humanity? We must pause to ask ourselves: Why do we tend to respond to the egregious crimes of our time with fear of personal loss? What about the elevation of human conscience, the protection of dharma in our community, society, and world? Would it not be the obvious, serene, and organic solution to many of our global problems simply to become vegetarians? More than half the problems that infect the heart, mind, body, spirit, community, and the environment would be eradicated if we became vegetarians. We could free the animals from their pain and degradation, and recreate healthful living environments that support the animals, forests, rivers, the sky, and ourselves. Now, more than ever before in our history, it is time we recognize the obvious solution.

Millions of dedicated organic dairy farmers are already out there hard at work to bring you fresh, wholesome milk from happy, thriving cows. Thousands of organic farmers in the West are discovering what the Hindus have been doing for thousands of years—using manure (which is produced from uncontaminated, non-drugged, healthful organic feed) as a farm-fresh energy source. The method of converting manure into alternative energy is just one benefit of the many gifts from the cow. Almost all organic-based dairies are family owned, and as active members of their communities, farm families take pride in maintaining natural resources—preserving the land where they live and work, protecting the air and water they share with neighbors, and providing the best care for their cows—the lifeblood of their business.

COSMIC MEMORY

Observing a peaceful lifestyle in harmony with the greater energies of the universe entails much more than not killing and eating animals: It demands retooling the mind to respect life, and relearning the abiding lesson that each and every creature in the world has the profound right to live its life to its natural end. As I move about the world on my peace-generating mission, I continually witness the sublime grace of the pristine state of innocence in which the animals live. I feel privileged to interact with them—the natural embodiment of earth's most ancient life forces—and recognize the cosmic memories that knit us together into one spectacular humanity. Indeed, my personal experiences with the animals have been great teaching metaphors, helping me to awaken to the heart of my own sentiency in ahimsa.

Through my profound and privileged journey into the subtle spheres of reality, I have discovered that each and every species serves as a guardian to a specific block of universal knowledge, a concept I call the Cosmic Memory Principle. The ongoing preservation of a block of cosmic memory is dependent on the well-being of the species that carries it. For instance, it is written in the Vedas that the elephant, Gaja, was sent to the earth as the cosmic guardian to the knowledge of all plants and herbs, playing a supreme role in the preservation of sustenance on the earth in accord with the Cosmic Memory Principle. In short, the elephants maintain the cosmic memory of all the earth's nourishment, plants, herbs, fruits, seeds, legumes, nuts, and minerals. If the elephants lose this vital information, it will be lost to all of us on the planet. For any species to thrive, including the human being, the whole network of cosmic memory must be retained in good order.

When a species becomes extinct as a result of the universe's natural course of evolution, its particular block of cosmic memory is then dissolved, no longer to be found within the vibratory field of memory in the universe. When the universe no longer needs a certain block of memory, the species that carries that knowledge naturally dies out and the memories that desist are no longer necessary to the welfare of the life forms still existing on the planet. In this dynamic creation, natural extinction occurs because the universe itself matures, transcending its dependency on certain blocks of cosmic memory, like when the snake no longer needs its worn out skin it is shed, and the snake is neither impaired nor enhanced as a result.

As I write from deep within the Nilgiri Hills in Tamil Nadu, India, I can hear scores of elephants thundering down the hillside. It is shortly before dusk, and the time has come once more for them to forage through the forest for their food. Elephants have been known to lead their caretakers on adventurous food "shopping sprees" through the forests and then supervise the careful preparation of their massive feasts. An elephant keeper in Bengal told me that his elephants' favorite meal was grain porridge wrapped in four-foot-long layers of a variety of large leaves shaped like a giant sushi roll!

Elephants have a remarkable sense of smell, so developed they can identify every plant, shrub, herb, creeper, bush, grass, and tree by smell alone—an extremely useful tool for the cosmic guardian of the plant world! Scientists claim that the elephant's sense of smell is one of the most acute of all mammals. Endowed with highly perceptive trunks comprised of nearly 60,000 muscles, elephants can also use their trunks to stack lumber, uproot enormous trees or clumps of grass, shake the coconuts off palm trees, powder their bodies with dust, or perform the delicate task of picking up a pin from the ground. Using its trunk as a snorkel, an elephant can tread water and swim for many miles almost completely under water. A woman in Chennai told me that she had witnessed an elephant save a drowning girl by carrying her to shore with its trunk.

Stories abound in India about this classically grand animal, but by far, the most heart-wrenching stories involve the devastating and hurtful actions, or himsa, committed against them by humans. The felling of the forests and hunting of these precious creatures for their tusks is rising with great rapidity. From the Vedic view, the more we deprive these magnificent creatures of their natural habitat, the less memory of earthly sustenance will prevail in the universe's network.

At present, you can find elephants in most unnatural states, roaming in a clouded daze, transfixed in confusion while invaders kill their calves in order to expand human territory. This noticeable confusion and fear indicates that the elephants are losing their innate memory, which does not bode well for any of us. As the universe loses more of its foundational memory, our human sentiency and sense of awareness also suffers.

Every day we confirm this ignoble reality by the hosts of new diseases and despairs that impugn and impinge the earth's maternal memory, reflected in the deteriorated state of nourishment and nurturance. We must adopt lifestyles that honor the significant role that even the tiniest animal has in preserving our cosmic memory and overall harmony on this planet if we truly want to heal and thrive! When you consider the Cosmic Memory Principal and the detrimental impact the mistreatment and slaughter of animals causes to our overall experience on this planet, it becomes evident that vegetarianism is not merely a dietary choice, but in truth, a profound path to peace.

DISPELLING MYTHS ABOUT VEGETARIANISM

The Myth that a Vegetarian Diet is Inadequate

There are myriad reasons to practice vegetarianism, yet I'd like to address some of the primary arguments or myths about this lifestyle that I encounter. Those considering a vegetarian lifestyle are generally concerned about getting sufficient nutrients, since the belief that meat is a requisite part of a daily diet for staying healthy is widespread. Some years ago, a group of eminent doctors called the Physician Committee for Responsible Medicine (PCRM), themselves members of the American Medical Association, decided to bring awareness about vegetarian nutrition to the medical community in the US. With years of nutritional research data in their grip, the PCRM is a well-informed organization that chooses to address these dietary concerns full force. *Hinduism Today* cited one of their reports:

> *The fact is, it is very easy to have a well-balanced diet with vegetarian foods. Vegetarian foods provide plenty of protein. Careful combining of foods is not necessary. Any normal variety of plant foods provides more than enough protein for the body's needs. Although there is somewhat less protein in a vegetarian diet than a meat-eater's diet, this is actually an advantage. Excess protein [from a meat diet] has been linked to kidney stones, osteoporosis, and possibly heart disease and some cancers.*

Scientists freshly emerging from their laboratory findings are ardent witnesses to the fact that food can mitigate or contribute to disease. Pancreatic cancer is most prevalent among populations that eat the most meat, caused largely by its high fat content. Numerous studies indicate that too much fried or barbecued meat, as well as smoked and cured pork, enhances chances of pancreatic cancer. In Japan, those who ate meat at least once daily were shown to have accelerated their pancreatic cancer risk by 50 percent.

Scientists are also now convinced that certain foods can cancel out the damaging and adverse effects caused by alien compounds in our foods. For several years, extensive research has been conducted to locate foods that are packed with anti-mutagens that can neutralize the cancer threat. Japanese scientists have discovered that cabbage, broccoli, shallots, green peppers, ginger, apples, pineapples, and eggplant all boast remarkable power to block cancer-promoting cell mutations. This is especially good news because our world food sources have become severely poisoned and impaired, and many foods contain mutagens that may cause genetic cell damage leading to cancer and other degenerative diseases. Vegetarians, however, are known to have lower rates of cancer, heart disease, stroke, and a number of other chronic diseases than meat-eaters.

The American National Cancer Institute recognizes the power of the vegetable and recommends eating at least five servings of vegetables and fruits every day. Green leafy vegetables (such as kale, collards, lettuces, spinach, arugula, bok choy, and chard) exhibit extraordinary anti-cancer power. These vegetables contain anti-oxidants including beta-carotene and folic acid, as well as lutein, a lesser-known antioxidant that many food researchers believe may be as potent as beta-carotene in mitigating and neutralizing cancer. Frederick Khachik, PhD, a research scientist at the Department of Agriculture, informs us that the darker the greens, the more cancer-inhibiting carotenoids they have. As Tolstoy puts it, "The garden of green is my best medicine chest."

Unlike Western approaches, Ayurveda's traditional system of medicine, which depends almost exclusively on plant medicine, does not dissect or fragmentize, or deconstruct a whole food in order to quantify its characteristics (calories, carotenoids, proteins, vitamin content, etc.). Through Ayurveda's understanding of the body's complex system of energy, we have a supreme way of seeing the whole nature of an entity, and therefore its parts. All traditional medicine systems honor the plant as the oldest form of medicine on earth. More and more, as we discover "new" herbs in the West, we find that traditional cultures all over the world have been using plant food as medicine for millennia. The *Taittiriya Upanishad* shares its perennial wisdom on the priceless healing power of plant foods for individuals and the planet: "Food is universal medicine. All life came into existence out of food. Food precedes all creatures in the order of creation."

The Myth that Humans Were "Designed" to Eat Meat

Some people argue that our human anatomy was developed to ingest meat, but our anatomy suggests otherwise. Our digestive systems are similar to those of other plant-eaters and totally unlike those of carnivores. If we were designed to eat meat why is it that the less meat someone eats, the greater their chances of leading a longer, healthier life free from diseases that will plague the meat-eater? Some also argue that humans should be classified as carnivores because we have canine teeth, but this does not take into account that other plant-eaters also have canine teeth, and that only plant-eaters have molars.

The Myth that Milk is Not Part of a Vegetarian Diet

Next, let's examine a question often asked by vegans, those who eat a vegetarian diet without milk products. Many groups of people refer to milk as an "animal food"—a term that implies that an animal is being exploited or slaughtered in order to secure the food—and ask how people who eat dairy products can consider themselves vegetarians. I would like to shed light on this erroneous perception of milk. We do not kill or harm the cow to gather its milk!

As you know, my ancient peace-generating tradition honors all animals, their memories, and their sacred right to life and living. Moreover, we feel gratitude for the abundance of gifts all the animals bring to the earth. One such gift is the *ojas*-packed food (immune boosting), milk. In fact, the cow is so venerated in my culture that it has been given the name *Go* in Sanskrit, also the name for the earth, as well as the Vedic scriptures. Lord Krishna is called *Gopala*, "the one who protects the cow." "Protecting the cow" is a common expression used by the Vedic seers to mean self-knowledge and/or the safeguarding of spiritual dharma. In ancient India, the cow was by far the most celebrated and adored of all the animals. Still today, in Kedarnath, a temple in the Himalayas, the rear hump of the bull is seen as the sacred lingam of Shiva, symbolizing one of Shiva's appearances in the form of a bull. It is touched by millions of Hindus in reverence.

The cow's essential nature is nurturing, solid, stoic, and mothering. Her milk can provide humans the same characteristics when cultivated in a peaceful and harmonious way from organic and humane dairy farming. In today's traditional dairies however, the intense abuse and victimization the cow endures in her captivity is being reflected in our present health conditions. It is no secret that many people today have a difficult time imbibing milk, are "lactose intolerant," (especially if they come from an ancestry which did not imbibe cow's milk) and for them it is understandable why they avoid milk for the benefit of their health.

In my tradition, the cow's milk reflects the milk of the eternal mother and is a vital part of our heritage. To enjoy the benefits of this powerful elixir, eradicate your health concerns, and at the same time safeguard the cow's welfare, the practical solution is to support organic dairy farmers and imbibe milk and milk products from animals we can be sure have been well cared for. In my estimation, if we were all to stop drinking milk, the cow would become an extinct species, eventually losing her ability to produce milk.

The Myth that Vegetarians Kill Plants

As I journey around the globe on my Living Ahimsa—The Power of Peace tour, I have been peppered a zillion times by vegans and meat-eaters alike with the same questions. Among these queries is a critical one: "By harvesting and eating a plant, aren't we also contributing to killing a life?" In short, no. In my tradition, we observe how the Great Goddess feeds and nourishes her universe through the universal law of yajna, sacrifice for the benefit of humanity. According to this law, the plant kingdom makes the greatest, most phenomenal sacrifice for the subsistence of life on earth. A plant's life is cosmically designed to be perennial, annual, or to last only for the span of a few months or a season. In the vegetable kingdom, plants such as carrots, beets, potatoes, and leeks, which we uproot to harvest, would not last out the season even if left untouched.

In contrast, I view senselessly felling a forest as an act of violence; the farming of cattle for the production of its meat as a death sentence to the prolific green earth; the unconscious, excessive exploitation of nature as a death sentence to the plant kingdom. We don't kill fruit trees or berry bushes when they bend in service to us with weighted offerings made to us year after year. They remain transfixed in dedicated service, with the single purpose of creating food for humanity and all earth's creatures. As the season of their bounty passes, they bow to the Mother, before shriveling, withering, and fading out of sight as they descend back into the bosom of the earth. Thusly, the cyclical, spiraling process of nurturance continues. The devoted plant continues to feed her mother, the Good Earth, after the vegetarian populations have had their fill. Most plants broadcast an infinite number of new lives through their seeds before they go under. We don't have to chase them, hunt them down with the fierce intention of wounding and killing them. They do not run from us, rather they are entirely at our disposal. They remain immobile as we reap their nourishment.

Plant food is a seasonal virtue. Plants have specific energy and nutrients that are most nourishing during their particular season, and when that season expires, so does the plant. By profound contrast, most animals do not die at the end of the season if they are not killed! They run for their lives when they are threatened. Hunters and butchers have to take them by force defying the cosmic principle of annam. The appropriate food for humanity does not run away from us; we do not have to claim it by force of will or shed living blood to obtain it. We can safely assume that the animals did not sign up with the Mother Goddess to make a sacrifice with their lives for human beings.

TRANSITIONING TO VEGETARIANISM

The good news is, that with the necessary effort, we can easily regain our human intelligence and ancestral memories—the innate cellular legacy inherited from our lineage. At the Mother Om Mission, 80 percent of our vegetarian converts find that their transition from a meat-eating diet was not as challenging as they had expected. I guide my students through an awareness program that cultivates understanding of the self—a foremost requisite before change at any level is possible. Many of my students come from Western and European backgrounds where eating meat is a perennial part of their ancestral diet. Taste, as you will see in later pages, is an intricate phenomenon that influences our choices in many different ways.

The inherent tastes of our ancestry are coded within the tissue memories of our bodies, and therefore play a paramount role in our likes and dislikes, especially our food preferences. Simply to will the mind to forego meat does not usually work. The Wise Earth Ayurveda method for transitioning is to cultivate the understanding necessary to grow into a more compassionate and peaceful human being. For this we must make a conscious commitment to harmony.

The following practice of Kapitthaka Mudra, or Smiling Buddha, is a simple and effective practice that takes very little time. It helps you open the pathway to your heart and create the necessary pause to contemplate what it means to live in ahimsa—a gentler, kinder life. Mudras were designed by Hindu seers in accord with the cosmic flow of energy. Various configurations of sacred hand postures create a circuit that allows energy to flow to different parts of the vital organs and brain. Each mudra has a specific purpose—such as creating mental serenity, physical and emotional healing, and deepening personal awareness. The Kapitthaka Mudra invokes a deep sense of security and serenity within.

THE PRACTICE: KAPITTHAKA MUDRA

OPTIMUM TIMING: Anytime.

INSTRUCTIONS:
- Sit comfortably in a chair or on the floor with crossed legs.
- Using your right hand, tuck your ring and pinky fingers inside your palms.
- Press your thumbs over the tucked fingers.
- Keep the index and middle fingers straight and extended with palms facing forward.
- Hold your elbows in toward your body, keeping about a 30° angle between your upper arms and forearms.

- Hold this mudra for 5-10 minutes as you visualize transitioning to a life of vegetarianism.

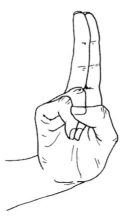

Figure 3.1 Smiling Buddha

Setting realistic time goals is important for the transition to a vegetarian lifestyle. The time it takes someone to completely eradicate meat from his or her diet varies greatly. I recommend a gradual transition, although more than 20 percent of my students stopped eating meat all at once. During the first six months, endeavor to stop eating red meat completely and slowly cut back on consuming poultry and fish with the intention of having a purely vegetarian diet by the end of twelve months. In this way, you can successfully stick with a realistic timetable for reaching your goal. Some may find it easier to begin this transition in the spring or summer when fruits and vegetables are more abundantly available and the weather is more conducive to lighter eating.

John's Story

The compelling reality of the power of ahimsa practice is elucidated by John, a young neighborhood farmer, who came to see me about his health concerns. He shares this amusing story about meeting me and his transition to vegetarianism.

> *Growing up in meat-and-potatoes country in Leicester, North Carolina, I was raised on meat from day one. I am a third generation cattle farmer; every weekend in the summer I joined my family for the usual barbecue outing in the backyard. Like most of my family, I was "a heart attack waiting to happen." In fact, my blood pressure and cholesterol got so high I started to fear for my life. My doctor told me that I had to go on a strict diet if I wished to control my blood*

pressure. He suggested I begin eating a lot of vegetables. The only vegetables I was accustomed to eating were some broccoli, collards, or turnip greens cooked in oil or lard. In fact, the only vegetarian person I knew in my area was a woman from India who had recently moved into the neighborhood. She was some kind of a spiritual person who liked to wear orange—a color that only the prison inmates around here wear.

I heard that she had given old Jenny some herbs from her garden to help heal her rheumatism. Jenny could hardly walk; the only thing that was in more pain than Jenny was her old bull, Henry. Apparently, after taking the herbs the Indian woman gave her, Jenny was pain-free and back on her farm tractor again. So I figured I would go visit her and ask for some help. It was about 8:30 in the morning when I got to her place and I found her in the field chanting to the cows in some foreign tongue. I couldn't help wondering if all vegetarian folks are that weird. I guess eating vegetables sure makes you happy. She walked over to greet me with a big smile.

As we walked up the hill to her cabin, a herd of deer came out from their resting place in the bamboo grove and greeted her by stretching their long necks as though they were throwing her kisses. I was born and raised in this valley; I have gone deer hunting with my father in these forests and have never seen anything like it. "How do you get them to do that?" I asked her. Her response blew me away, "They recognize the energy of harmony; they know they are safe with me, that I could never hunt or hurt or eat them!"

With some help from her, I became a vegetarian. She recommended her books to read, A Life of Balance *and* The Path of Practice, *and I have been a vegetarian for six months now. My mother was so impressed by the excellent health report of my cholesterol and blood pressure checkup that she decided to become a vegetarian too. To my family's surprise, I stopped hunting. Every time I see a deer, I now think of the amazing moment with the Indian woman. I am hoping that one day they will trust me enough to come up to me and throw kisses.*

For a split moment, John had experienced the profound effect of being in harmony with the Mother Consciousness, and that was all it took to shift his awareness into becoming a gentler being.

MAKING A CONSCIOUS CHOICE

Many of you have spent a lifetime eating meat without ever being introduced to the ideas that I am presenting to you now. Like all new ideas, they may take a little getting used to. I suggest letting the words you've just read sink into your body and soul. How does your body feel when you consider freeing it from the burden, both physical and emotional, of consuming meat? Do you envision your life as being more whole and light if you were to become a vegetarian? Essentially, does it feel right to you?

When you get to the point where you feel you are ready to embark on this new path toward greater health, harmony, and awareness—leading the life of a shakahari—I encourage you to honor your decision by taking The Shakahari Oath, part of the ceremony I perform at the Wise Earth School with my vegetarian converts. You may recite this alone (out loud or in your mind); write it down in a special journal or on beautiful paper you keep on your altar; or make this oath in the presence of your family, or like-minded people who will support and embrace your loving decision.

THE SHAKAHARI OATH: COMMITMENT TO A WHOLE & SACRED LIFE

- *I take The Shakahari Oath with full awareness. I am making a commitment to Inner Harmony and a Whole and Sacred Life.*

- *From this moment onward, I will not eat the animals, nor contribute to killing, harming, or hurting them in any way.*

- *From this moment onward, I will be conscious of my life fire, agni, and remember that it transports and connects me in Oneness to a Whole and Sacred Life.*

- *From this moment onward, I will protect and preserve the sanctity of all life in mind, body, and spirit.*

- *From this moment onward, I will strive to be the best instrument of the Mother Consciousness that I can be.*

Chapter Four

FASTING BODY, FEASTING SPIRIT

What empties the body feasts the spirit;
what feasts the body fuels the mind.

HEALING JOURNEY

Over the years, I have been asked numerous times what my diet consisted of during the critical six months I retreated into the depths of the Vermont winter and healed myself of ovarian cancer, after being handed down a death sentence from my physicians. Was it a miracle diet? Was it a vegetarian diet, a raw foods diet, or a brown rice diet? What Ayurveda remedies did I take? What holistic therapies did I endure?

The answer in short: Apart from a one-pot meal of mostly rice and mung bean *kichadi*, my primary food regimen was one of fasting. I not only fasted the body by eating very little, I fasted the mind by observing silence in the solitude of spirit, and I fasted the spirit by weeping my tears while writing voluminous pages to air out and neutralize the conflicts I had experienced from childhood and beyond. Unbeknownst to me at that time, during those tumultuous days, the act of fasting thinned out my fears and grief. I was transported high into the realm of the Mother Consciousness—transcending emotional and physical pain—touching her luminous serenity. I did not know then what I now share with you: The Mother Consciousness was within me all the while, and the incidental act of fasting allowed her light to swell within my entire being. In essence, I know without a doubt that this is the power that reignited my life force and helped me overcome the terminal cancer diagnosis.

In this timeless grasp with eternal memory, I had separated myself from the norm—the daily rituals of life and the living—to find a semblance of peace within; to reconcile unbearable ancestral grief; and to complete a farewell letter I was writing to my father and mother before leaving the earth and journeying to the higher ethers. In the swell of so doing, I came up short with death and regained not only my life, but my sacred purpose on this journey. Fasting body, mind, and spirit is the primary Living Ahimsa practice that gave me back my blessed life. Indeed, I experienced a miracle; not the kind of miracle we search for outside of ourselves, but the greatest miracle of all: the living energy within that is the Mother Consciousness; the awakening to the heart of ahimsa that reinforces our prana, our life force; and the power of Inner Medicine healing. I discovered that in unintentionally fasting the body, I had feasted the mind and filled the spirit. I discovered my purpose and thereby the means of reconciling my karmas.

LESS IS MORE

The understanding behind what makes us feel, think, and live wholesomely requires earnest inquiry into what feeds, nourishes, and nurtures the whole foundation of the body, mind, and spirit. Learning to live each and every moment in concert with the cyclical rhythms of the universe provides a solid foundation for building a rich and wholesome life. All internal functions—the movements of the body and mind and the desires and intentions we hold as sacred—are shaped by nature's rhythms. There are distinct lunar, seasonal, and cyclical fluctuations of life that foster a state of healthful balance.

For example, there are critical times when we can easily secure a deep sense of nourishment, feel abundant and fat and happy inside. There are other times when we are cyclically supported in feeling cosseted in our deep and private spaces within; and there are times when our best Inner Medicine is to be sparse, light, and silent. Within the intelligence of the cosmic rhythms, there is a time to feast and a time to fast, and a time for everything in between. Remember this Inner Medicine rule: *What empties the body feasts the spirit; what feasts the body fuels the mind.*

To learn to appreciate how "less is more," we must learn to flow in harmony with the cosmic rhythms and live in tune with the universally friendly days to feast or fast. We must learn when to be meditative or active, celebrate or retreat, cleanse or pamper. Living in accord with nature's dynamic rhythms, we know when to strip down or adorn the body, mind, and psyche. You will be amazed to learn that the most powerful effect of our sacred food can be found after fasting. In *Living Ahimsa Diet: Nourishing Love & Life,* you will learn that sometimes your best feast lies in the fast.

Twice monthly on *Ekadashi*, (the lunar time for fasting, as you will soon discover) I sit within myself in the sublime space of fasting, at home or wherever my travels take me. I marvel at the palpable sense of clarity I experience as the body and mind become unfettered from the busy world that bustles around me. My spirit lightens and soars in meditation and all things come to a point of pause. Thoughts that disturb my mind resolve; prayers for the well-being of all disciples are instantly answered. My life force celebrates its renewal—rebirthing itself into profound joy.

We all have the ability to reach this point of pause within. One way of so doing is to take time during Ekadashi to sit within ourselves, observe fasting, and empty the density of the self. As many have discovered, fasting can be challenging when the mind and spirit are out of alignment with the greater energies of nature. To fast the body, we must release toxic thoughts, conflicts, and unresolved feelings that tend to fill our lives. When breath, mind, and psyche are invoked to flow in harmony, the art of fasting becomes first nature. In order to awaken our inner healing capacity, we engage in sadhanas—abundant health-generating practices—that facilitate recovery of our resonant space within. Each one of us can find, recover, and awaken our inner serenity. Sumati's story illuminates this truth.

Sumati's Story

After recovering from her four-year bout with breast cancer, Sumati returned to her ancestral ground in the foothills of the Rocky Mountains to enter a period of stillness. In a note to me she said that these mountains were the first vision that came to her when her oncologist announced she was free of cancer. She understood this priceless metaphor: The mountain represented the force of stability within her. The sacred atmosphere of her mountain climate induced her own sense of serenity, which she was able to regain by embracing her ability to be at peace with absolute stillness. As she prepared to enter a period of fasting in stillness, she heard ethereal sounds from within. She fasted for one month, and found abundant energy and lightness after her fast. She said that she felt and looked 10 years younger and had much more clarity than she has ever had in her life! Fasting in sublime solitude is the armor that safeguards the spirit and provides an absolute sense of security.

Before we explore the simple ways in which we can successfully perform the act of fasting, let us focus our attention on calming the mind. Since the mind has the greatest impact on our physical desires, urges, and responses, it is essential that we learn how to take pause and make the inner environs of the mind and psyche tranquil.

SILENCING THE MIND

There is no greater medicine than the silence of the mind. In the same way that the body needs rest, the mind and senses must also be allayed from time to time. To reap the major benefits of fasting, you must be prepared to take pause and create the necessary space around you to invite the critical experience of inner tranquillity. As you approach a fast in the ideal way, you are entering the cosmic realm of nurturance. Silence is a profound way to help the mind and senses withdraw themselves from the external world so that you become aware of the center of the world within yourself—the *terra incognito*—a place most people are fearful to enter. This fear of being in the immutable presence of ourselves—reaching into the less traversed territory of the inner self—stems from the accumulation of cultural habits and societal education which teach us to use our mind and senses in the exact opposite way that serves humanity, wholeness, and wellness. For this reason, the brilliant sentiency of the self is hidden from us, and has become the unknown terrain we are afraid to tread.

But, we no longer have to fear. In this Living Ahimsa work, you will learn how to effectively use your mind and find perfect guidance on the journey of exploring the inner self to recover your Inner Medicine and heal! Practicing inner quietude is a perfect method for loosening the mind and sensory organs from their external activities. It is easier for the body to endure a fast when you can first allay the busy mind. Silence is a way of fasting the mind and senses, and once accomplished, it makes the sojourn of the fast an illumined affair.

There are countless ways to ease the mind and senses during fasting. To reach your destination of inner serenity, you must empty your mind of pressure. Given all the stress and demands we face each day, how do we make time in our lives to access the profound inner silence that unites us with the universal greater consciousness? A daily meditation practice is the foundation upon which we build a quiet mind.

THE PRACTICE OF MEDITATION

As you develop your practice and your inner awareness grows, the mind and senses receive the signal to take a break—hunger and desire abate and bodily functions become still. As you keep up your practice, you go beyond imagination and mental fluctuations. The realm you are trying to enter is formless and wordless. It is the state of enlightenment that the Vedas call *samadhi*—complete meditative absorption that lies beyond the spiritual states of contemplation and concentration. With continuous practice you can enter this less traversed space, but in the meantime, the goal at hand is to secure a point of pause and calmness. As time goes by, you will discover that only your personal awareness can sustain your physical, mental, and emotional well-being. Practice the art of fasting mind and body, and you'll find the center of support and stability within your spirit. Taking leisure at the appropriate times is imperative if you are to start exploring your inner realm of sentiency where all healing forces are held.

When I enter into silence, I sit in meditation for six or seven hours at a stretch. When my body gets tired, I stand up and stretch. When I am not fasting, I prepare myself the simplest of meals—a pot of kichadi, and perhaps some greens that I pick from my garden. I minimize physical activity, although I take a short walk every day, because if my mind is preoccupied with a thought or feeling, the walking meditation will help to dissolve it. I look at the deer grazing in the fields and the crows and hawks flying overhead. I notice the green grass, the buds coming up in the fields, or the river flowing higher than normal this year. I take in the sights and sounds of nature around me, but I do not hold on to the perceptions. My mind observes and then moves on. I leave the deer where they are, the birds in flight, and the river where it is. I do not take them with me when I return to sit in my cabin. My mind becomes immersed in the realm of *inner* awareness—thought without thoughts. Sometimes I see visions or lights, and other times I experience absolute tranquillity. There is no pushing or doing. I am simply there, simply present.

SHANTI MUDRA—THE PATH TO INNER SILENCE

A profound way to fast the body and mind while feasting the spirit is to enjoin silence. You may enter into this process through the practice of Shanti Mudra, the hand gesture for peace and tranquillity, which will deepen and replenish your inner silence. This simple practice can be done anywhere and at any time.

THE PRACTICE: SHANTI MUDRA—THE PATH TO INNER SILENCE

OPTIMUM TIMING: Anytime.

INSTRUCTIONS:
1. Facing north, sit in a comfortable posture with your legs crossed or in a meditative pose. Rest your hands in your lap and close your eyes.
2. Relax your hands and connect the tips of the thumb and index fingers to form a circle. While keeping this posture, rest the hands on your knees, palms up.
3. Breathe normally and hold the Shanti Mudra for 5 minutes.
4. Open your eyes. Maintain the mudra position for a few more minutes before releasing it, and sit for a few moments in silence.

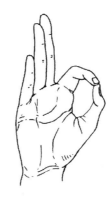

Figure 4.1 Shanti Mudra

THE VITALITY OF BREATH

There is a breath for feasting and a breath for fasting. The stronger your breath force, the greater the degree of awareness and inner harmony you will harvest. Breathing should not be taken for granted. It is a highly evolved science of life and longevity. When you breathe in accord with the cosmic energies, you enhance the quality of your life, happiness, and wellness. This science is called *pranayama.* Your breath force is the manifestation of cosmic energy. Did you know that, according to the ancient Hindu seers, your life is defined not by the number of years you live, but by the number of breaths you are given for your journey? Ninety-nine percent of your life exists in a cosmic quantum field that is invisible and intangible energy; it is no surprise that the invisible breath plays such a significant role in our everyday lives.

Learning the art of enhancing your awareness through yogic breathing promotes unification of body and nature, mind and cosmos, individual and community. Consider these Vedic principles regarding the way in which fasting affects our physical, physiological, and spiritual bodies. It increases inner tranquillity and thereby produces more oxygen and internal prana—the vital life force that sustains health and immunity.

Health and harmony respond to the many layers of prana in the body. The 72,000 or so *nadis* (nerve channels through which prana flows) that exist in the body are vibration sensitive; they function strictly through vibrational energy. Therefore, good breathing practices increase the vitality of these prana conduits. Prana that is flowing through the nadis also becomes robust with vigor. When the prana is healthy and filled with vitality, it stimulates healthy vital tissue and organ activity so that good health is achieved and maintained.

Vital prana and a harmonious mind work hand-in-hand. They travel through the body like a great wave, revitalizing the cells of the brain and inspiring the mind to produce fluent, clear, and happy thoughts. Breathe well and you'll transcend obstacles and distractions in your path to move into the light of your greater awareness. Mircea Eliade, one of the 20th century's preeminent philosophers of religious traditions, says yogic practice "is an attention directed upon one's organic life, a knowledge through action, a calm and lucid entrance into the very essence of life."

Joe's Story

At a recent book signing event at a Barnes & Noble bookstore, Joe, an elderly gentleman in his 90s who sat attentively but slightly slumped over in the front row, wanted to know what to do about his life-long asthmatic condition. He framed his question to me, "I know I may not have much longer to live, but I'd like to experience what it's like to live for one day without this dreadful condition." I marveled at his sheer sense of aliveness during my talk, especially given his seemingly frail condition. In fact, I told him I thought he was a saint to sit through a long talk on women's conditions at his age!

Recognizing that all conditions involve the body and mind, and that most are rooted in our family ancestry or stem from the relationships we forge and how we respond to them, I asked him, "How is your mother, is she still alive?" The audience laughed loudly and Joe laughed along with them. Obviously, she would have had to be about 120 years old if she were alive! "No she is not," he responded, "but funny you should bring her up because she, herself, suffered profoundly from asthma." To which I responded, "She may be gone, but she is still alive within you in more ways than you know." All of a sudden, the silence in the room was palpable. You could see Joe's face lit by a lightening bolt of clarity from instant recognition of the root of his condition. His face softened, his posture now erect, he nodded his head in understanding.

"How are you feeling? Are you breathing more easily?" I showed him how to perform the Lunar Breath for Fasting detailed in the pages that follow. After about a minute or so of practice, he was astonished to find that his breath was no longer constricted and was in a state of perfect balance. "I feel an ease inside myself the likes of which I haven't felt before." I asked a final question: "Is your mother still alive within you?" He pondered for a moment and said, "Yes, I feel I'm holding her now in a gentler way." Bingo! He had found the Inner Medicine link to his asthma. "Now, Mr. Joe, how do you maintain the gentle love of the maternal spirit?" He became emotional. You could almost "see" him turning the pages of his life's book from the last pages going backward to the present. "I feel at peace," he said with a contemplative nod.

The kindness of the universe is always at our beck and call. This eventful encounter with Joe actually occurred during *Pitri Paksha*—the time of the ancestors, which I explore further in chapter thirteen, "Autumn Practices for Harvesting Nurturance." As we will explore in later pages, this is the most fitting time of the year to heal the wounds of our ancestors and the legacy of pain that we may have inherited from our lineage. I guided the audience through a mantra for the welfare of the forebears, and asked Joe to keep a gentle focus on his mother's face, honoring her during his recitation of the mantra.

I have no doubt that by shifting his awareness about his asthma condition and his relationship to his mother, Joe will be able to experience blissful forgiveness and relief from his condition. He promised to keep up the Lunar Breath for Fasting Practice, a gentle practice that will remind him to maintain his newly discovered awareness in the secured space of vibrant memory. The solutions to all challenges are conspicuous when you learn to access and use your Inner Medicine.

THE PRACTICE: LUNAR BREATH FOR FASTING

OPTIMUM TIMING:
- All year, during fasting and meditation.
- In the early morning.

Contra-indications: Do not practice this breath during menstruation or when bleeding.

The Lunar Breath for Fasting is a simple, contemplative practice you may do during fasting or meditation to deepen inner balance. We have 2 primary channels of breath in the body: Lunar Breath, propagated by the moon's energies, and Solar Breath, influenced by the sun's energies. The Lunar Breath is channeled through the subtle energy conduit of the body called *Ida*, and flows through your left nostril. The solar breath courses through the subtle energy channel of the body called *Pingala*, and flows through your right nostril.

Our Solar Breath is strong and powerful like the sun, and our Lunar Breath is calm and introspective like the influence of the moon. It is important to note that as a general rule, the Lunar Breath is naturally stronger in the daytime and the Solar Breath is stronger in the evening to assist the body and mind maintain a state of equilibrium. During the day, our calming Lunar Breath prevails to balance the natural solar cycle we experience externally, and during the evening, our Solar Breath dominates to help us balance the introspective energies of the moon.

If our Solar Breath were stronger during the day, we would find ourselves in a state of being overheated, angry, or aggressive. Conditions such as violence, anger, hatred, and jealously are related to an imbalance in the Solar Breath. Conversely, if our Lunar Breath were stronger in the evening when the moon's energy dominates, we would find ourselves in a depressed, lethargic, or restless state. In fact, conditions like insomnia and depression also point to the misalignment of our natural breathing mechanism. When the body is in good health, the Lunar and Solar Breaths will perform as they should.

For the purpose of this practice, we will concentrate only on the workings of the Lunar Breath. Harnessing the Lunar Breath supports contemplative activities such as fasting and meditating, or simply taking a restful reprieve. It increases ojas (our body's immunity) and aids the mind in maintaining a sense of fulfillment and clarity.

In this practice, the classical formula for length of inhalation versus exhalation is to hold the breath for 4 times as long as the inhalation, then exhale for twice the length of the inhalation. Once you feel comfortable with the mechanics of the practice, you may want to silently count the seconds of your inhalation, and then try to extend your exhalation for twice that count. As you become more adept, work your way up to inhaling for 8 counts, exhaling for 16. You may then incorporate the more classical technique which involves holding your breath between inhalation and exhalation. Begin with a ratio of 4:16:8 (so that the holding is 4 times the length of the inhalation, and the exhalation is twice the length of the inhalation), and work your way up to a ratio of 8:32:16.

ALTERNATE NOSTRIL BREATHING:

Start with a few minutes of exhaling your breath from the belly. Then continue by alternating your breath from one nostril to the other in this way:

1. Block your left nostril with your right ring and pinky fingers, and inhale through your right nostril.
2. Then block your right nostril with your right thumb, and exhale through your left nostril.
3. Continue alternating right and left nostrils for approximately 3 minutes. Be sure always to inhale through the same nostril from which you just exhaled.

NEXT STEPS:

4. Make a fist with your left hand and place it securely under your right armpit. This invokes the meridians that control the workings of Ida and Pingala, the 2 main channels of prana.
5. Proceed by alternating right and left nostrils for another 3 minutes or so. Be sure always to inhale through the same nostril from which you just exhaled.
6. Release the hands, and check your breath by using your hand to close 1 nostril at a time, expelling the air out of the other into your palm to gauge which breath is stronger.
7. Your Lunar Breath should now be the stronger breath, coming out with more force through your left nostril.
8. If the right breath is stronger, do not repeat the practice. Sometimes it takes a while for the breath to find its place of stasis. Trust that it will eventually shift to the left, or lunar, side during your fasting observance.

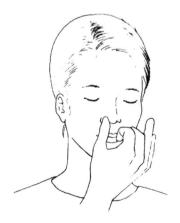

Figure 4.2 Lunar Breath for Fasting

YOUR COSMIC VIBRATION

As we strengthen our breath power we increase our resonant field of ahimsa—intuition, power, beauty, and healing that is waiting in contentment within us. It is through this resonant field that one attracts the person she marries, children she carries, and discovers love and comfort in relationships. This cosmic vibration also influences the objects, sciences, arts, and professions to which we are drawn. As we refine the power of our breath, we will discover the vast energy of cosmic resonance that supports body, mind, and spirit, and by extension, our life purpose and journey.

As you may know from my other writings, cosmic resonance is the primary Inner Medicine means for healing that each and every human possesses. This powerful protocol includes Sound Medicine—a system of healing Wise Earth Ayurveda education has effectively implemented. Ways and means of Sound Medicine are numerous: listening and chanting Sanskrit mantras; emulating nature's sounds; reciting Vedic chants; playing raga music; listening to classical music or to the expert playing of nature-made instruments such as the Himalayan singing bowl, the Hindu *damaru*, an Indian or African handmade drum, an Aboriginal *didgeridoo*, or the Japanese bamboo flute. But of all of nature's sublime instruments of cosmic sound, the most powerful one is the human voice.

Herman's Story

Herman, a middle-aged gentleman I met at my recent book signing event at East West Books in New York, eagerly came up to meet me with his wife to get his book signed. He said that they had both wanted to meet me for so long that when they heard I'd be in New York they seized the opportunity to come, even though they lived in Romania, over 4,500 miles away! "Such a long journey," I exclaimed, and gave them both a hug. Herman began to choke on his words, and with tears in his eyes, he whispered, "I will cherish this hug forever!"

At the end of the three-hour long event, Herman and Gloria came back up to see me. Apparently, they had sat patiently waiting until most of the participants had left. Suspecting that they must have had something of urgency to share with me, I invited them to walk with me back to my lodgings which were nearby. Gloria told me that four years ago Herman was diagnosed with throat cancer; his oncologist told him the condition was so advanced that there wasn't much they could do for him. They sought the help of an Ayurveda physician from India who was visiting their hometown in Romania. Among the recommendations he gave them was my book, *Ayurveda: A Life of Balance,* and my Vedic Chanting CD, *Darshana.* After listening to the CD "Herman took to the Vedic chants like a fish to water," effused Gloria with pride and passion in her beautiful accent, even though he had never heard a word of Sanskrit before.

"I can't believe I'm here walking on Fifth Avenue with you in person!" Herman exclaimed. Gloria went on to tell Herman's riveting story of healing. They cooked "every recipe in the Pitta-Kapha category (Herman's Body Type) while Herman chanted along with my CD for three hours every day for four months. Six months after the grim diagnosis from his oncologist, Herman returned to see him. His oncologist was shocked, although neither Herman nor Gloria were surprised to find that the results of his tests showed no sign of cancer. When we had reached my destination, and as I said goodbye to both, Herman began to chant the *Mrtyunjaya* mantras from *Darshana*. "Mother, how is my chanting?" he asked shyly. "*Desaversit*," I responded, "Perfect indeed!"

FEASTING THE SPIRIT ON COSMIC RESONANCE

In the final exploration of our power to heal through fasting, let us examine how fasting our physical organism can be a feast for our immutable spirit. In practicing fasting during Ekadashi, we rest the instruments of our body, mind, and psyche, and along with them, the burdens of ancestral karma. Garnering the Lunar Breath releases stress and toxicity and awakens the primordial resonant field of the body. At the very least, the tension from our body and mind eases. In so doing, we connect to the rhythm and memory of our individual power and creativity.

Each and every one of us carries this primeval potential for healing through our inner sound—a sound that expresses itself a million times over every time we use our voice. Regardless of our tradition, when we use our personal sound as a mantra—the raw cosmic expression of inner harmony—the intrinsic sounds of the body's chakras, or energy centers, become entrained and suddenly our sense of awareness grows in leaps and bounds.

Each one of our inner sounds, when nurtured and expressed, can direct us toward the natural, vibratory balance of body, mind, and spirit that gives us clarity and purpose in our daily lives. As we strengthen our practice through the art of fasting, we feast on the brilliance of our inner sounds and perhaps discover the sacred power of our voice. The human voice is one of our most misunderstood and misused possessions. We take our voices for granted; we use and abuse it for the most mundane, trivial, and hurtful communications—forgetting to honor it as the divine instrument of cosmic truth within us. This is why I encourage you to take The Vow of Ahimsa in your speech, as well as in your thoughts and actions.

The Vedic seers emulated the primordial sound in order to fashion the first human expression, called *sruti*, the cosmic revelation as heard by the rishis. Sruti is also referred to as "the Word," and the song of *Sama Veda* informs us that, "Verily, if there were no Word, there would be no knowledge of right or wrong, or of truth and untruth, or of the pleasing and unpleasing. The Word makes all this known." The voice as a sacred human instrument is one of our most powerful Inner Medicine tools for healing. The rishis revealed that the rhythmic speech of the human voice was the first life-generating Sound Medicine. From the onset of time, we humans have used rhythmic speech and music to transcend the physical, mental, and emotional planes. This explains why television shows like "American Idol" or music concerts can draw phenomenal crowds of people who are captivated by rich human sound, and being held together in a bond of common unity for that all too brief moment in time. Sanskrit mantras and Vedic chants take us a cosmic step further. These mediums of sound engineered by the rishis themselves, enable us to transcend even the spiritual climes.

Following is a Devi Mantra venerating the Mother Consciousness. The sounds of this mantra are empowered with Mother's Grace to feast your spirit with cosmic resonance as the words reverberate through and awaken the sentiency of Living Ahimsa in your heart, your infinite source of personal awareness. This potent mantra can be used during your fasting observance or at any time throughout your life. Recite the mantra 108 times directly before dusk.

Om Dahar'Akasha-Rupinyai Namah
(Pronounced: OOM DA-HAR AAKAA-SHA RUH-PIN-YAI NAH-MAH-HA)

Reverence onto Her who is the Subtle Self in the heart of humans
(Referring to the Supreme Goddess, Lalita Maha Tripurasundari)

Stephanie's Triumphant Story
As you become accustomed to sitting within yourself and celebrating your inner sound, you'll discover your own unique, inner vibrational tempo—the wellspring of Inner Medicine for your healing. You alone will hear the distinct sounds of your innermost being. In the case of Stephanie, the sounds that arose conveyed an important message about her childhood—memories that she could not otherwise access.

Stephanie, a 40-year-old American woman with breast cancer, had been told by her oncologist that her prognosis was grim—her tumor had metastasized to her lungs. He recommended she immediately begin an intensive regimen of chemotherapy, but she did not want to undergo the treatment. Stephanie felt she needed time to compose herself, time to catch her breath before making decisions about a course of treatment. It was clear to me that she needed to reconnect with her roots—with the familiar sensory experiences that had nourished her as a child and were part of her heritage. She took my advice and retreated to a serene space where she could find solitude.

She found a cabin in the forest of Virginia about 100 miles from where she grew up and stayed there for two weeks. It was springtime in the beautiful countryside and although Stephanie had always been surrounded by rolling hills and the fresh smell of hay throughout her life, she had barely noticed these wholesome scents before. As she began her time in solitude, she noticed that her sense of smell became so strong that she could distinguish between the scent of buttercups, daffodils, and freshly cut grass. The forest where she sat was filled with tall pines and hemlocks, oaks and birches, squirrels and raccoons, cardinals and hummingbirds, and a myriad of other creatures that live in the woodlands.

Almost immediately following her arrival to the forest cabin, she became acutely aware of the fullness of her breath and her increased stamina. As a result her senses became vibrant. She could clearly hear the ambient sounds of nature around her: the winds howling through the trees at night, the scurrying sounds of the squirrels, the flight of the hawks above her, and the crackling of winter's last leaves as the deer foraged for their morning repast. Her sense of vision also became clearer. It was as though she had witnessed the sun rising in the morning for the very first time in the half century of her life. She told me she was pulled by an irresistible force into nature.

As she settled into the space of her inner quietude, aided by her Wise Earth Ayurveda regimen, she committed herself to the practice of fasting and resting to rejuvenate her spirits. Her daily Wise Earth Ayurveda routine included the practice of Vedic Chanting, Living Ahimsa Meditation, and a Semi-Fast (on pages 73-77) with fruits, nuts, seeds, fruit juices, and water. Each morning she met the dewy dawn with a sense of reprieve and deep serenity. Her physical pain continued for a while as the angry memories of her tense relationship with her mother and unhappiness in her marriage floated to her consciousness. As she began the painful examination of her joyless relationship with her mother and husband, she spent several days weeping and releasing the pain she had imprisoned within herself. After the first week of being sequestered, her mind became crystal clear. The sense of inured fear and anger she had experienced earlier had been vanquished.

Was it the practices that brought her the inner calm she needed or was it her discipline of fasting? Was it the clean air of the forest, the shimmering light of dawn, or the peaceful vibrations of the forest's vegetation? One could say it was the sum total of all of these ahimsa forces held together by the great grace of the Mother Consciousness. Once we make inner harmony our first commitment, we can summon our Inner Medicine to help us heal and claim our healthful destiny through many means. Through her Semi-Fast, and her breath and sound practices, Stephanie was able to quickly access her own private stock of Inner Medicine healing energy when she needed it most.

Two weeks later, she returned to the small city where she lived, feeling strong and revived in spirit. Her brief time in solitude had helped her discover the wounds in her heart and spirit—the loneliness in her marriage and the bitterness toward her mother that she had held tightly in her heart. When she returned she had emotionally purged these life-threatening emotions and was stronger for it. She was ready to move forward with her healing journey and returned to her oncologist with a fortified intuition to guide the process of her own treatment.

She underwent three of the seven chemotherapy treatments recommended by her doctor, and became so physically and mentally ill from the toxic side effects that she decided to curtail the remaining therapy protocol. Once again, she turned to the Living Ahimsa practices she had embraced during her time in the forest, but instead of fasting I advised her to continue with the practices of organically prepared, warm, freshly-cooked whole grains, beans and vegetables, fruits, seeds, nuts, and ghee. Yum!

Two weeks later she had regained her semblance of strength and returned once again to see her doctor and continue her Western medicine treatments. After conducting the usual tests, her doctor and his colleagues were surprised to find that the tumor that had metastasized to her lungs had disappeared, and that the one in her breast had shrunk to half of its size. After working closely with her doctor, she ended up taking one more round of chemotherapy, and still continues to practice her Living Ahimsa healing regimens to this day. It is now a year later, and Stephanie is free and clear of cancer.

It is never surprising to witness the miracle of the body's potential to heal itself when we create the appropriate conditions and environment for nurturing the mind and spirit—unfastening it from the strictures and stresses of the overdriven lives we lead. As you will see in the next chapter, any of us can create a milieu of peace and serenity around us and thereby invoke our primordial Inner Medicine power to nourish, nurture, and heal. In my ancient, peace-generating tradition, emptying the body of its toxic baggage, clearing the mind of its clutter, and simply sitting in the profoundly magnificent quietude of the self are the proven paths to cultivating the greatest gift of abundant health and well-being. When breath, mind, and psyche are invoked to flow in harmony, the art of fasting becomes first nature.

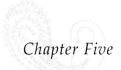
THE ART OF THE FAST

*Counting the eleven days from the day of the
new moon, and the day of the full moon, you will
discover Ekadashi—the optimum time to create
space for your reprieve—a time to observe fasting,
inner silence, cleansing, and recuperation.*

LUNAR DAYS TO LIGHTEN THE BODY, MIND & SPIRIT

The rishis tell us that observing fast, silence, rest, and other states of austerity during the appropriate lunar days are practices that strengthen our sense of personal discipline and cosmic lawfulness. In other words, when we learn to live in the embrace of dharma, we attract spiritual, emotional, and physical health and fulfillment.

As human beings we are equipped with a cosmic anatomy which functions in accord with the cyclical rhythms of Mother Nature, and in particular, the turn of the lunar wheel of time. According to the Vedas, each month brings with it two optimum days when the lunar energies support our efforts to cultivate excellent health; a period when fasting, cleansing, and other recuperative measures are greatly enhanced. We call these days Ekadashi—days when we can effortlessly coax the mind and spirit back into their divine source of silence to discover the fullness, anandam, of our spiritual beings.

The Vedic Calendar is based on the movement of the *Kala Chakra*, or cosmic lunar wheel. According to this calendar system, each year has 12 lunar months, each lasting approximately 30 days. Each lunar cycle, or 30-day period, is calculated by tracking a waxing and waning phase of the moon, with approximately 15 days in each phase.

In Sanskrit, *eka* means "one," and *dashi* means "ten," adding up to the number eleven. The word Ekadashi refers to the eleventh day of both the waxing moon phase and the waning moon phase. In each month, these two days have the same numerical energies and are the auspicious days to observe fasting and other austere acts of healing.

In Vedic numerology, each number contains a specific elemental potential, or *Shakti*. The number eleven represents the sum total of our cosmic anatomy: the five sense organs (eyes, ears, nose, tongue, and skin); the five motor organs (hands, feet, mouth, reproductive and excretory organs); and the mind. Ultimately,

Ekadashi is a cosmic metaphor for the workings of the mind, as the mind has the greatest impact on our cosmic anatomy as a whole. As such, the natural vibrations held in the cosmos during Ekadashi enhance the mind's state of equanimity when we fast at this auspicious time each month.

For the most part, Ekadashi occurs 11 days following the new moon (counting the new moon day) and 12 days following the full moon (not counting the full moon day). However, this is not always the case, depending on many lunar factors which cannot be easily systematized from month to month or year to year; it can also occur 12 days from the new or full moons. The best course of action is to purchase a Vedic Calendar, which you can easily find online. It is important to remember that in general, every month has—more or less—two "eleventh days," so there are 24 Ekadashi days in a year. It is believed that on the eleventh day, the sattva, or peace-generating quality of the universe, is vastly increased in all living organisms if we honor the Ekadashi credo. Hence, if you observe a spiritual cleansing practice during this time, you can unleash your sattva potential and reap abundant energy and inner harmony.

One day of each lunar phase is best dedicated to the disciplined practice of emptying and resuscitating the mind and the mental plane. As the optimum time for remembering our inner divinity and cultivating the spirit of ahimsa, honoring Ekadashi provides a necessary pause from our laden lives and mundane tasks. It's a rejuvenating time to free ourselves from shopping, cooking, eating, cleaning, talking on the telephone, worrying, working, studying, and other activities that fill most of our waking lives. Imagine spending a period of time in perfect tranquillity, embracing your children with serenity, and making time to feel deep gratitude to the Mother for the trillions of bountiful gifts that she gives to us freely. Such a feeling of serenity has a far-reaching and profound healing effect on everything and everyone around us, inadvertently permeating the pores of your family and community with a palpable sense of harmony. (You may recall that I explore *The Art of Taking Pause* in great detail in my book *Women's Power to Heal*.)

SECURING THE INNER SPACE FOR FASTING

To support our energies for retreat, it is important to create harmony in the space around us so our outer world becomes a reflection of the peace we are cultivating within ourselves during this time. You will also want to clear a room or area that is not used a lot, preferably in the northeast corner of your home, to designate as a reflective area during your fast. Set up a small Living Ahimsa altar space there on which you keep a ghee lamp, also called a *dipa*, or a beeswax candle, as a sacred reflection of the illumined spirit within you. You may place an image of a traditional deity, or an ancestor, or a photograph of your Guru or a family elder with whom you feel a deep connection on your altar. By doing this, you are preparing yourself to reconcile the karmas of your ancestors whose patterns of behavior you carry in your tissue memories. Spread out a simple, clean, cotton or woolen mat on the floor with a meditation pillow, symbolic of the simplicity you seek and the bare comfort that enlightens the heart. Light your ghee lamp and offer water, fruit, and fresh flowers (if available) each time you sit for meditation—gestures of gratitude that remind us of our divine source of nourishment in the Mother. It is easier to make room in your busy life for silent contemplation when you dedicate a physical space to retreat into. What you create around yourself will permeate into your inner space of being.

If your schedule is as full as those of the women and men I meet during my travels, chances are you would be hard-pressed to find time to spend a day in silence. If your spouse's schedule does not allow him or her to care for the children so that you can spend some hours alone in silence, try to find like-minded women or men within your community who are willing to trade for one day (or even an afternoon) a month.

Once you have emptied your calendar of all responsibilities, you may be tempted to read, write letters, or pay bills. Instead, see how it feels to spend a long time soaking in a bath, meditating, practicing breathing exercises, playing the drums, grinding spices, taking a hike in nature, or doing some yoga poses. Practice the art of simply being. Observe the movements around you; notice and detach.

Once your sense of inner quietude strengthens, your senses will soar. You will hear the faint beating of your heart against the tapestry of a deep, rich, inner vibration. You will see specks of light you have never noticed before, you will hear the hawks cooing from a far distance, you will feel your children's presence, especially when they need your guidance, and you will smell your favorite spices or fragrances. Many of my disciples smell lavender when they think of me or need my help although they do not know that I frequently use lavender essential oil in my bath. These experiences can happen to you when you make your own resonant field of intuition strong through the act of simply being.

EMPTYING THE BODY

Fasting is a profound means to recover tranquillity of the body, mind, and senses in order to reach the deeper spiritual recess within you, and it is a practice that I will be recommending during each of the six seasons throughout the course of this book. More than limiting or eliminating your food intake, fasting is about consciously healing yourself; it's about taking an imperative pause. Slowing down your metabolism and digestion and letting your vital tissues and organs rest from time to time is necessary if you are to maintain excellent physical, emotional, and spiritual health. It will help you add years of vibrancy to your life!

Observing a fast during both the "eleventh days" in a month is ideal. However,

if this is not possible, try to practice a fast on the eleventh day of the bright fortnight when the moon is waxing. If your body is not accustomed to doing a complete fast (where no food or liquids are imbibed), you will want to drink plenty of
warm water, a few cups of herbal tea, or water mixed with dried ginger powder
and Sucanat or jaggery. If you are unable to fast on liquids alone, you may fast on
water, fruits, nuts, and organic cow's milk. (See the section at the end of this chapter on Semi-Fasting for more details.) Also be sure to practice the Lunar Breath
for Fasting, which I detail on pages 59-61 in chapter four, "Fasting Body, Feasting
Spirit." The Practice: Observing a Fast on Ekadashi details how fasting should be
observed on all the Ekadashi days throughout the year and will serve as a refer-
ence for you throughout this book.

THE PRACTICE: OBSERVING A FAST ON EKADASHI

OPTIMUM TIMING:
- 2 times each month.
- 11th day following the waxing moon (generally).*
- 11th day following the waning moon (generally).*

*I highly recommend purchasing a Vedic Calendar to calculate the exact timing of the
new and full moons of the Ekadashi days.*

Contra-indications: Do not fast during severe illness, menstruation, or when bleeding.
The elderly and young children should also avoid fasting.

Optimum Observance: Complete fasting.

Water Fasting: If you are unable to do a complete fast, fasting with water alone is
encouraged. You may also imbibe water with dried ginger powder and Sucanat or jaggery.

Semi-Fasting: If unable to fast on liquids alone, you may fast on water, fruits, nuts, and
organic cow's milk (if allergic to lactose, do not use milk). (See the section at the end of
this chapter on Semi-Fasting.)

PREPARATIONS:
To effectively make your transition from the world of activity and noise into the serene
sanctuary of the self, I would recommend you apply the Four Pillars of Living Ahimsa
Practice we teach in Wise Earth Ayurveda:

- Simplify
- Organize
- Complete tasks
- Do nothing

Before taking your pause for fasting, complete any unfinished tasks that may be weighing on your mind so you will be physically and emotionally poised to sit in yourself and be at one with harmony. As you fast, you will be practicing the art of "simply being." As you may know, the act of "simply being" can be a very difficult one for most of us. Before you can entice the mind into its container of serenity and transcend the routine of activity and noise you will be leaving behind, I highly recommend you engage in non-mental work that needs to be done. In this way, you can gradually, but emphatically, shift into the present moment while you fast.

A great place to begin is by clearing your kitchen cupboards and closets. Clean out unnecessary utensils, stale packaged foods, and electric appliances you are no longer using. Vigorously clean the kitchen walls, shelves, countertops, sinks, and floor; scrub the pots, pans, and ladles. Allow this act of cleaning the space that nourishes you within your home to be one of sankalpa—blessing—affirming your sacred intention to open your internal pathways for cleansing and nourishment during the fast. As you engage in your space clearing activities, you will find a surge of energy coursing though your limbs, and your mind will begin to feel light, joyful, and eager to partake in the spirit of the fast.

INSTRUCTIONS:
Beginning Your Fast

- Begin your Ekadashi day by doing the Lunar Breath for Fasting Practice (see pages 59-61 in chapter four) in the early morning before starting your fast. This exercise will create the prana, life force, necessary to support the body and mind in reclaiming its stored sense of abundance, and more importantly, in letting go of its food cravings and alleviating any feelings of fear, anxiety, discontentment, and grief.
- Light your ghee lamp and offer water, fruit, and fresh flowers to affirm your intention on this day.

During Your Fast

- Avoid all grains, beans, vegetables, spices, oils, ghee, and sugars.
- Avoid all cooked foods.
- Use this time to let go and "simply be." Bear witness to the feelings or thoughts that may come up during your fast and let them go, effortlessly drawing in the healing energies that are abundant during this time.

- Also use this time to engage in deep and fruitful meditation. Doing nothing can be especially difficult, therefore you must make peace with the mind. In so doing, you do not engage the mind, combat it, or try to negotiate it, nor can you ignore it. What you can do is stay fixed on your intention to sit in meditation regardless of what's happening within and around you, except, of course, in a dire emergency. Whatever thoughts occur, remember your sakshi ability to bear witness to them by silently addressing them in the following way:

I acknowledge you.
I bear witness to you.
I am resolved to continue my sitting.

Breaking the Fast

- On the morning after your Ekadashi observance, break your fast by starting your day with a rejuvenating warm bath.
- Afterward, sit in contemplation for a few moments, and if you desire, recite this mantra for remembering the Mother Consciousness within, either out loud or in prayer:

Om Shantyai Namah
(Pronounced: OOM SHAANT-YAI NAH-MAH-HA)

Om Svasti Matyai Namah
(Pronounced: OOM SWAS-TEA MAAT-YAI NAH-MAH-HA)

Om Kantyai Namah
(Pronounced: OOM KAANT-YAI NAH-MAH-HA)

Reverence onto Her who is Serenity
Reverence onto Her who is Benediction
Reverence onto Her who is Luminosity

- It is ideal to break your fast by taking a light meal of kichadi made from white basmati rice, split yellow mung beans, and ghee.

Alternate Cleansing to End the Fast

Alternatively, you can choose to break your fast with this simple Wise Earth Ayurveda cleansing routine wherein the body's toxins, *malas* and *ama*, are expelled. (You may observe this mild purgation as necessary at any time during the year.)

- Drink 2 cups of organic cow's milk diluted in 2 cups of hot water. You may spice it up

with 1/2 teaspoon of ginger powder.
- Within 30 minutes, your bowels should be completely evacuated, and an immediate sense of lightness will ensue.

AHIMSA MEALS FOR SEMI-FASTING

If doing a complete fast or water fast proves to be challenging, you can start by observing a week-long or fortnight-long Semi-Fast in lieu of the twice monthly Ekadashi Fast. Within a few months of semi-fasting, you will find your resolve strengthening and will probably be able to secure the stamina you need to accomplish a full day, or even a full week, of fasting.

Alternatively, if you are unable to observe a complete day or more of fasting, you can orient yourself each month to conduct an incremental fast in the following way: As the moon begins to wax on the day following the new moon, take one mouthful of food. Increase it incrementally each day until you reach 15 mouthfuls on full moon day. If possible, you can observe a full day of fast on the new moon day prior to starting your 15-day incremental Semi-Fast. The recipes that follow are appropriate meals for your semi-fasting sojourn.

THE PRACTICE: OBSERVING A SEMI-FAST

For your Semi-Fast follow the instructions in the preceding practice Observing an Ekadashi Fast, but with the addition of teas and light foods that will help support you as you get accustomed to fasting.

WARM TEAS FOR SEMI-FASTING:
The following tonics and teas will be particularly nurturing during your Semi-Fast.
- Take 1 teaspoon or more of lemon or lime juice in 1 large cup of warm water each morning to help cleanse your system.
- If feelings of nervousness arise, use bala, lemon balm, catnip, chamomile, organic rose petal, or nutmeg teas.
- Also for nervousness, you may steep 10 fresh basil leaves in a large cup of hot water for 10 minutes or so, then strain and drink. You may also simply eat the fresh basil leaves.
- If a sense of lethargy or fatigue sets in, use cardamom, clove, ginger, cinnamon, or lemon tea spiced with a pinch of black pepper. You may add a smidgeon of honey.
- For mental and physical ease, drink nurturing teas such as licorice, peppermint, or raspberry. You may also drink 1 tablespoon of edible quality aloe vera gel in 1 cup of warm water.
- To relieve gaseousness during the Ekadashi Fast or Semi-Fast, take 1 tablespoon of

grated ginger with 1 tablespoon of edible quality aloe vera gel in 1 cup of warm water.

LIGHT & NOURISHING FOODS FOR SEMI-FASTING:
The following recipes are healing and nutritious meals that will help sustain you during your fast or at any other time of the year.

Gluten-free recipes are indicated by ♡

WHITE BASMATI KICHADI ♡
Season: All Year
Serves: 2
1 cup white basmati rice
1/2 cup split mung beans
1 pinch turmeric powder
1 pinch asafetida
1 tablespoon organic ghee (recipe on pages 150-151)
6 cups boiling water

Wash rice and beans thoroughly. Sauté the turmeric and asafetida in ghee over medium heat for a few minutes, then add rice and mung beans. Sauté on low heat for 3 minutes. Add boiling water. (Reduce amount of water for a thicker kichadi.) Stir, cover, and simmer gently on low heat for 35 minutes.

COUSCOUS & CARROTS
Season: All Year
Serves: 2
2 1/2 cups water
1 cup couscous
1/2 cup diced carrots

Bring water to a boil; add couscous and carrots. Cover and simmer for 5-8 minutes. Garnish with fresh cilantro or roasted cumin seeds. Serve warm.

WHITE BASMATI RICE & MILLET ♡
Season: All Year
Serves: 2
3 cups water
1/2 cup white basmati rice

1/2 cup millet

6 curry leaves

1 pinch rock salt

Wash grains thoroughly. Bring water to a boil in a saucepan; add rice and millet, curry leaves, and salt. Cover and simmer for 20 minutes, until grains swell. Remove from heat and serve.

BROWN RICE KICHADI ♡

Season: All Year

Serves: 2

1 cup brown basmati rice or short-grain brown rice

1/2 cup whole mung beans

1 teaspoon whole peppercorns

1 tablespoon cumin seeds

1/2 teaspoon ginger, minced

1 tablespoon organic ghee (recipe on pages 150-151)

8 cups boiling water

1 pinch turmeric powder

1 pinch rock salt

Wash rice and beans thoroughly. In a large pot, sauté the peppercorns, cumin seeds, and ginger in ghee for a few minutes over medium heat. Add rice and beans. Sauté on low heat for 3 minutes. Add boiling water, turmeric, and salt. Stir, cover, and simmer gently for 1 hour on low heat, stirring occasionally. Serve warm.

SOFT MILLET & CARROTS ♡

Season: All Year

Serves: 2

1 cup millet

4 cups water

1/2 cup diced carrots

1/2 teaspoon rock salt

1 teaspoon organic ghee (recipe on pages 150-151)

Wash millet thoroughly and parch until dry in a large cast-iron skillet. Bring water to a boil in a saucepan. Add millet, carrots, and salt. Cover and simmer on medium heat for 40 minutes. Add water to soften further, if necessary. Add ghee, stir, and serve warm.

CARROT & SNOW PEA KIMPIRA ♡

Season: All Year

Serves: 2

3 carrots

1 handful snow peas

1/2 teaspoon sunflower oil

3 tablespoons water

1 pinch rock salt

Scrub carrots and snow peas; cut carrots into matchsticks. Heat sunflower oil in a stainless-steel pan and sauté vegetables over medium heat. Add water and cover; simmer on low heat for a few minutes. Add salt and continue to simmer for another 5 minutes. (This dish can be made with other vegetable combinations; cut root vegetables into matchsticks and cut all other vegetables into long slivers.)

STEAMED BROCCOLI, CAULIFLOWER & CARROTS ♡

Season: All Year

Serves: 2

1 head broccoli

1 head cauliflower

3 carrots

1 tablespoon ginger, grated

1 teaspoon organic ghee (recipe on pages 150-151)

Wash and cut broccoli into long, thin spears. Cut cauliflower into florets. Scrub and quarter carrots into 4-inch long strips. Sprinkle the grated ginger over the vegetables, place in a steamer, and steam for 10 minutes. Arrange on plate, alternating the broccoli and carrot strips, and place cauliflower florets across the top. Add ghee and serve warm.

STEAMED SNOW PEAS & ACORN SQUASH ♡

Season: Early Winter

Serves: 2

1 acorn squash

1 handful snow peas

Scrub squash and cut into thin strips along its indentations. Steam for 20 minutes until firmly tender. Add snow peas to steamer for the last 3 minutes.

SUMMER SQUASH & BABY ONIONS 🖤

Season: Summer

Serves: 2

3 yellow squash

6 baby onions, peeled

1 tablespoon sunflower oil

1 pinch rock salt

1 pinch turmeric powder

3 tablespoons water

Cut squash into 1/4-inch slices on a slant. Sauté whole onions in sunflower oil in a skillet over medium heat for 3 minutes. Add squash, salt, turmeric, and water. Cover and simmer for another 10 minutes. Serve warm.

DILL & PARSLEY SWEET POTATOES 🖤

Season: Winter

Serves: 2

2 medium sweet potatoes

1 teaspoon sunflower oil

2 teaspoons cumin seeds

1 green chili, minced

1 onion, diced

1/4 teaspoon cayenne powder

8 tablespoons water

1 tablespoon fresh dill, minced

3 tablespoons fresh parsley, minced

Scrub the sweet potatoes and cut into 1-inch cubes. In a large skillet, heat sunflower oil and brown the cumin seeds, chili, and onion for 4 minutes over medium heat. Add cayenne and potatoes. Stir, cover, and sauté for a few minutes. Add water, lower heat, and simmer for 10 minutes. Add drops of water and stir occasionally to loosen potatoes from pan. Cook for 30 minutes. Serve warm with minced fresh dill and parsley.

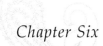

Chapter Six

LIVING IN HARMONY WITH THE SEASONS

When we bring awareness to the divine luminosity
of the winter's full moons; or thrive in the rustling
sounds and warm colors of the autumnal leaves; or
pause to appreciate the significant babble of the brook
after the heavy rains; we are taking the necessary pause
to consciously synchronize our vital tissues and cells
and their memory of the divinity that is health.

ATTUNING TO THE RHYTHMS OF THE SEASONS

In Living Ahimsa, we live in accord with the rhythms and cycles of the seasons. As you learn to pay attention to the workings of your inner rhythms, you will discover that like the plants, all of your experiences are linked to the cycle of the seasons down to the day, week, month, and year. Each and every life is connected to nature's indefatigable energies and tempos. As you learn to honor the cyclical rhythms of the sun, moon, and earth in your daily life, you will begin to move in tandem with the Mother Consciousness. You will discover that the center of the universe resides within the self, and this truth will allow you to flow with the graceful rhythms of nature. The seasons are nature's messengers, delivering the cyclical ebb and flow of health and healing that significantly impacts our well-being.

Our ancient ancestors recognized that nature has her own imperishable rhythm. She methodically sequences her edible sustenance for her plant-loving creatures: First comes the perennial herbs, then the berries, followed by succulent fruits and vegetables, then the beans and leafy vegetables, roots, and autumnal fruits. Nature's bounty is not happenstance. She fulfills our nutritional needs and feeds our vital tissues in accord with seasonal intelligence, thereby enlivening our eternal core memory of love and harmony. That is, when we are in reverent attunement with her generosity. As we become attuned to Mother's rhythms, our journey also becomes more seamless; we begin to mitigate negative influences and help nature restore her balance. Each one of us has the immutable power to build, fortify, and strengthen the pervasive energy of love in everything we do—in our responses to prana, movement, thought, word, and deed. Essentially, good health is about strengthening and preserving the foundation of harmony!

As noted earlier, your vital tissues are created from nature's seasonal rhythms and provisions, therefore your health depends on them for your most basic sustenance and nourishment. By imbibing nature's foods, you are able to transport nature's essential nutrients into the minutest cells of your mind and body. Thus, your mood, memory, and health are directly affected by the biorhythms held within each and every tissue of your body. This is why we must remain attentive to the cyclical changes of our inner rhythms during each season and its transition into another.

Throughout human existence, people have traced the circle of time and its passing by marking the seasons and cycles of nature. Many cultures knew with certainty that when a season ended the body experienced its greatest vulnerability. They understood that when the full moon arrived, the ocean swelled; when the animals gathered their sustenance, the winter was near; and when the hawks flew in circles, the brilliant sun was about to dip into the horizon.

The ancients carved into wood, bone, and stone, calendrical renditions of the recurring astronomical cycles. They kept abreast of the changing positions of the stars and constellations, the daily and annual movements of the sun and moon, and the changing of the seasons. Recently, for example, elaborate woodcarvings of astronomical reckonings made by a tribe of hominids in India around two million BCE were discovered. Their carvings depicted time as a circle. They seemed to know that the circular interworkings of the universe bore a direct and yet dynamic relation to all life, and appeared to recognize that all things, within and without, move inside the spiraling, cyclical rhythm of the universe. In Latin, the word *circulus* refers to "a circuit of time." In old Celtic tradition, the passage of time was symbolized by a wheel, and its solar calendar was called *bleidonii*. Native American shamans refer to this wheel of life as "the sacred hoop."

THE PERSONALITY OF EACH SEASON

Like the Western Calendar, in the Hindu Calendar a solar year has 365 days and 12 months, and a leap year has 366 days. But unlike the Western Calendar, the Vedic solar year is divided into six seasons of two months each: spring, summer, rainy season/early fall, autumn, early winter, and late winter. One solar month consists of the number of days taken by the sun to move from one sign of the zodiac, or *rashi*, to another, and each rashi is identified with its corresponding Gregorian zodiac sign. In this system of measuring time, Hindu months will straddle two months of the Western Calendar.

According to the Hindu Calendar the year begins with the month of *Chaitra* (March-April) when the sun enters the zodiac sign of Aries on the day after the spring equinox. (See appendix two, "The Six Seasons of the Vedic Calendar," for additional information.)

THE SIX SEASONS OF THE VEDIC CALENDAR		
SEASON	SANSKRIT NAME OF SEASON	OCCURS IN
Spring	Vasanta	March–April
Summer	Grishma	May–June
Rainy Season/Early Fall	Varsha	July–August
Autumn	Sharada	September–October
Early Winter	Hemanta	November–December
Late Winter	Shishira	January–February

Table 6.1

It is important that you make a commitment to learning the awesome splendor of each season for the simple reason that what you love or dislike in each season precisely speaks to your inner condition. Your vital personal rhythms emulate seasonal characteristics. When we bring awareness to the divine luminosity of the winter's full moons; or thrive in the rustling sounds and warm colors of the autumnal leaves; or pause to appreciate the significant babble of the brook after the heavy rains; we are taking the necessary pause to consciously synchronize our vital tissues and cells and their memory of the divinity that is health. Likewise, when we experience fear from the pounding sounds of the thunder; or despise the raw coldness of the late winter; or get angry with the rains; or in general, do not recognize the need to protect the trillion or more gifts of the Mother Consciousness, these untoward emotions can be traced back, not to the seasons or the weather, but to our lack of awareness of specific conditions within ourselves.

Ayurveda sages understood that a primary means of learning our inherent nature of ahimsa—joy and love and fullness—is through attunement of the self to the recurrent cycles of the seasons. Our vital tissues are created from the same five elements that created the seasons and their rhythms; we share a symbiotic nature with the earth, created as we are from the same cosmic blueprint of memory, energy, and rhythm. Only the rhythms of the seasons have the power to fully restore our vital tissues and their innate memories that guide their form and function to perfect health. We experience distinct emotions and energies associated with each and every season although we may not be aware of them.

Spring–Rebirth
All life awakens. We experience increased vulnerability during this time. Spring is a time of rebirth for all creatures, and therefore a feeling of rawness and fearfulness prevails. Paying careful attention to your choice of foods and activities is very important during this season. Making affirmations and seeking self-reinforcement are good steps to take. Recognize that this is a time of vulnerability and rebirth at

every level. Embrace your vulnerability. It is only during this period that growth and personal transformation can occur. When you face whatever arises, you are no longer vulnerable.

Summer–Celebration

Trees are laden with fruits and nature's wholesome sustenance. Naturally, we experience fullness, fulfillment, and leisure in the rich and profuse personality of summer. The whole universe appears to be on our vibrational wave of playfulness and enjoyment of summer's abundance. Seize every chance to celebrate the spirit of family, community, and togetherness as the golden sun gives its prismatic light and warmth to the earth. This is a time to reinforce your stamina, to take advantage of your abundant energy, and to lessen ambitious goals and mental activities.

Rainy Season/Early Fall–Reorganization

The rainy season brings the ideal atmosphere to nudge the mind into reorganizing its surrounding space. It's a good time to clean out the files and closets and catch up on neglected paperwork. Clean house, reevaluate your choices, reexamine your motivations. Since the entire universe is experiencing the energy of reform and reorganization, it helps the mind to be in harmony with the vibration of these greater cosmic energies.

Autumn–Harvesting

Autumn is the season of the harvest, reaping the fruits of your labor, and paying homage to Mother Nature by receiving her bountiful foods and honoring the ancestors. This is a good time for harvesting your "gold" internally by simplifying your living and working spaces, and your whole life in general. The harvest season brings a sense of completion to your year's hard work and provides an abundance of energy and invigorating weather while you transition from the warmth of summer days into the frosty winter months ahead. Go into nature and experience the majestic sounds and colors of this remarkable season which transitions us into the coldness of the winter. This season provides the last opportunity to reap the earth's fresh, bountiful foods—give yourself permission to reap the benefits from the year's hard work.

Early Winter–Gathering

Like the squirrels that dwell in the forest, in early winter you want to gather your resources, and take stock of "food" (everything that nourishes body, mind, senses and spirit) before the harsh rhythms of late winter set in. Stock up on your dried goods: grains, legumes and seeds, and dried fruits and root vegetables (if you keep a root cellar). The energies of the earth are scattered and fragmented at this time, and have significant impact on the mind and emotions. This is a good time to gather yourself in all ways.

Late Winter–Resting

Rest, reflection, and introspection are the activities to indulge in during this austere period of the year: the optimum time to cogitate and perfect your Living Ahimsa spirit within. Like the bear that hibernates in its cave, we humans desperately need to acknowledge the winter's rhythms and their demands on our physical, mental, and spiritual bodies. Retreat inward to revise the spirit. Moderate your work schedule, reduce all activities, and do restful, wholesome practices that serve to refuel body, mind, and spirit.

From the Living Ahimsa perspective, fatigue syndrome is a direct result of our disregard for the winter rhythms, living out of sync with them. Rest and reprieve are necessary for human strength and endurance, and these innate qualities are fed and nurtured when we align ourselves with the greater energies of the seasons and, in particular, the winter.

THE ENERGY OF THE SEASONS	
SEASON	ENERGY
Spring	Rebirth
Summer	Celebration
Rainy Season/Early Fall	Reorganization
Autumn	Harvesting
Early Winter	Gathering
Late Winter	Resting

Table 6.2

THE TASTES OF THE SEASONS

Taste goes far beyond the preparation and consumption of food. Each one of us has a vast spectrum of aesthetics and experiences that influence our emotional, physical, psychic, and spiritual "taste," called *rasa*. Our choices are largely influenced by our unique rasa: how we express our emotions, the clothing we wear, the art we prefer, the careers we are drawn to, the people we love, and the spouses we marry. In Wise Earth Ayurveda, the mechanism of rasa engages long before we actually taste a food on our tongues and plays a prodigious role in the process of healing.

Rasa controls the palate and the way in which an herb or food is absorbed into the body and then projected as nourishment into the vital tissues. When the correct blend of unadulterated, natural ingredients is received on the tongue in a manner that promotes digestion, rasa responds positively. Our rasa transforms the ingredients and sends their medicine deep into impaired body tissues to prod good health and restore their memory of perfection. When we do not fully experience our food, rasa cannot do its job, and a food's essence arrives unannounced through the process of digestion into our vital tissues. Like an uninvited guest, our tissues are taken by surprise and are not prepared to take in the vital essences of the food.

Each of the six seasons of Ayurveda—spring, summer, early fall, autumn, early winter, and late winter—produces a specific taste which enhances rasa: astringent, pungent, sour, salty, sweet, and bitter. The six tastes should be enjoyed proportionately, and as a general rule, the sweet taste should be the most dominant taste in our daily nourishment. Pungent, salty, and sour tastes should be secondary tastes, depending on the season. Bitter and astringent tastes should always be minor or remedial tastes. Following are the descriptions of each of the six tastes and their qualities, listed according to their predominance in the universe:

Sweet is the dominant taste of all nourishment and sustenance. Almost all foods contain some degree of sweetness. The water and earth elements produce the sweet taste, which includes all carbohydrates, sugars, fats, and amino acids. The primary element of life, which is water, is considered sweet, as are milk and all sugars. The sweet taste enhances bodily tissues, nurtures the body, and relieves hunger, and is most beneficial for Pitta types. Our diets should therefore be proportionately high in good quality "sweet" foods, including whole grains, root vegetables, and fruits. Herbs such as corn silk, cotton root, lily, and marshmallow are naturally sweet in taste.

Pungent is the taste formed from the elements of air and fire. It helps stimulate appetite, maintain metabolism, and balance the secretions in the body. The pungent taste is most beneficial for Kapha types, and includes such foods as garlic, ginger, kale, mustard, tomatoes, and peppers. Examples of pungent herbs are cloves, eucalyptus, dill, horseradish, and lavender.

Salty is the most beneficial taste for Vata types, although it may be used in small quantities by all types to cleanse bodily tissues and activate digestion. The third most dominant taste, it is formed from the elements of water and fire and is found in all salts and seaweeds. Most watery vegetables, such as tomatoes (also pungent), zucchinis, and cucumbers are naturally high in saline. Few herbs boast the salty taste. Moss, kelp, seaweed, and rock salt are predominantly salty.

Sour is the taste formed from the earth and fire elements and helps digestion and the elimination of wastes from the body. This taste may be used in small quantities by everyone, although it is most beneficial for Vata types. Most fruits are considered somewhat sour, with lemons, limes, and tamarind considered the sourest. All organic acids and fermented foods, such as yogurt, soy sauce, and pickles, are considered sour. This taste may be found in hawthorn and rose hips.

Bitter is a taste that should be used by everyone in small quantities, and is especially good for Pitta and Kapha types. Bitter detoxifies the blood, controls skin ailments, and tones the organs. This taste is formed from the elements of air and space. It exists in all medicines, alkaloids, glycosides, and bitter foods such as aloe vera, arugula, radicchio, dandelion greens, and the spice turmeric. Examples of bitter herbs are blessed thistle, chaparral, chicory, and passion flower.

Astringent taste is formed from the elements of earth and air and is intended for medicinal use by all types. The astringent taste reduces bodily secretions and constricts bodily tissues. Examples of astringent foods are those high in tannins, such as dried legumes and bark teas. Herbs such as bistort, blackberry, cramp bark, hibiscus, raspberry, and uva ursi are highly astringent in quality.

THE TASTES OF THE SEASONS	
SEASON	TASTE
Spring	Astringent
Summer	Pungent
Rainy Season/Early Fall	Sour
Autumn	Salty
Early Winter	Sweet
Late Winter	Bitter

Table 6.3

AHIMSA GARDEN OF GRATITUDE

I have been growing most of my own foods by maintaining a natural herb, fruit, and vegetable garden for 30 years. My garden is comprised of 16 acres of unadulterated forest in the Pisgah Mountains. It is a serene space created in accord with the wisdom of the *Vastu Sastra*—the Vedic art of placement—laid out in precise architectural splendor in symphony with my environment. As a result, all who eat from my garden are nourished by the enhanced influences of the six seasons and five elements. The pine forest naturally mulches ginseng and ashwagandha, herbs which thrive in the shade, and the tall river grasses siphon the breezes to provide the necessary coolness for the indigenous fiddlestick ferns.

Central to this exquisite ahimsa garden is personal gratitude; a simple act of yajna—a rite or a sacrifice. A firepot is strategically set out in the northeast corner of my garden. Before planting organic seeds in the earth, I make seasonal offerings to the Mother Goddess with water from a pristine mountain spring, fragrant dried herbs from the preceding season, along with ghee made from the raw milk of the "chanting" cows in the neighboring organic dairy farm, and pine sticks gleaned from the fallen branches of the white pines. I use these salubrious ingredients to nourish the fire of life, agni, by taking pause and lighting a fire with prayers of gratitude for the Mother's bountiful yield. As informed by the *Katha Upanishad*, agni, 'hidden in the two fire sticks and well guarded by its mother like a child in the womb,' is venerated day after day by people who are awakened to the spirit of ahimsa and by those who offer oblations in the sacrificial fire. This Living Ahimsa practice helps me to safeguard my inner power of agni, and therefore remember my devout purpose and cultivate a sense of gratefulness for the deities who manifest the rains and sun, winds and light, and the cooling shade of night.

In order for my garden to be in accord with the energetic patterns of the land, I plant it in the way of companionship by not fidgeting with the topsoil or creating raised beds; by sprinkling spinach and/or mustard seeds (rich in minerals) over the dirt in the sparse winter season when the earth is resting and revitalizing herself; and by sowing seeds that grow into plants that like to live with and support each other. Like a person, a plant also has an individual prakriti, or disposition, and thus its preference in neighbors—it too thrives in the company of some and suffers from fatigue in the company of others.

The animals that live in Pisgah Forest are all keenly aware of the prayerful space which surrounds them. The herd of deer, for example, frequently attend my early morning ceremonies and meditation. If the meditation bell sounds later than usual, the bucks will climb the stairs to my cabin and wait on the landing until the bell is rung.

They are also eager to receive blessings following our ceremonial happenings—*pujas*—and seem to understand the significance of them. Often I will offer them the blessing water as well as place traditional *bindi* on their foreheads, which they proudly sport as they spend the morning grazing and feasting on the young barley grasses.

GIFTS OF THE GODDESS

The complete definition of *annam* is: "food which grows on the earth for humans and creatures so that they may be fed, nourished, and nurtured and thereby preserve the life force," and this implicitly tells us that there is energy beyond the pragmatic function of nature. This energy is ahimsa—offspring of the Mother Consciousness. Imagine the care, love, and devotion an earthly mother pays to her child, the magical mystery she experiences in the process of nurturing her children, whether or not she believes in her innate power to heal. Multiply that equation by zillions of trillions of billions and you will discover the infinite sacrifices that our Mother makes to care for her entire universe. Each day, the Great Mother lavishes her priceless gifts on humanity—her sun, moon, earth, light, air, space, water, forests, herbs, vegetables, fruits, and plants. Because we have always enjoyed her splendid bounty, we often do not recognize her generosity. Rarely do we stop to give gratitude to her, and we almost never acknowledge her many sacrifices.

My tradition believes that the proper function of the whole universe depends on the acts of sublime sacrifice performed continuously by the Great Mother. As I mentioned in chapter three, it is a principle called yajna, which means "rites and sacrifices." The universe thrives on sacrifice—this is how Mother Earth provides abundant love, stimuli, inspiration, nourishment, food, and purpose for all her creatures, including the microscopic ones. As Hindus, we honor this centrifugal belief by making sacrifices in the form of peaceful offerings through ritual and ceremony. We make these offerings to communicate our gratitude to the Mother and to advance personal awareness and collective consciousness. We honor her through prayers, mantras, mudras, yajnas, and yoga, and we make precious food offerings of milk, honey, jaggery, ghee, khus grass, coconuts, raisins, saffron, and betel nuts—foods that we believe are imbued with the energy of gratitude and humility.

These rituals are thoughtfully designed to mirror specific, natural patterns of energy that continually transform, serve, sustain, and preserve the whole universe. Contrary to what some may believe, Hindu ceremonies are not about idol worship or mindless ritual. The Vedic rishis bestowed humanity with the precise knowledge and practices that propitiate and honor the living universe through rituals that pay respect to each of its component parts. In fact, each image or form of a Hindu deity embodies a set of characteristics that exist in the configuration of the cosmic memory code, the same set of codes embedded in the human form of body, breath, mind, memory, and soul.

THE AHIMSA KITCHEN

As I look around my sacred cooking space, I see a Vedic fire pot, organic camphor cubes, and tiny pieces of pine kindling set on a shelf, my food offering altar. A small statue of Ganesha, the elephant-headed god, sits next to the fire pot. Before every meal, I put pieces of camphor and pine, along with a tiny amount of whatever I am eating, into the pot, light a fire, and say my prayers. Glancing around my own ahimsa kitchen temple, I savor the profusion of sensory stimuli with which I am surrounded: the fragrant aroma of roasted coriander seeds as I grind them with my mortar and pestle; the aroma of cumin seeds roasting in ghee; the soothing "shush" sound as I pour the hot seeds into a soup pot. I never tire of hearing the hissing sound of mustard seeds popping in the hot skillet, of the wafting aroma of saffron and cinnamon and clove boiling in milk, or of watching the play of effervescent light flooding into my kitchen.

My kitchen holds ample evidence of my own ancestry. There are intricately decorated brass *talis* (trays), and the *sil batta* (spice-grinding stone) is laid out with spring greens and herbs fresh from my garden: violet-flowered oregano, white-flowered arugula, dandelion leaves, spring mustard, the season's first cilantro leaves, licorice, and mint. My shelves are lined with ceramic jars filled with yellow mung beans, red aduki beans, black rice, white basmati rice, golden-orange corn, and all varieties of ivory, tan, and buff-colored rices. (I love every variety of rice; it is after all my ancestral grain!) An open cabinet displays jars of my favorite tea leaves—lavender, rose petals, rose hips, hawthorn berries, dried orange peels, and raspberry leaves. In the summer, my window sills are laid out with bunches of mint, thyme, marjoram, Indian basil, parsley, cilantro, comfrey, and tansy. Several wind chimes hang in the window and provide me with echoes of nature's music in the eternal mountain breezes.

The greatest act of nourishing the body comes from the shrine that is your kitchen. Transform this space into a goddess sanctuary for the energized preparation of meals that will heal and nurture all who taste them. This goddess sanctuary is yours; the goddess is you. Can you envision yourself as a goddess? See the kitchen as a spiritual place for healing, complete with nature's utensils made from natural materials like stone, clay, straw, leaves, bamboo, and wood. Each utensil is a means for extending your Shakti power into the creation of Inner Medicine healing foods. Choose a few good quality, heavy stainless-steel and enamel pots and pans, as well as several cast-iron skillets. I recommend that you use utensils made from a variety of non-toxic materials because they all lend different energies to food. You will want some clay and wooden bowls; stainless-steel and wooden ladles; a ceramic hand grater for your ginger, turmeric, and garlic; and most importantly, a grinding stone or mortar and pestle for your herbs, seeds, and remedies. And of course, every kitchen must have a sharp knife or two!

Chapter Seven

LIVING AHIMSA FOOD PRACTICES

My hand is the Lord.
Boundlessly blissful is my hand.
This hand holds all healing secrets
Which makes whole with its gentle touch.
— Rig Veda

EATING WITH THE HANDS OF AHIMSA

Eating is a wonderful act of ahimsa—when we do it with consciousness. When we touch nature's foods with our hands it brings the universe's fire through our fingers into the food and then joins it with agni, the transformational fire of digestion within each of us working to digest, assimilate, and refine the potent memory of ahimsa within our mind, body, and spirit. Its heat flows through our vital organism to eliminate physical, mental, and emotional toxicity, giving way to the clear pathways of inner luminosity and light within our being. If we are aware of awakening the fire of agni within ourselves, we digest the food and our life experiences healthfully. As you are learning in this work, only when the digestive system is awry can disease arise in the mind, memory, and body.

The ancient Vedic people knew the power of agni held within the hand. We touch the universe, elements, and nature with our hands as we extend them to give and receive, to heal and express compassion. Hands are our most precious organs of action. We use them hundreds of times a day for scores of applications, but now I want you to take a long look at them, and recognize them to be the hands of awareness, attached to you. Since most of us do not have the opportunity to experience firsthand the harvesting of golden fields, the feel of delicate blades of rice or wheat grasses, the threshing of the harvest, and the ethereal sounds of the earth, wind, and sun as they intertwine in dance, we must not miss any chance that arises to use our hands to give thanks for Mother's nourishment.

A hand that is energized is a hand that heals; a healing hand replaces the need for medicine. We use them in different ways every day without knowing the nature of the profound energy they hold. Conscious use of our hands directs each and every movement into a spectacularly choreographed dance wherein we are harmoniously exchanging and transforming energy with the breathing, living earth. This rich palpable energy infuses everything you touch into a blessing of nurturance.

Hands and feet are conduits of nature's elements—space, air, fire, water, and earth. In Vedic anatomy, each element predominantly flows through each finger.

THE FIVE FINGERS & THEIR CORRESPONDING ELEMENTS	
FINGER	ELEMENT
Thumb	Space
Index Finger	Air
Middle Finger	Fire
Ring Finger	Water
Little Finger	Earth

Table 7.1

When we use our bodies with awareness, we are serving and honoring the Mother Consciousness. In my tradition, we eat with our hands because the five elements expressed through them help to transform food and make it digestible even before it reaches the mouth. Eating is a wonderful, sacred ritual of nourishment. It brings the fire from the Mother Consciousness through our hands and fingers into the food, and then combines it with the fire of digestion. When you eat with awareness—unhappiness and disease will diminish and ultimately disappear.

Vedic tradition is informed by the wisdom and sanctity of life with infinite numbers of mantras and mudras and rites and rituals—all symbolizing the intricate patterns of Mother's energy that permeate and support the living universe. We feed our babies by directing the flow of the mother's milk with our hand into their mouths; we gather the maternal Shakti energy from the earth's bounty by using our hands to measure, prepare, and sanctify our foods. Living Ahimsa food practices provide you infinite opportunities to reconnect with your precious Inner Medicine by recognizing the blissful instrument of peace, love, and joy that *is* your hands.

When we use our hands in the action of ahimsa, we can actually touch upon a palpable divinity. Mudras (derived from the root *mud*, "to delight" or "to gladden")—special hand gestures—were used to receive and gather the universe's energy and to seal off negative influences from entering the body and mind. Today these hand mudras are used in many ways. In Hindu rituals, the priests use these sacred mudras to worship deities. Thousands of Hindus bring the palms of their hands together in front of the heart in prayer, called Anjali Mudra, and utter the sacred word "Namaste." In meditation practice, the most commonly used mudra is Chin Mudra (also called Jnana Mudra or "Wisdom Seal").

The ancient tradition of eating food with the hands is derived from mudra practice. Gathering the fingertips as they touch the food stimulates the five elements and invites agni to stoke our digestive juices. Each finger is an extension of one of the five elements; each serves to aid in the transformation of food before it passes on to internal digestion. The sadhana of feeding yourself from hand to mouth enhances your vital memory and inner balance.

An extension of the practice of eating with the hands is to use the body as the ruler and measuring cup for all our needs. In keeping with this principle, it is good to become comfortable using your hands and eyes for your culinary measurements (however, the recipes in this book use standard measurements). In addition to the mudra by the same name, the term *anjali* also refers to the volume that can be held by your two hands cupped together. Two anjalis of grain or vegetables from your hands is designed by nature to fill your own stomach. When you are cooking for others, prepare two anjalis for each adult and one anjali for each child. Likewise gauge your spices or accents with your own pinch. Like your handful, it is tailored to provide a suitable amount for your own personal body needs. *Angula* refers to the distance between the joints of each finger. This unit of measure is used in Ayurveda cooking and is naturally designed to gauge the amounts of spices and herbs such as cinnamon sticks and ginger.

As you become accustomed to preparing the recipes in this book, start using only those tools that are absolutely necessary. As soon as possible, give up measuring cups, spoons, and useless kitchen paraphernalia. These adjuncts are distracting and interrupt your direct energetic exchange with the food. It may be difficult at first to take this conscious step to trust the accuracy of your own physical-spiritual apparatus. With time, you will become comfortable enough to return to the original and most natural system of measurement.

Your hands should partake fully in all food preparation. Knead your energy into the dough, massage your hands with the grains, pat the chapatis and roll the rice balls between your palms. Allow the universal energy to mix with and transmute your own energy. Puree sauces and mash potatoes with your hands. Tear leafy greens gently with your fingertips. When the hands must have a medium, use the grinding stone, mortar and pestle, or the suribachi for the positive energy provided by clockwise motion. This is sadhana. The closer to nature each utensil or apparatus, the more connected the prepared food will be to the energy of the cosmos. Using your limbs as an instrument of lightness automatically demonstrates your gratitude to the Mother Consciousness for all that is given to you, each and every day.

One way to show your gratitude for food is to take a handful of grain and offer blessings for it. Remember this is a gift from nature, her elements, the farmers, and the good earth. Grains are the basis of the earth's sustenance for humans. In my culture, each morsel of grain is a deity of the Mother Consciousness. Another way of honoring the abundance of food given to us is to prepare the ultimate feast by learning to attract potent cosmic energies into our hands and infuse their healing energies into our nourishment.

Sophie's Story

Sophie was a 22-year-old young woman who developed an aversion to food. Her parents tried all kinds of therapies but could not get Sophie to eat, and she was wasting away. In desperation, her mother brought Sophie to one of my Living Ahimsa food workshops at the Open Center in New York. They remained after the workshop to seek my help. Having helped many people recover from eating disorders, I understood that an aversion to food is a sign that one is feeling separated, alienated from joy, love, and life itself. I inquired about the foods that Sophie once liked and advised her mother not to force her to eat, but to demonstrate instead the simple art of eating with one's hands.

Sophie's favorite meal used to be hot dogs and potato salad, so I advised them to spend quality time in the kitchen together, transforming it into an ahimsa shrine that is pristine and inviting. Sophie perked up at my description of an ahimsa kitchen filled with light and freshness and kindness. Since she once loved hot dogs, I recommended she buy tofu hot dogs from the nearby health food store. In using animal-free food that did not imbue the suffering or killing of an animal, she would feel more connected to her foods and at peace with her nourishment. Before they left, I asked Sophie if she would consider preparing her own foods and taught her to use her hands in the way of preparing her meals in the spirit of ahimsa.

Some months later, I got a letter from Sophie. She was ecstatic about being able to eat, celebrate, and enjoy her meals. Apparently, she had taken to cooking her own meals and found a new joy in washing and peeling and mashing potatoes with her hands, sautéing onions in freshly-made ghee, popping mustard seeds and cumin seeds while roasting them, and grilling tofu dogs to her heart's content. She confessed to loving the feel of the food on her hands while she fed herself in her ahimsa shrine. This is how Sophie began to eat again. Through the sacred instrument of her own hands, she was able to reconnect to the energy of life.

IMBIBING HARMONY

Most people still pay very little attention to the harmony of eating, digesting, and assimilating the nectar of a meal. They skip breakfast, eat a less-than-nutritious lunch on the run, and sit down to dinner at nine o'clock at night. How can proper digestion occur when we force the system to put up with such abuse year after year? It's no wonder that we have such a high incidence of cancer and heart disease in the West, when we refuse to observe the integrity of our physiology by nourishing our bodies and souls with dignity and respect.

Here are some simple guidelines to help honor the ahimsa of food and facilitate digestion:

• Maintain a consistent mealtime schedule.
• Be mindful of your conversations during meals. While it is best to observe

silence, you may choose to engage in calm, soothing conversations.

- Experiment with the experience of eating with your own hands—from hand to mouth.
- Chew your food well and be aware of its smells, tastes, textures, and the sounds it makes while you are ingesting it.
- Be attentive to your digestion during meals. Never eat when you are upset. Wholesome foods turn sour in our digestive tracts when influenced by negative emotions.
- Allow a few hours to pass between meals and bedtime.
- Sit on your heels for 15 minutes after meals, or take a gentle walk to encourage proper digestion.
- Never eat and run.
- Never eat while standing up or lying down.

THE SACRED ART OF SPICE GRINDING

At this point, you are becoming aware of how important your intention and the attention paid to your ahimsa practice are in the preparation of your healing meals. You will find that many of the recipes in this book use whole, fragrant spices that I urge you to grind as you create a particular dish. Spice grinding is more than a means for making truly delicious *masalas,* or spice blends, although the flavors that result from freshly ground spices are unparalleled! The art of spice grinding is a magnificent meditation in motion, a wholesome practice that helps us grow into maturity and splendor. It is an ancient ahimsa practice valued by women from every corner of the world. The spice grinding stone that my grandmother bequeathed to my mother was so important that she carried it with her (one of few possessions) when she fled from Guyana during the civil war.

The grinding stone and mortar and pestle are ancient symbols of the power of male and female energies. My tradition recognizes the mortar, or base, to be symbolic of *Parashakti,* the primordial feminine power that brought forth manifestation. The pestle represents the lingam, or *Parashiva,* the masculine force that represents Divine Consciousness. When we grind our spices, we bring our feminine and masculine forces into a state of balance, and reenact the forces of divine creation.

Grinding stones, in various shapes made from all kinds of materials, have been in use worldwide for ages, and are still easily found today: the *suribachi* and *surikogi,* an unglazed pottery bowl and a wooden pestle from Japan; the earthenware mortar and pestle in Thailand; the *molcajete,* large, fluted stone mortar and pestle used in Mexico and Peru; and the porcelain apothecary-style mortar and pestle used in England and in much of Europe. No Vedic kitchen is complete without at least one mortar and pestle. The most popular type is the sil batta. *Sil* is the flat stone base, and *batta* is the handheld stone roller which is worked back and forth across the base.

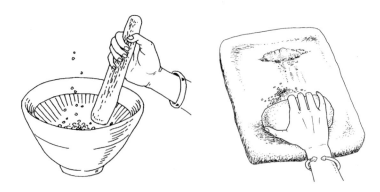

Figures 7.1 & 7.2 Suribachi & Sil Batta

The grinding stone you use will become a symbol of your stability and purpose. Look for a base stone that represents who you are, and a hand stone that fits comfortably in your palm. Before your first use, wash the stones with a non-toxic detergent and use a scrub brush to remove loose dirt and pieces of sediment. If possible, place them in the sun to dry; otherwise, wipe them off well with cloth made of natural fibers. After the rocks are thoroughly dried, rub them with sunflower oil, and leave them in the sun for an hour. Wash your stones well after each use.

A young medical practitioner and a dedicated student of mine, Laura, healed herself into cancer remission through Wise Earth Ayurveda's Food, Breath, and Sound teachings. She has created a thriving community around her by sharing the ahimsa food practices in this book with her students, many of whom enjoy scouting the nearby dessert climes to find their own precious grinding blocks and hand stones straight from the earth for their spice grinding.

Hand tools are the preferred method for grinding spices in the true spirit of ahimsa because these tools allow us to imbue the healing energies of our hands right into the foods and spices. Since mechanical grinding tools have been widely used, the vital connection of hand on stone or hand on clay has been lost. The healing in this alchemical process derives from the rhythm of stone grinding on stone, earth on earth, which renews our deepest cellular memories of our connection to the earth. This profound process helps us recall our ancestral pasts; each spice triggers a cosmic memory and aligns us with a particular rhythm of nature.

Beatrice's Story

The potent and ancient ritual of spice grinding can be an ancestral bridge between generations, healing us at our deepest levels where we are free from the tethers and complexities of verbal communication that can so often come between two people. Another student of mine, Beatrice, had difficulty communicating with her daughter, Anne, who had recently gone through a divorce. Beatrice felt estranged from Anne. She wanted to support her but didn't know how. So she sought my advice as to how she could mend the emotional chasm between them.

I had noticed Beatrice enjoying grinding spices during a Living Ahimsa work-shop, so when she came to me with her dilemma I said, "You love using the suri-bachi, so offer one as a gift to Anne along with a good assortment of spice seeds like coriander, cloves, cumin, ajwain, and cardamom—perfect spices that herald the arrival of autumn." I also told her to buy a *katori*—a round, covered, Indian spice container made of wood or stainless-steel, with seven little compartments for storing ground spices. "If Anne receives the gift well, you can invite her to help you make a masala for the season."

At first Beatrice was skeptical about this recommendation for healing her prob-lems with her daughter. But I had every confidence in the power of ahimsa in our food: Anne was an artist and I knew that working with the sheer beauty of colors, sounds, and smells of the spice seeds while grinding them would help both mother and daughter to grind away their angst and differences with each other. Aware of this, I said, "You'd be surprised. Your daughter probably has more connection to the aesthetic act of ahimsa and food than you do."

Beatrice bravely accepted my suggestion, and went to see her daughter with this simple offering of peace in her hands. As she later wrote me, "Anne was so moved by my gift that she broke down into tears when she opened it. Now we have a date every month to make masala while we grind away our conflicts with love and a new appreciation for each other."

THE SACRED GRAIN

Humans are bound together by their dependence on grain, the earth's most sacred food and the foundation of every known culture: rice fortified Asians, millet sus-tained Africans, quinoa strengthened the Incas, wheat nourished the Europeans and buckwheat the Eastern Europeans, and corn nurtured the indigenous people of the Americas.

We must begin to see all plants and the ahimsa practices that sustain them as reaching as far as the galaxies and stars. These practices are not only about composting, sowing, and then reaping the bounty of nature, they are also about recognizing the divine life carried by each seed and grain, life they give to us as sustenance and memory.

Grain is so revered in the cultures of the East that when the harvest is especially abundant, it is believed that even the gods can become jealous. At such times, the village elders will distract the gods from the magnificent bounty by hopping around the fields shouting, "Bad rice, bad rice!" My ancestors learned to cook their grain hundreds of different ways and valued it as one of the most important offer-ings made during any religious ceremony.

Rice is the first food a Hindu bride offers to her husband during her nuptial ceremony. It is also the first solid food an Indian mother offers her infant. The Chinese word for rice is the same word as *food*. A common greeting in China translates to, "Have you had rice today?" Japanese mothers encourage their children to eat all their rice by calling each grain "a little Buddha." In Thailand the dinner bell is tolled accompanied by the exclamation, "Eat rice!"

Keep the following practice in your awareness the next time you create a meal using any kind of grain. You will notice a remarkable difference in the aromas, flavors, and satisfaction you experience as you partake of your energy-filled meal.

THE PRACTICE: WASHING GRAINS

- Begin by massaging your hands with the grains as you wash them, rubbing the grains between your palms and infusing them with your healing energies.
- Feel the energy of the sun and wind within their seed-memory soaking into your being.
- Notice the stimulating touch and vibrancy of your hands as you wash the grains.
- After you cook the grains, savor their rich energy-filled taste.

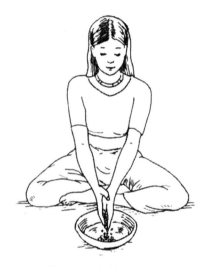

Figure 7.3 Washing Grains

THE BOUNTY OF BREAD

Chapati is without a doubt the most popular of all Indian breads. It is traditionally made from *atta*, a finely milled wheat flour, although barley, buckwheat, spelt, soy, or corn flours may also be used. Chapati is baked on a hot griddle, called a *tava*, until it is cooked three quarters of the way through, with light brown spots and small pockets of air on the surface. Then it is held with tongs over an open gas flame where it swells into a scrumptious, steaming balloon.

Although it was my father who primarily taught me to cook, I learned the fine art of rolling and cooking chapati from my mother, who is an exceptional Vedic cook. It took me months of practice to achieve the proper consistency in my dough and to roll out a perfectly round and thin chapati. As my skills grew, so did my patience. Now, I love to watch the light, delicate bread swell over the open fire of my wood stove. Your first batch of chapati will most likely be all sorts of odd shapes and sizes and may not puff up, but don't be discouraged: You will be amazed at how effortless this wonderful sadhana becomes with practice, after just a few tries. This is a marvelous practice for the family to do together, and children especially will delight in helping knead and roll out the chapati dough.

To start your practice, wash your hands and knead dough for bread or chapati from freshly ground flour. Feel the texture of the dough as you knead your energy into it. Be aware of the touch, sights, sounds, and smell of the bread as it passes through all the phases of its preparation. Then marvel at its delicious taste. You'll find chapati recipes in the section called *Flavorful Flatbreads & Indian Chapatis* on pages 176–179.

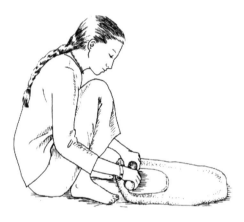

Figure 7.4 Rolling Chapati

HONORING THE LIFE-LINE OF A VEGETABLE

Did you know that each and every plant, herb, and fruit carries a distinct life-line through which the vital cosmic life forces of prana and agni flow, nurture, and sustain that organism? Through this viaduct, the universe and her five elements nurse and feed the seedling until she is nourished enough to serve as your food. By taking conscious pause to observe the natural grain or life-line of a plant, its roots and leaves, we are more likely to cultivate an ahimsa awareness of our foods. In so doing, we become aware of the great sacrifice the plant makes for our subsistence and as a result, an awesome feeling of gratitude overcomes the mind. Showing respect for the plant's sacrifice to feed and sustain us, we recognize each seed, vegetable, herb, fruit, and grain carries the profound will of the Mother Consciousness within.

The Vedic culture approached foods and their preparation with great reverence and a serene disposition. How we handle each food is reflected in its power to heal as well as its awesome taste. There is no chopping, tossing, throwing, or unruly scrambling associated with a Living Ahimsa meal. Cooking is a profound act of healing. It brings great serenity of mind when you discover how easy it is to be poised in your awareness. First though, put away the busy mind, shouting at your children, or chatting on the phone and bring your attention to the sacred act of cooking in the shrine that is your kitchen.

In keeping with the principle of Living Ahimsa, the first cut of any fruit or vegetable must be done by acknowledging its life force which flows along its distinct life-line. This action develops greater poise within the mind. Vegetables which grow on a stalk, such as broccoli and celery, need to be cut lengthwise. In the event small pieces are needed, they are further cut horizontally. Leafy greens are to be cut along the grains of the leaves, and their stems may be diced horizontally. Avoid using the coarse or purplish parts of stems. Elongated root vegetables such as carrots, daikon, and parsnips may be cut in many ways, but the initial approach needs to be one of cutting on a horizontal slant. The slant cut incorporates both the air (top) and earth (bottom) energies of the root, as well as the element of fire, which exists in the middle of the vegetable. Rounded root vegetables such as rutabagas, potatoes, and onions have a grain which runs along the center length of the vegetable. Onions and tomatoes endure the most unjust handling as they are generally cut opposite to their grain—most people seem fascinated by creating circular rings rather than the proper lengthy slices (which taste much sweeter than the incorrect ring-cuts).

It is a marvel to observe foods more closely and to proceed with the mind of ahimsa—with harmony and thoughtfulness—in our food preparation. These considerations will add much more joy and a connection to your cooking.

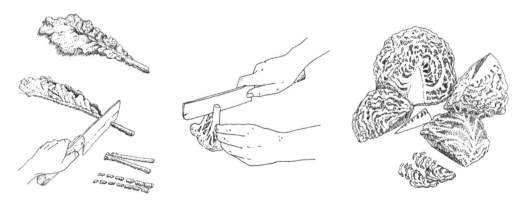

Figure 7.5 Vegetable Prepping

THE LOVE OF CHUTNEY

Chutneys are a celebration of the creativity, joy, and freshness of the human spirit, and making chutney is a lavish sadhana which celebrates the perennial youthfulness of our spirit and replenishes our vitality. Although chutneys can be made all year long, we can take special delight in this sadhana during the summer months, when we enjoy an abundance of fresh fruits.

According to Indian tradition, before a young man marries, his mother will put the prospective bride's homemaking skills to the test by having her make some chutney. If the bride makes a chutney well, it indicates that her power to love will be strong and that she will be a good wife and mother. The groom's happy mother proclaims, "A bride who makes a fine chutney has a good womb for bearing my grandchildren." In ahimsa practice, each activity we do is done with love. But to make a good chutney, the ingredient of love is imperative. Maya's story exemplifies this truth.

Maya's mother is a fantastic Indian vegetarian cook. She grew up in Pune, India in a home filled with affection and joy. The kitchen was the heart of the home, from which the aroma of spices continually wafted from her mother's chutney making. She looked forward to helping her mother prepare the ripened mangoes, oranges, dates, and currants for the chutney while sharing stories and laughter together. Maya is now bringing up her 7-year-old daughter in the same tradition of joy and love while teaching her the art of chutney making—a perfect ahimsa activity for mother and daughter bonding.

Fresh chutneys are ground daily in large stone mortars in most Indian households. They can be accents to the most lavish meals, or, as in South India, are often served as a main dish. There are literally hundreds of delicious combinations, from the traditional sweet mango or coconut chutneys to the hot, piquant ginger, lemon, tamarind, and chili mixtures. The more extravagant preparations are made from fresh and dried fruits such as mangoes, peaches, plums, cherries, dates, and currants and are spiced with masalas and fresh herbs, and marinated in ghee or jaggery (unprocessed brown sugar). No Vedic meal is complete without a dab of this luscious concoction.

You will find these delicious chutney recipes within this book:
- Ginger Pear Chutney (p 209)
- Savory Mango Chutney (p 179)
- Spring Strawberry & Mint Chutney (p 370)
- Summer Cherry & Tangerine Chutney (p 370-371)
- Early Fall Date & Coconut Chutney (p 371)
- Autumn Currant & Plum Chutney (p 371)
- Early Winter Ginger Chutney (p 372)
- Winter Fig & Currant Chutney (p 372)

BECOMING AWARE OF QUANTITY

The quantity of food you eat plays as important a role in maintaining good health as food quality. Generally, eat enough food to satisfy your system without feeling heavy. Ayurveda recommends filling half of your stomach with solid food, one quarter with liquid, and leaving the remaining quarter empty to ease digestion.

A simple way to determine the appropriate amount of solid food to enjoy at each meal is to cup your hands together and measure the amount of food that would fill this "cup" to the brim. As noted earlier, the "cup" of your hands is referred to as anjali and is the perfect measure for your particular stomach. A single cupped handful of liquid is the ideal ration of liquid at each meal. The smaller your hands, the less food and drink you need to sustain yourself when you are in perfect balance.

However, when you are doing hard physical work you will want to eat a larger amount of food. When you are exerting very little energy throughout the day, you will want to reduce the quantity of food proportionately. During illness or the transition between seasons, it's best to reduce your food intake to one-third the size of a normal meal. Decreasing the amount of food allows the digestive system to reorganize itself by reducing its workload so the body is nourished without unduly disturbing agni. The appropriate quantity of food allows *apana*, the breath responsible for evacuation of wastes from the body, to move downward while agni is encouraged to rekindle.

CHOOSING WHOLESOME QUALITY FOODS

The Ayurveda sage Charaka taught, "For food to be digested in a timely manner, thus promoting energy, healthy complexion, strength, and longevity, it must not only be imbibed in proper measure, but also must be of wholesome quality."

Ways to Ensure Good Food Quality:
- Strive to choose seasonal foods harvested in the climate you find yourself in. This is especially important when eating fruits, vegetables, legumes, and nuts. If this food is unavailable to you, your next best choice is food grown in the neighboring climatic region, or foods harvested from the preceding season.
- When possible, eat foods that are organic.
- Support your local organic farmers as much as possible, thereby encouraging the resurgence of community spirit.
- Avoid foods with preservatives or those that have been genetically engineered or altered in any way.
- Discard all old spices (older than one month), frozen foods, and commercially canned foods from your kitchen entirely.
- Use only organic or certified milk and dairy products.

- Use pure ghee made from sweet butter, not from vegetable oil.
- Only use naturally processed oils. Avoid hydrogenated or commercial brands.
- Use pure spring, well, or rainwater (avoid rainwater if you live in an area of the world where there is acid rain).
- Whenever sugar is called for in a traditional recipe, substitute brown sugar, jaggery (unrefined Indian palm sugar), Sucanat (specially processed brown sugar made from the juice of sugarcane), raw honey, or pure maple syrup. Never use white sugar, commercial brands of brown sugar, or sugar substitutes.
- Use Ayurveda rock salt or sea salt. Never use commercial salt, iodized salt, or salt substitutes.
- Use fresh organic fruits, not waxed or sprayed with chemical pesticides, and dried fruits that have not been sulfurized or processed with sugars or chemicals.
- Use whole fruits and minimize the use of fruit juices.

In order to benefit most from the recipes and practices you'll find in this book, I suggest that you avoid certain foods and minimize practices that contribute to depleting your energy of ahimsa.

Avoid the Following:
- Aluminum cookware
- Microwave ovens
- Electric stoves (use gas or wood-burning stoves)
- Teflon, Tefal, or non-stick cookware
- Margarine and other hydrogenated fats
- Refined salt, table salt
- Chlorinated water
- Antibiotics
- Aspartame
- Monosodium glutamate, MSG
- Pesticides
- Carcinogens
- Mass-produced, commercial quality milk (drink organic, small dairy farm, bottled milk)
- Food additives, like hormones
- Refined sugar, corn syrup, and other foods containing concentrated sweeteners
- Refined oils
- Baking powder
- Hard and dry bovine milk cheeses (parmesan, asiago)
- Junk foods (hamburgers, pizza, hot dogs, tacos, nachos)
- Fried, smoked, or grilled foods
- Soft drinks and alcoholic drinks

Those on a gluten-free diet will find dozens of appropriate recipes throughout this book. In general, avoid all nuts and dry-roasted nuts, except for peanuts and tree nuts that are considered legumes.

Grains to Avoid on a Gluten-Free Diet:
- Wheat
- Rye
- Barley
- Commercial Oats
- Oat Bran
- Oat Fiber
- Malt
- Couscous
- Durum
- Spelt
- Kamut
- Bulgur
- Farina
- Semolina

Grains Allowed on a Gluten-Free Diet:
- Rice
- Potatoes
- Corn
- Pure, uncontaminated oats
- Quinoa
- Tapioca
- Buckwheat
- Millet
- Yams
- Teff
- Amaranth
- Arrowroot flour
- Gelatin
- Xanthan gum
- Guar gum
- Sorghum

Storing Food Grains, Herbs & Spices:
Always use glass or ceramic containers with airtight seals to store spices, grains, and herbs. Be sure to place containers in a pristine, dry, and cool place away from direct sunlight and moonlight. Replenish dried herbs and spices frequently, storing only enough for a fortnight's use at a time.

In the second part of this book we will explore the six seasons in depth. I recommend you put aside some time to observe each season as it passes, and take note of the remarkable sense of transformation that is naturally occurring within you with the changing of each season. You will find that your emotions and desires, as well as your sense of taste, smell, and touch, change radically as your body, mind, and spirit reach out to embrace the distinct elements each season brings with it. Seize the chance to make your journey through the seasons a partnership with nature; a Living Ahimsa experience—an act of innocence, wholeness, and joyfulness as you experience the shifting landscape within while consciously garnering the vast resource of Inner Medicine that each one of Mother's magnificent seasons bring.

Part Two

SPRING

I take The Vow of Ahimsa

I make inner harmony my first priority

Chapter Eight

SPRING PRACTICES FOR REBIRTHING AHIMSA ENERGY

The winds in fragrance move;
The lakes are bright with lotuses;
The women luminous with love;
The days are soft, the evenings fair
And charming; everything
That moves and lives and blossoms, dear,
Is sweeter, in the Spring.
— Kalidasa

THE EARTH'S OFFICIAL NEW YEAR

Spring is a time of rebirth and regeneration for all earth's creatures. Life begins to thaw out, reemerging from the safe bosom of the earth, and a feeling of fragility and wonder for the profound beauty of Mother Nature prevails. Her blossoms of hazelnut, cherry, plum, and dogwood trees; her sprouting green foliage of the tulips, daffodils, and irises; and the songs of her finches, cardinals, sparrows, and blackbirds fill the atmosphere of spring with awe and quiet delight. Harsh snows and rains give way to a budding, soon-to-be-thriving earth. Animals begin to give birth and the earth awakens to the scent of fruit tree blossoms carried by the invigorating winds. Spring is nature's youth, a time when we can embrace the childlike impulses that are aroused at this time.

According to the Vedic Calendar, spring begins when the full moon sits in the Vedic constellation of *Chaitra* during the month of March. Unlike the Western Calendar of counting time, Vedic astronomers cite the month of March as the earth's official New Year. This is when the sun enters Aries according to Western astrology. This is also the day after the spring equinox.

Considered one of the most auspicious times of the year, we also celebrate *Rama Navami*—the birthday of Lord Rama, the god of dharma (righteous action)—at the top of the Hindu New Year, which also marks the complete annual rotation of the six seasons. This occurs each year on the ninth lunar day of the month, which generally falls in April.

The celebration of *Vasanta Panchami* marks the first day of the spring season.

It occurs on the fifth day of the waxing moon of *Magha*. Saraswati—the goddess of wisdom, art, and learning—is venerated on this day. Mirth, gaiety, sweetness, and fragrance are the day's essences. Yellow clothing is worn and saffron rice is prepared, representing the golden hue of maturity and spirituality. The goddess is worshipped through music and poetry, and children are initiated into learning the alphabet on this day. Students bearing food, flowers, and ornaments tend to the temple. Books, pens, and writing tablets are placed on Saraswati's altar to be blessed.

In Vedic culture, festivals, fasts, feasts, and religious ceremonies are intimately connected to the seasons and their transitions. Many traditions have developed holiday rituals and celebrations tied closely to geographical and cultural themes. These seasonal holidays often correlate with agricultural cycles, religious and mythical traditions, historical events, or rites of passage.

In my tradition, spring is called the "King of the Seasons." It is the most celebrated season throughout the world. Christians in India and the world over observe a fast for 40 days prior to the period known as Lent, which comes from the old English word for spring. Masses and prayers are held during this time of penitence and fasting. Easter arrives, marking the resurrection of Christ, and is celebrated with exuberance. In the spring, the Mayan culture worshiped Acat, the god of fruitfulness; Aima, the goddess of fertility, was worshipped by the ancient Hebrews; and the sun goddess Amaterasu is celebrated in Japan during this time. The ancient Romans and Greeks celebrated springtime by worshipping Apollo, god of abundance and health, and the Chinese honor Tien Kuan, god of gladness and health. Lono, the goddess of productivity, is celebrated in the spring by Polynesians. Throughout the world, farming communities bless and honor the earth with fervent supplication for divine favor for the forthcoming bounty of food.

AWAKENING TO SPRING'S RHYTHMS

With all of its glory, spring can be a time of profound extremes, so I encourage you to remain aware during this significant time of transition. Your physical body is emerging from its winter hibernation, experiencing a feeling of rawness and vulnerability heightened by the naked beauty of spring's nature. Coughs, colds, fevers, chicken pox, and measles are some of the body's responses to this season of rebirth.

Ayurveda informs us that spring is predominantly Kapha in nature and a vulnerable time. Purifying and cleansing the system of toxicity accumulated during the winter is necessary at the onset of spring. The Pitta dosha is also affected during the spring, which can result in a weakened digestive fire and feverish conditions. Pay careful attention to your choice of foods and activities throughout this season. Eating foods that are excessively sweet, sour, or astringent is discouraged. Excess fluids and cold, stale, or oily foods should also be avoided.

Excellent foods and herbs for spring are: apples, arugula, asparagus, barley, blackberries, blueberries, broccoli, buckwheat, carrots, chickpeas, cilantro, collard greens, endive, kale, lettuces, millet, mung beans, oregano, parsley, raspberries, sage, scallions, snow peas, spinach, split peas, thyme, and wheat. A light and warming diet along with regular exercise, meditation, and yoga practice is especially beneficial. Exercising moderation in sleep and cohabitation serve to safeguard the body and mind and prevent the accumulation of Kapha during the spring season.

The following are user-friendly guidelines for the appropriate activities during this season. These time-tested lunar observances are more than symbolic—they help you psychologically prepare to move through the cycle of time, negotiating its challenges and the ever-generating energy each season brings. Learning and adhering to these seasonal healing practices will help you to alleviate the vulnerability, anxiety, and depression that pervade the atmosphere during this season. These practices will help you nourish your spirit of rebirth.

THE ENERGY OF SPRING

PRIMARY ACTIVITY	PREDOMINANT TASTE	PREDOMINANT ELEMENTS	TIME OF YEAR	DOSHIC NATURE
Rebirth	Astringent	Air and Earth	Mid to late-March through mid to late-May (Northern Hemisphere)	Vata and Kapha
			Mid to late-September through mid to late-November (Southern Hemisphere)	

Table 8.1

REBIRTHING AHIMSA ENERGY

Spring Moon Fast

As you learned in chapter five, "The Art of the Fast," fasting in all of its glory constitutes an inseparable part of the Vedic wisdom tradition. These timeless Living

Ahimsa practices are empowered by centuries of dedicated observance to help us move through the denseness of ill health and despair we experience in our lives today. There are numerous ways to fast and lighten the body, mind, and spirit. The core intention behind all forms of Vedic spiritual austerity is to honor the magnificent wisdom we carry within—to know that we are one with the Mother Consciousness.

To purify and cleanse the body, mind, and spirit, Hindus everywhere celebrate the Goddess Mother Parvati—consort of Shiva—by observing a nine-day fast called *Vasanta Navaratra*. This occasion—which venerates the Goddess Mother and marks the beginning of the warm seasons—is quietly observed. Traditionally, we fast on two cloves, lemon water, fruit, and/or saltless food each day for nine days.

On the fifth day of the bright fortnight, or waxing moon, in *Chaitra*, the month of April, we observe a fast to venerate the refreshing vitality of nature. This day marks the sanctity of our first nourishment of the official New Year imbibed as *navanna*, symbolized by the sheaves of grain from the new harvest that are offered to the deity at home. It is a day to reawaken our ability to learn, know, and understand. The goddess of wisdom, Saraswati, is revered as the deity of this day since it is believed to be the day she first manifested her energies in the universe.

Navaratri celebrations honoring the goddess occur twice annually: At the start of the cold seasons in the autumn, the goddess is again celebrated, but with great pomp and ceremony. The beginning of spring and the beginning of autumn are two very important junctions of climactic and solar influence. These two periods are seen as sacred opportunities for the worship of the Divine Mother. The dates of the festivals are determined according to the Vedic Lunar Calendar. Through popular venerations and sacred practices of the goddess, the disciple is helped to invoke the divine power of Goddess Shakti—the feminine aspect of cosmic energy that perpetuates all life.

Although an age-old practice, fasting in harmony with the lunar rhythms is one of the most powerful sadhanas we can perform to reclaim our wisdom, peace, and well-being. To this end, the rishis developed imperative vratas—nurturing practices—to foster excellent health, communal harmony, and the Mind of Wisdom. The Sanskrit word *vrata* means "vow." It is derived from the root *vru*, which means "to honor and worship; to resolve a desire; to invite good health and prosperity." In essence, a vrata is a specific spiritual observance—a certain restriction in our daily routine—corresponding with a lunar day and time, which venerates a particular deity in order to fulfill a specific desire or cultivate awareness.

All fasts are spiritual commitments and have one overriding purpose—to cleanse the body and mind in order to free the spirit so awareness and consciousness can soar. Ultimately, fasting is an act of devotion to the divine energies, which enhances the memory of our sacred origins. The side effects of a fast are many: it lightens the body, relieves toxins, cleanses and nourishes tissues, revitalizes cells, and strengthens intelligence. Fasting also provides necessary rest to the digestive system and agni, its fire power: It is an organic and powerful Inner Medicine way of healing all diseases.

In the Vedic tradition, there are a variety of fasts, each one initiated in accord with a specific phase of the moon, and therefore possessing profound healing value. You may choose any of the number of appropriate vratas that follow to fast in accord with the lunar cycle. Even if you are skeptical, I encourage you to put this system of lunar living to the test at least once. Try fasting on an Ekadashi day (detailed on pages 70-73) focusing on a specific challenge you wish to have resolved in your life, then see if you find resolution after your fast.

There are various traditional forms of fasting, and each ultimately addresses the need to cleanse disharmonious conditions from our lives while diminishing hurtful actions and challenging karmas. Each type of fast is specific to the result you wish to achieve.

For example, *Ayachit Vrata*—one of the more arduous acts of fasting—is a vow that helps you cultivate a sense of gratitude for everything, including conditions you perceive as negative. In this practice one remains content with meals that are freely offered to them. In this vowed intention, one is forbidden from requesting meals or from eating during certain junctures of the day (dawn, noontime, dusk, midnight) and other times deemed cosmically inappropriate. Obviously, this would be a difficult practice for most people to do.

In the observance of *Prajapatya Vrata*, a 12-day nourishment discipline, you regulate mouthfuls of food incrementally every three days until the last three days when a complete fast is practiced. For instance, in the first quarter (or three days) you take 22 mouthfuls of food, in the second quarter 26 mouthfuls of food, in the third quarter 24 mouthfuls of food, and in the last quarter you fast. This deep austerity enhances fertility and is said to fulfill the desire for progeny.

Hindu ascetics and widows perform *Nakta Vrata*; having fasted throughout the day, they break fast right before sunset. This observance is practiced as a way of life; the evening meal is imbibed while viewing the constellation *Nakta Vrata*. This fast helps to attain the state of One Consciousness with the Absolute Reality, suitable in preparation for renunciation of the material world.

Ekabhukta Vrata is the act of imbibing only one meal a day, a more attainable practice for everyone to do at least once a week to maintain personal health and wellness.

Chandrayan Vrata concerns the making of a promise to eat in accord with the phases of the moon. This fast, which generally can be practiced for a fortnight or throughout an entire month, serves to cleanse ancestral karmas of hurtful patterns of behavior. For this practice we will fast in accord with the moon by observing an Ekadashi Fast, which I also call Spring Moon Fast.

THE PRACTICE: SPRING MOON FAST

To maintain good health of body, mind, and spirit, the spring season is one of the two primary seasons of the year when fasting is imperative. (The other season is autumn.) The Spring Moon Fast comprises 4 days of fasting during Ekadashi.

OPTIMUM TIMING:*
Northern Hemisphere:
- 12 days following the full moon in early March (not counting the full moon day).
- 11 days following the new moon around mid-March (counting the new moon day).
- 12 days following the full moon in early April (not counting the full moon day).
- 11 days following the new moon around mid-April (counting the new moon day).

Southern Hemisphere:
- 12 days following the full moon in early September (not counting the full moon day).
- 11 days following the new moon around mid-September (counting the new moon day).
- 12 days following the full moon in early October (not counting the full moon day).
- 11 days following the new moon around mid-October (counting the new moon day).

*I highly recommend purchasing a Vedic Calendar to calculate the exact timing of the new and full moons of the Ekadashi days.

Contra-indications: Do not fast during severe illness, menstruation, or when bleeding. The elderly and young children should also avoid fasting.

INSTRUCTIONS:
- On the optimum Ekadashi days noted above, begin a 4-day Spring Moon Fast.
- Ekadashi generally occurs twice monthly and you must seize each and every opportunity to observe at least one Ekadashi fasting day in each month.
- Refer to instructions in The Practice: Observing a Fast on Ekadashi on pages 70-73.

This sacred lunar observance is practiced to reclaim your state of inner balance with cyclical rhythms and reclaim your grace with nature, thereby healing and nullifying personal health and familial challenges. This fortnight of practice is aligned with the waxing and waning tempo of the moon. (Remember, if you are unable to complete a full fast, try to observe a modified Semi-Fast, detailed on pages 73-77.)

SPRING MOON FEAST

Once the body is empty, illumed with space and the grace of fasting, we continue to flow in tandem with the Mother Consciousness and look forward to fostering a life of balance. Where there is a fast, a feast is certain to follow. A harvest of creative ideas, and a feast of wellness, love, joy, and abundance is waiting to reign in the empty space you created during your fast.

As noted earlier, the Hindu New Year is celebrated throughout India at the beginning of spring. The woman's festival of *Ganguara*, "fresh spring moon," is celebrated at this time, on the third day of the waxing cycle of the moon. It is where young and elder women alike venerate Goddess Gauri who bestows marital happiness and familial bliss.

The first day of spring is also a day to celebrate your riches of joy, prosperity, and wellness, because the birthday (the day the goddess was made manifest) of Goddess Lakshmi—giver of family bliss and prosperity—is also commemorated at this time. In Vedic astronomy, the world was created on this day, and the computation of time started from the sunrise of this day many epochs ago.

THE PRACTICE: SPRING MOON FEAST

OPTIMUM TIMING:
- Northern Hemisphere: On the 3rd day of the waxing moon (following the new moon occurring at the end of March).
- Southern Hemisphere: On the 3rd day of the waxing moon (following the new moon occurring at the end of September).

INSTRUCTIONS & PREPARATIONS:
- Celebrate the Great Goddess on this day in whichever cultural form you perceive her.
- Start this glorious day with a warm, nurturing, aromatic bath filled with love and drops of lavender, jasmine, or other essential oils.
- Dress in new and colorful clothing.
- Offer prayers of gratitude to the Divine Mother.
- Clean your living space and decorate it with fresh flowers and fruits.
- Prepare a scrumptious feast for your family and friends. (Use the recipes set out in the next chapter, "Fragrant Nourishment for Spring."
- Invite your friends to join you in making fresh Spring Masala to use in your feast if you desire (recipe on page 374).
- Give thoughtful gifts to your employees, friends, and neighbors to show gratitude for their support.
- Invite your women friends and daughters to stay on for a Spring Moon Celebration on the auspicious third night of the waxing moon (which follows).

THE PRACTICE: SPRING MOON CELEBRATION

OPTIMUM TIMING:

- **Northern Hemisphere:** On the 3rd night of the waxing moon from 8:00–10:00 p.m. (following the new moon occurring at the end of March).
- **Southern Hemisphere:** On the 3rd night of the waxing moon from 8:00–10:00 p.m. (following the new moon occurring at the end of September).

INSTRUCTIONS & PREPARATIONS:

- Set out a number of small bowls filled with water (1 bowl for each participant) in a perfect circle on a flat space on the ground or on an outdoor deck.
- Place a natural candle or ghee lamp on a flat stone in the center of the circle.
- Bring your shawls, sweaters, flasks of tea, drums, or any percussion instruments you have to the gathering.
- Sit in a circle around the bowls of water.
- Watch the waxing moon reflect in the bowls as she rises in the skies.
- Bask in her splendor; celebrate with songs of your tradition, telling stories of your everyday womanly lives.
- Invoke your female ancestors to bless you.
- With a pure heart, declare your wishes to the beautiful moon, and let her hear them.
- Your wish will most likely be fulfilled.

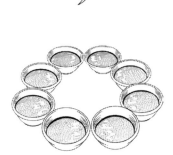

Figure 8.1 Water Bowls & Moon

CONTEMPLATING THE LUMINOUS GODDESS OF WISDOM

As I mentioned earlier, Goddess Saraswati is venerated during this splendid time of year. In Vedic iconography, Goddess Saraswati is depicted as a beautiful, luminous, fair-skinned deity who is simply dressed in pure white and seated on a white lotus. Although she is often depicted on a white lotus, her actual *vahana*, or cosmic vehicle, is known to be a white swan representing the Absolute Truth, inferring that Saraswati has experienced the Absolute Reality. The swan symbolizes discrimination between the good and the untoward; the eternal and the evanescent. In fact, it is believed that the sacred swan, if offered a mixture of milk and water, is able to drink the milk alone. Due to her association with the swan, Goddess Saraswati is also referred to as *Hamsa-vahini*, which means "she who has a swan as her vehicle."

She is also depicted standing near a flowing river which relates to her early history as a river goddess. The swan and Saraswati's association with the lotus flower remind us of her ancient primordial origins. Also often portrayed sitting on a peacock, the goddess teaches her disciples to tame their material ambitions. The peacock is symbolic of feeling arrogance and pride about one's physical beauty. By *sitting* on this aspect of the human self, we can control our base instincts and emotional desires—transcend our physical moorings to attain a state of wisdom and knowledge of the eternal truth.

Saraswati's white dress signifies the purity of true knowledge. Occasionally she will be robed in yellow, representing her embodiment of spiritual nourishment reflected by the spring season and its flowers. Saraswati exudes the absolute simplicity that is inculcated by knowledge. She has four arms, which symbolize the four aspects of learning for the human personality: mind, intellect, awareness, and ego. Alternatively, these four arms also represent the four Vedas, the primary sacred books for Hindus. She is depicted holding the following items in her four hands:

- A book, which is the sacred Vedas, representing the divine, eternal, and true knowledge of the universe, as well as her perfect knowledge of the scriptures.
- A mala, or rosary of crystals, representing the power of meditation or the taming of the mind.
- A pot of sacred water, representing creative and purificatory powers.
- The *vina*, or stringed musical instrument, represents her perfection of all arts and sciences. Saraswati is also associated with *anuraga*, the love for and rhythm of music, representing the emotions expressed through speech or music.

Set aside some time in your spring meditations to contemplate the resplendent goddess Saraswati. Obtain a portrait of her for your altar and contemplate each of her aspects as described above.

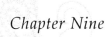

Chapter Nine

FRAGRANT OFFERINGS OF SPRING

The light and warming repast of the spring season offers you the golden chance to invoke your Living Ahimsa power to lessen the stresses and burdens of daily life. You will find a deeper sense of satisfaction with the more fragrant, light meals of this profound season of rebirth and rejuvenation. Feast yourself with spring's gentle greens, berries, and legumes—bolstered by revitalizing fresh salads, invigorating grains, and scrumptiously delicate desserts such as Vedic Rose Pudding and Almond Lime Squares.

SPRING MENU PLANNING

The Spring Season:
- Northern Hemisphere: Mid-to-late March through mid-to-late May.
- Southern Hemisphere: Mid-to-late September through mid-to-late November.

Vulnerable Time: For Kapha and Pitta Types*
- Kapha: Avoid excess sweet, sugars, refined carbohydrates and fatty foods.
- Pitta: Avoid excess sour and salty tastes, oily, fatty foods, and intoxicants.
- * To learn your body type, see appendix one, "Wise Earth Ayurveda Body Types."

SPRING MENU: DO's & DON'T's	
APPROPRIATE FOODS FOR SPRING	**FOODS TO AVOID IN SPRING**
Pungent, bitter, and moderately salty tastes	Astringent or excess sweet or sour tastes
Light, warm, fresh, and stimulating foods	Cold, heavy, stale, unctuous foods
Barley, millet, wheat, buckwheat, and seasonal fruits, herbs, vegetables, legumes	Animal flesh products: meats, fowl, fish, and eggs

Table 9.1

SAMPLE SPRING MENU

Spring Breakfast:
- Kapha: Breakfast is not recommended.
- Pitta and Vata: See appendix three, "Breakfast of Champions," for a wide array of breakfast choices that can be enjoyed throughout the year.

Spring Lunch:
- Healing Ginger & Scallion Soup (p 133)
- Classic Soft Millet (p 120)
- Almond Lime Squares (p 138)
- Cinnamon Mint Tea (p 140)

Spring Dinner:
- Sublime Spinach Masala (p 128)
- Lively Steamed Asparagus (p 125)
- Sweet Bulgur with Lotus Seeds (p 124)
- Vedic Rose Pudding Cake (p 137)

Gluten-free recipes are indicated by ♡

REVITALIZING SPRING SALADS

ESCAROLE & TAMARIND SALAD ♡
Serves: 6

2 tablespoons tamarind paste

1/4 cup warm water

1 teaspoon corn oil

1 teaspoon rock salt

1 head escarole

Dilute the tamarind paste in water, then add the corn oil and salt and set aside. Wash the escarole and tear it apart, separating the whole leaves. Arrange the leaves on a platter and pour the tamarind dressing over them. Use a flat-bottomed plate weighted down with a large stone to press the salad for 1 hour. Serve in small quantities.

MEDITERRANEAN BUCKWHEAT SALAD
Serves: 6

2 cups buckwheat groats, cooked

1/4 cup fresh Italian parsley, minced

4 sun-dried tomatoes, thinly sliced

1 tablespoon sunflower oil

I teaspoon rock salt

I/2 teaspoon black pepper, finely ground

I teaspoon tamarind paste

I/4 cup warm water

Belgium endives, to garnish

In a large bowl, combine and toss the buckwheat groats, Italian parsley, sun-dried tomatoes, sunflower oil, salt, and pepper. Dilute the tamarind paste with warm water and pour
over the salad. Decorate the outside of a platter with whole endive leaves and arrange the
salad in the center of the leaves. Serve at once.

MIZUNA & ORANGE SALAD ♥
Serves: 6

I orange

2 teaspoons rock salt

I lime, freshly juiced

I large bunch mizuna leaves

Wash and thinly slice the orange with the peel still on. Season the orange slices with the
salt and all of the lime juice. Arrange the seasoned orange slices on top of the mizuna
leaves and serve.

ZESTY MILLET ♥
Serves: 6

I tablespoon sunflower oil

I tablespoon cumin seeds

2 cups millet, cooked

2 small red onions, thinly sliced

I tablespoon fresh thyme, minced

I tablespoon fresh oregano, minced

I lemon, freshly juiced

I tablespoon orange zest

I teaspoon rock salt

Heat the sunflower oil in a large skillet over medium heat and roast the cumin seeds until
they are golden brown. Add the cooked millet and cook on medium heat for 5 minutes.
Remove from heat and allow to cool. Use your clean hands to make small plum-size balls
with the cooled millet by wetting your hands and rolling the millet between your palms. In
a large bowl, combine raw onions, thyme, oregano, lemon juice, orange zest, and salt. Add
the millet balls to the salad. Toss and serve at once.

WATERCRESS & LEMON SALAD ♡

Serves: 6

2 lemons

I teaspoon corn oil

I teaspoon rock salt

I teaspoon fresh garlic, minced

I/4 cup warm water

3 small bunches watercress

Wash and thinly slice the lemons with the peels still on. In a small bowl combine the lemon slices, corn oil, salt, garlic, and water. Wash the watercress and arrange it on a platter. Pour the dressing over it and place a flat-bottomed plate, weighted down with a large rock, on to the salad to press for I hour. Serve in small quantities.

BARLEY & PEA SALAD

Serves: 6

2 cups pearl barley, cooked and still warm

I/2 cup fresh peas

I tablespoon fresh marjoram, minced

I tablespoon fresh Mexican basil, minced

I tablespoon corn oil

I/2 lime, freshly juiced

I teaspoon rock salt

Combine and toss all the ingredients in a large salad bowl. Serve warm.

SPROUTED MUNG BEANS ♡

Serves: 6

I cup whole mung beans

4 cups warm water (80 degrees)

I lemon, freshly juiced

In a large glass jar, combine the beans and water. Cover securely with plastic wrap and allow to sit overnight. Drain well, and then divide equally among 4 clean quart jars. Cover each with a piece of cheesecloth secured with a rubber band around the rim. Keep the jars in a warm, dark place. Twice daily, fill the jars with warm water and shake them gently to make sure all the beans are moistened. Drain the water out of the jars through the cheese-cloth. Let the jars stand until the small white shoots of the sprouts appear. Garnish with lemon juice and serve.

COCONUT & SNOW PEA SALAD ♡

Serves: 6

1 cup fresh snow peas

3 cups Sprouted Mung Beans (recipe on page 118)

1/2 cup fresh coconut, grated

(if fresh coconut is unavailable, substitute with dried coconut)

1 large head oak leaf lettuce

1 tablespoon corn oil

1/4 cup warm apple juice

1 teaspoon rock salt

1/2 teaspoon mustard powder

Blanch the snow peas and combine them with the sprouted mung beans and grated coconut in a large bowl. Tear the lettuce into large pieces and add it to the snow pea and coconut mixture. Combine the corn oil, apple juice, salt, and mustard powder in a tightly covered jar and shake to mix. Pour over the salad and serve at once.

ARUGULA & STRAWBERRY SALAD ♡

Serves: 6

1 tablespoon organic ghee (recipe on pages 150-151)

1 tablespoon fennel seeds

1 quart fresh strawberries, halved

2 bunches arugula

2 tablespoons honey

1 lemon, freshly juiced

2 tablespoons warm water

1/2 teaspoon black pepper, finely ground

Heat the ghee in a small skillet over medium heat. Add the fennel seeds and roast them until they are golden brown. Combine the ghee and fennel mixture with the strawberries in a salad bowl. Wash the arugula, tear it into bite-size pieces, and toss it with the seasoned strawberries. Combine the honey, lemon juice, water, and black pepper in a tightly covered jar and shake well to mix the dressing. Pour over the salad and serve immediately.

AROMATIC ARAME RICE SALAD ♡

Serves: 6

1 cup arame seaweed

1 teaspoon sunflower oil

2 cups long-grain brown rice, cooked

1/2 cup shallots, chopped
1 tablespoon rice vinegar
Green leaf lettuce, to garnish

Wash and drain the arame. Add sunflower oil to the skillet and lightly sauté the arame for 3 to 4 minutes. Toss in a large bowl with brown rice, shallots, and rice vinegar. Tear the green leaf lettuce into bite-size pieces and use to garnish the rice salad. Serve at once.

INSPIRING GRAINS

CLASSIC SOFT MILLET ♥

Serves: 4

2 cups millet
5 cups boiling water
1 pinch sea salt

Wash millet until water runs clear and add to the boiling water. Add salt. Cover and simmer over medium-low heat for 25 minutes. Serve warm.

BASMATI & WILD RICE ♥

Serves: 6

3 1/2 cups water
1 1/4 cups basmati white rice
1/4 cup wild rice
1/2 teaspoon rock salt
1 tablespoon fresh tarragon, minced

Bring water to a boil in a medium-size saucepan. Wash the basmati and wild rice and add to the boiling water, along with the salt. Cover and simmer on medium-low heat for 35 minutes until the wild rice bursts open. Mix in the fresh tarragon and remove from heat. Cover and let stand for 5 minutes before serving.

CRACKED SPELT WITH CHERRIES

Serves: 4

3 cups water
2 cups cracked spelt berries
1/4 cup dried cherries, pitted and halved
8 cardamom pods
2 cinnamon sticks

1 teaspoon fresh ginger, grated
1/2 teaspoon rock salt
Yogurt, to garnish

Bring water to a boil in a medium-size saucepan. Wash the cracked spelt berries and add to the water, along with dried cherries, cardamom pods, cinnamon sticks, fresh ginger, and salt. Cover and simmer on medium heat for 18 minutes until the spelt is cooked. Remove from heat and let stand for 10 minutes. Remove the cardamom pods and cinnamon sticks before serving. Garnish each serving with a dollop of yogurt.

ZUCCHINI & LEMONGRASS RICE ♡

Serves: 4

4 cups water
1 tablespoon dried lemongrass
2 cups basmati white rice
1 teaspoon rock salt
1/2 teaspoon black pepper, finely ground
1 tablespoon corn oil
1 tablespoon cumin seeds
1 large zucchini, finely cubed

Bring water to a boil in a medium-size saucepan. Steep the lemongrass for 10 minutes in 1 cup of the boiling water; strain the tea, discarding the lemongrass. Wash the basmati rice and add to the remaining water. Pour in the tea. Add salt and pepper, cover, and simmer on medium heat for 12 minutes. Remove from heat and set aside. Heat corn oil in a medium-size skillet. Roast the cumin seeds for 1 minute over medium heat and then stir in zucchini. Cover and cook on medium-high heat for about 3 minutes until zucchini begins to char. Remove from heat. Fold the cooked rice mixture into zucchini. Serve at once.

MATAJI'S RICE PILAF ♡

Serves: 4

3 1/2 cups water
1/2 cup rice milk
2 cups long-grain brown rice
1/2 cup fresh peas
1 teaspoon rock salt
1/4 cup raisins
2 tablespoons fresh basil, minced
1/2 lemon, freshly juiced

1 tablespoon honey
12 strands saffron
1 teaspoon sunflower oil
1/4 cup chopped cashews

Bring water and rice milk to a boil in a medium-size saucepan. Wash the brown rice and peas and add them to boiling water-rice milk mixture. Then add salt and raisins. Stir, cover, and simmer for 20 minutes on medium heat until rice is cooked. Remove from heat and set aside. Combine the basil, lemon juice, honey, and saffron in a small bowl and gently stir into the warm cooked rice. Coat skillet with sunflower oil and roast the cashews over medium heat until golden brown. Garnish rice pilaf with cashews and serve warm.

LOTUS SEEDS & BARLEY
Serves: 4
3 1/2 cups water
2 cups pearl barley
1/4 cup dried lotus seeds
1 teaspoon sunflower oil
1 pinch rock salt

Bring water to a boil in a medium-size saucepan. Wash the barley and lotus seeds and add to the boiling water. Add the oil and salt. Stir, cover, and simmer over medium-low heat for 20 minutes. Remove from heat and let stand for 10 minutes. Serve warm.

HEALING SPRING BARLEY
Serves: 4
4 1/2 cups water
2 cups pearled barley
1 teaspoon rock salt
1/2 teaspoon turmeric powder
1 teaspoon coriander powder
1/4 cup scallions, chopped
1 teaspoon organic ghee (recipe on pages 150-151)
1/4 cup roasted sunflower seeds

Bring water to a boil in a medium-size saucepan. Wash barley and add to boiling water. Add salt, turmeric, coriander powder, scallions, and ghee. Stir, cover, and simmer on medium-low heat for 45 minutes until the barley is very soft. Garnish with roasted sunflower seeds and serve warm.

MILLET & PEA SUPREME ♡

Serves: 4

3 1/2 cups water

2 cups millet

1/4 cup fresh peas

1/2 teaspoon turmeric powder

1/2 teaspoon cumin powder

1/2 teaspoon ajwain seeds

1 teaspoon rock salt

1 tablespoon sunflower oil

1/4 cup currants

1/4 cup roasted almonds, slivered

1/2 lemon, freshly juiced

1 teaspoon orange zest

Bring water to a boil in a medium-size saucepan. Thoroughly wash the millet and add it to the boiling water, along with the peas, turmeric, cumin powder, ajwain seeds, and salt. Cover and simmer on medium heat for 20 minutes. Heat the sunflower oil in a small skillet, and add the currants and almonds. Stir for a few minutes until the currants begin to swell. Add the lemon juice and orange zest. Combine this mixture with the millet and continue cooking for 10 minutes. Serve warm.

SPRING KICHADI ♡

Serves: 4

Kichadi is a classical Ayurveda dish, gentle and rich in its healing properties. It has been used for centuries as a primary Ayurveda meal while cleansing the body or semi-fasting. Generally, kichadi is a combination of basmati rice and mung beans seasoned with ghee and medicinal spices such as coriander, cumin, ajwain, and turmeric—although you may use a multitude of variations of grains and beans. When combining the grain and the bean, be sure to choose a grain and bean that have an affinity for each other. The best way to determine compatibility is by taste and timing: Choose pairings that would create a wholesome, rich tasting meal.

3 1/2 cups water

2 cups basmati white rice

1/4 cup red lentils

1 teaspoon rock salt

1 teaspoon corn oil

1 teaspoon fresh garlic, grated

1 teaspoon cumin seeds

Bibb lettuce, for garnish

Bring water to a boil in a medium-size saucepan. Wash rice and lentils and add to the water, along with the salt. Cover and simmer on medium-low heat for 12 minutes or until the kichadi turns fluffy. Remove from heat and set aside. Heat the corn oil in a small skillet over medium heat. Roast the garlic and cumin seeds for a few minutes until golden brown. Gently stir the roasted seeds and garlic into the kichadi. Serve at once over whole Bibb lettuce leaves.

THREE GRAIN MEDLEY ♡
Serves: 4

3 1/2 cups water
1 cup millet
1/2 cup basmati white rice
1/2 cup quinoa
1 teaspoon rock salt
1 teaspoon black pepper, coarsely ground
1/4 cup sunflower seeds

Bring water to a boil in a medium-size saucepan. Wash the millet, basmati rice, and quinoa separately and then add each to the boiling water. Cover and simmer on medium-low heat for 12 minutes until the grains are swelled and fluffy. Remove from heat and set aside. In a small skillet, dry roast the sunflower seeds over medium heat stirring frequently until they are almost golden brown. Add the salt and black pepper. Garnish each serving of the grains with a tablespoon of the seasoned sunflower seeds.

SWEET BULGUR WITH LOTUS SEEDS
Serves: 4

3 1/2 cups water
2 cups bulgur
1/4 cup dried lotus seeds
1/2 teaspoon cardamom powder
1 teaspoon coriander powder
1 teaspoon sunflower oil
1 pinch rock salt
1 pint fresh strawberries, halved
1 tablespoon maple syrup

Bring water to a boil in a medium-size saucepan. Wash the bulgur and lotus seeds and add to the boiling water. Add the cardamom, coriander, oil, and salt. Stir, cover, and simmer over medium-low heat for 15 minutes. Remove from heat and let stand for 10 minutes. Lightly

daub the strawberries with maple syrup. Amply garnish each serving with the fresh strawberries and serve at once.

STRENGTHENING SPRING GREENS

LIVELY STEAMED ASPARAGUS ♥

Serves: 6

24 asparagus spears
1 tablespoon organic ghee (recipe on pages 150-151)
1/2 fresh lime
1 teaspoon black pepper, finely ground
1/2 teaspoon rock salt

Trim the ends off the asparagus, place asparagus spears in a steamer over boiling water,
and steam for 3 to 4 minutes. Remove from steamer and place in a serving dish. Pour
melted ghee over asparagus spears, squeeze lime over them, then sprinkle with black
pepper and salt. Serve at once with a cooked grain of your choice.

SWEET BABY TURNIPS ♥

Serves: 6

24 baby turnips
2 tablespoons corn oil
1 tablespoon Wise Earth Garam Masala (recipe on page 373)
1 tablespoon unprocessed brown sugar
1 cup water
1 cup apple juice

Peel turnips, retaining 2 inches of their green tops. Heat corn oil in a large saucepan,
and lightly roast the garam masala for 1 minute over medium-high heat until it begins to
sizzle. Add the baby turnips and sugar, along with the water and apple juice. Cover and
simmer on medium heat for 15 minutes until turnips are very tender. Serve warm over
cooked basmati white rice.

ESCAROLE & ZUCCHINI ♥

Serves: 6

2 red bell peppers
1 tablespoon sunflower oil
1 teaspoon cumin seeds
5 zucchini

2 green onions, chopped
1 teaspoon rock salt
1 pound fresh escarole

Wash and spear whole red bell peppers with a long fork. Grill over an open flame, gradually turning the peppers to completely blacken the skins. Remove from heat, and run cold water over them. Carefully peel off the charred skins. Slice the peppers lengthwise in thin strips, discarding the core and seeds. Set aside. Heat the sunflower oil in a large skillet over medium heat and roast cumin seeds until golden. Wash zucchini and cut into thin diagonal slices. Add to the roasted cumin seeds, along with the green onions and salt. Sauté over medium heat for 2 minutes until zucchini slices are slightly braised. Wash and tear escarole into large pieces, then stir into the zucchini mixture. Remove from heat. Garnish with red peppers, and serve at once with a cooked grain of your choice.

BROCCOLI RABE WITH GARLIC ♥
Serves: 6
2 pounds broccoli rabe
2 tablespoons olive oil
4 cloves garlic, peeled and crushed
1 pinch rock salt
1/4 cup roasted sunflower seeds

Wash and dry the broccoli rabe, then trim and discard stems. Heat olive oil in a large skillet over medium heat and sauté the crushed garlic for a few minutes until golden. Be careful not to brown the garlic. Add whole leaves and shoots of broccoli rabe. Add salt, stir, cover, and let simmer on medium heat until leaves become limp. Garnish with roasted sunflower seeds and serve at once over cooked pasta of your choice.

BABY CARROTS IN LEMON GHEE ♥
Serves: 6
2 pounds baby carrots
1 tablespoon organic ghee (recipe on pages 150-151)
1/2 lemon, freshly juiced
1 tablespoon corn oil
2 tablespoons fresh lemon thyme, minced
1 teaspoon coriander powder
1 teaspoon rock salt
2 handfuls dandelion leaves, for garnish

Wash the whole baby carrots (trim and discard the stems) and then blanch them for 5 minutes in boiling water. Drain and put in a large bowl, then add the ghee and lemon juice. Heat the corn oil in a small skillet and sauté the lemon thyme for 30 seconds over medium heat. Add the coriander powder and salt. Remove from heat and add to carrots. Toss and serve over a cooked grain of your choice. Garnish with dandelion leaves, if desired.

PEA & NEW POTATO CURRY ♡
Serves: 6
2 cups fresh peas
12 new potatoes
1 tablespoon coriander seeds
1 tablespoon ajwain seeds
1 tablespoon sunflower oil
1 teaspoon turmeric powder
1 teaspoon cumin powder
1/2 teaspoon cardamom powder
2 dried red chilis
1 teaspoon rock salt
1/2 cup water
1/2 cup organic yogurt

Wash peas and set aside. Scrub potatoes and cut into quarters. Dry roast coriander and ajwain seeds for 2 minutes in a large cast-iron skillet over medium heat until golden brown. Remove from heat and crush seeds with a mortar and pestle. Heat the sunflower oil in the same skillet, and add the seeds along with the peas and potatoes. Add the turmeric, cumin, and cardamom powders, along with the chilis and salt. Stir together and simmer for 3 minutes, before adding the water. Cover and simmer on medium heat for 15 minutes until potatoes are very soft. Remove from heat and immediately fold in yogurt. Serve at once over cooked long-grain basmati brown rice.

STRING BEAN, ASPARAGUS & CARROT MÉLANGE ♡
Serves: 6
1 pound string beans
1 pound asparagus spears
1 pound thin carrots
1 cup chickpea flour
1 tablespoon sunflower oil
1 tablespoon yellow mustard seeds
1 teaspoon black pepper, finely ground

I teaspoon rock salt
I cup soy milk
1/2 cup warm water

Wash vegetables, then trim and discard ends. Cut each carrot lengthwise, then in half. Arrange vegetables in a large steamer, with carrots on the bottom, string beans in the middle, and asparagus on top. Place steamer over boiling water and steam for 7 to 8 minutes. Remove from heat, place in a large serving dish, and set aside. Parch chickpea flour in a large cast-iron skillet over medium heat for a few minutes until it begins to turn golden brown. Put the flour in a bowl and set aside. Dust off skillet and heat sunflower oil over medium heat, then roast mustard seeds until they begin to pop. Add black pepper, salt, parched flour, milk, and water. Stir until mixture is smooth. Continue simmering for 3 to 4 minutes until mixture is thick and creamy. Pour the sauce over steamed vegetables, and serve at once over a cooked grain of your choice.

SUBLIME SPINACH MASALA ♡
Serves: 4
2 bunches spinach
I tablespoon organic ghee (recipe on pages 150-151)
I tablespoon Spring Masala (recipe on pages 374)
I teaspoon tamarind paste
1/4 cup warm water
I teaspoon unrefined brown sugar
I teaspoon rock salt

Wash the spinach and trim the stems. Melt ghee in a large skillet, and roast the spring masala for 30 seconds over medium heat until the ghee starts to bubble. Add the wet spinach. Stir, cover, and let simmer for 3 minutes until the leaves turn limp. Dilute the tamarind paste in the warm water, and add to the spinach mixture, along with the brown sugar and salt. Stir, cover, and simmer for 3 minutes more. Serve warm with Lively Steamed Asparagus and Lotus Seeds & Barley (recipes on pages 125, 122).

POLE BEANS IN ALMOND SAUCE ♡
Serves: 6
2 pounds pole beans
I tablespoon sunflower oil
1/4 cup slivered almonds
I teaspoon cayenne powder
I teaspoon rock salt
2 tablespoons almond butter

1/4 cup warm water

1 tablespoon curry powder (recipe on page 134)

1/4 cup chopped scallions, for garnish

Wash pole beans, and remove ends and strings. Cut each diagonally into 2 pieces. Blanch beans in boiling water for 5 minutes. Drain and set aside. Heat sunflower oil in a large skillet, and roast almonds for a few minutes over medium heat until golden brown. Add cayenne powder and salt. Dilute almond butter in warm water, then combine it with the seasoned almonds. Add curry powder and stir until mixture begins to bubble. Pour the curry-almond sauce over the pole beans. Garnish with scallions and serve over soft cooked millet.

KALYANI'S GREEN FEAST ♡

Serves: 6

1 bunch broad leaf mustard

1 bunch spinach

1 tablespoon corn oil

12 white baby onions, peeled

1/2 teaspoon black pepper, finely ground

1 pinch rock salt

Wash greens and trim off stems. Do not dry them. Heat corn oil in a large skillet and add the onions. Sauté onions on high heat for 3 minutes until they become slightly braised. Then add wet greens. Cover and simmer on medium heat for 3 minutes until greens become limp. Season with pepper and salt, and serve over cooked quinoa.

NEW POTATOES & FRESH FENNEL ♡

Serves: 6

16 new potatoes

2 medium fennel bulbs

3 tablespoons corn oil

4 sprigs fresh rosemary

1 tablespoon fresh marjoram, minced

1 teaspoon cumin powder

1 teaspoon rock salt

1/4 cup water

1/4 cup fresh fennel herb, minced

Scrub potatoes and cut into thin slices. Wash fennel bulbs, cut into matchsticks, and set aside. Heat corn oil in a large skillet on medium heat. Slightly bruise rosemary with your fingers and add to the oil along with the marjoram. Sauté for 30 seconds, and add the cumin powder and salt. Add potatoes and fennel sticks, stir, and simmer for 3 minutes until fennel sticks begin to turn slightly brown. Add the water, stir, cover, and simmer on medium heat for 8 minutes until potatoes are tender. Serve warm over bulgur, garnished with fresh fennel herb.

SPINACH & MUNG MASALA ♥

Serves: 6

2 bunches spinach
1 tablespoon organic ghee (recipe on ages 150-151)
1 tablespoon Wise Earth Garam Masala (recipe on page 373)
2 cups Sprouted Mung Beans (recipe on page 118)
1 teaspoon tamarind paste
1/4 cup warm water
1 tablespoon maple syrup
1 teaspoon rock salt

Wash spinach, and trim and discard stems. Do not dry. Melt ghee in a large skillet, and roast Garam Masala for 30 seconds over medium heat until ghee starts to bubble. Add wet spinach and mung bean sprouts. Stir, cover, and let simmer for 3 minutes until leaves turn limp. Dilute tamarind paste in the warm water, and add to spinach mixture along with maple syrup and salt. Stir, cover, and simmer for 3 minutes more. Serve warm over a cooked grain of your choice.

MARINATED SNOW PEAS & TOFU ♥

Serves: 6

1 pound snow peas
2 pounds semi-firm tofu
3 tablespoons tamari
1 1/2 cups hot water
1 lemon, freshly juiced
1 tablespoon fresh ginger, grated
2 scallions, chopped
2 tablespoons cashew butter
1/2 teaspoon turmeric powder
1 teaspoon coriander powder
1 small bunch dandelion greens, for garnish

Wash snow peas, and cut tofu into 1-inch cubes. Blanch both in boiling water for 5 minutes, drain, and set aside. In a large bowl, combine tamari, hot water, lemon juice, ginger, scallions, cashew butter, and spice powders. Stir until cashew butter is dissolved. Add blanched snow peas and tofu to the seasoned tamari sauce. Cover and let marinate for 2 hours. Pour mixture into a large saucepan, and simmer on medium heat for about 7 minutes. Serve over long-grain brown rice, garnished with dandelion greens.

ZESTY ZUCCHINI FRITTERS ♡

Serves: 6

8 zucchini

1/4 cup soy flour

1/4 cup chickpea flour

1 tablespoon coriander powder

1 teaspoon cumin powder

1/2 teaspoon mustard powder

1 teaspoon kudzu powder

1/2 teaspoon black pepper, finely ground

1 teaspoon rock salt

1/2 cup water

1/4 cup corn oil

Wash zucchini and cut diagonally into thin slices. Set aside. In a large bowl, combine flours, spice powders, pepper, salt, and water. Mix into a thick batter. Dip zucchini slices into the batter, coating each slice well. Heat corn oil in a large skillet over medium heat. Carefully lay slices in a single layer and fry for 3 minutes until slices are browned. Use a flat ladle to turn slices, and brown for about another 3 minutes. Remove from heat, and repeat the procedure until all zucchini have been cooked. Serve warm over cooked Basmati & Wild Rice (recipe on page 120).

STRING BEAN & COCONUT STEW ♡

Serves: 6

1 pound red runner beans

1/2 pound string beans

1 cup water

1/2 cup red lentils

1/2 cup fresh coconut, grated (if unavailable, substitute with dried coconut)

1/2 cup fresh coconut milk

1 tablespoon coconut oil

1 tablespoon brown mustard seeds

1 tablespoon cumin seeds

1 teaspoon coriander powder

2 mild green chilis, minced

1 teaspoon rock salt

1 small bunch fresh cilantro, minced

Wash beans and remove the strings. Cut diagonally into 1-inch pieces. Set aside. Bring water to a boil in a large saucepan. Wash lentils and add to water. Cover and simmer on medium heat for 5 minutes. Add the beans, coconut, and coconut milk, and continue simmering. Heat coconut oil in a separate skillet over medium heat, and roast spice seeds until the mustard seeds begin to pop. Add to the bean and coconut mixture, along with chilis and salt. Stir, cover, and simmer for 10 minutes more until the stew thickens. Add cilantro and remove from heat. Cover and let stand for 5 minutes, then serve with a cooked grain of your choice.

SAUTÉED SPRING GREENS ♥
Serves: 6

1 small bunch dandelion

1 small bunch escarole

1 small bunch chicory

2 tablespoons corn oil

1/4 cup sesame seeds

1/2 lemon, freshly juiced

1 pinch rock salt

Wash greens, then trim and discard stems. Heat corn oil in a large skillet over medium heat and roast sesame seeds for 30 seconds, before adding the wet greens. Sauté for about 2 minutes until greens turn limp. Remove from heat. Add lemon juice and salt. Serve as a side dish.

SCINTILLATING SOUPS

CREAMY ASPARAGUS SOUP ♥
Serves: 6

1/2 gallon water

1/4 cup soy flour

2 tablespoons sunflower oil

1 teaspoon black pepper, finely ground

1 teaspoon coriander powder

1/2 teaspoon cayenne pepper

1/2 teaspoon turmeric powder

2 green onions, chopped

1 tablespoon rock salt

12 asparagus spears

1 quart soy milk

Pour water into a large soup pot. Dissolve soy flour into water and bring to a boil. Heat sunflower oil in a small skillet and roast the spice powders for 15 seconds over medium heat. Then add spice mixture to the soup by stirring the soup pot with the small skillet (if possible). Add green onions and salt. Cover and simmer on medium heat for 5 minutes. Wash and trim asparagus spears, diagonally cutting each into 3 pieces. Add to the broth, along with the soy milk. Cover and continue simmering for 5 minutes more. Serve at once.

HEALING GINGER & SCALLION SOUP

Serves: 6

1 1/4 gallons water

1/4 cup quinoa

1/2 cup oat bran

3 tablespoons fresh, minced ginger

1 clove of garlic, crushed

1 teaspoon white pepper, finely ground

1 tablespoon rock salt

6 scallions, chopped

1 tablespoon organic ghee (recipe on pages 150-151)

1 bunch watercress, for garnish

Bring water to a boil in a large heavy-bottomed soup pot. Add quinoa, oat bran, ginger, garlic, white pepper, and salt. Stir, cover, and simmer on medium-low heat for 25 minutes. Add scallions and ghee, and continue to simmer for 10 minutes. Serve at once over a handful of cooked noodles. Garnish with sprigs of watercress.

CURRY YOGURT SOUP ♥

Serves: 6

1 gallon water

2 tablespoons curry powder (recipe on page 134)

1 tablespoon rock salt

1 tablespoon sunflower oil

1 tablespoon yellow mustard seeds

1 tablespoon cumin seeds

1 quart organic yogurt

3 handfuls of land cress, for garnish

Bring water to a boil in a large soup pot. Add curry powder and salt. Heat sunflower oil in a small skillet and roast the spice seeds over medium heat until the mustard seeds begin to pop. Add to the soup water by stirring the soup with the small skillet (if possible). Fold in yogurt, stirring frequently to prevent it from curdling. Wash the land cress, tear into bite-size pieces, and add to the soup. Remove from heat, cover, and let stand for 5 minutes before serving. Serve each bowl with a handful of bijun noodles that turn translucent when cooked.

TAMARIND CURRY SOUP
Serves: 6

1 1/2 gallons water

1/2 cup barley

1/2 cup millet

1/2 cup green lentils

4 large potatoes

1 large yellow onion, chopped

1 tablespoon curry powder (recipe follows)

1 tablespoon coriander powder

1 teaspoon cumin seeds

1 teaspoon black mustard seeds

1 tablespoon tamarind paste

1 tablespoon dried parsley

1 teaspoon fresh ginger, minced

1 tablespoon rock salt

1 tablespoon organic ghee (recipe on pages 150-151)

Bring water to a boil in a large heavy-bottomed soup pot. Wash grains and lentils and add to boiling water. Wash and peel potatoes and cut into quarters. Add to soup, along with onion, curry and coriander powders, cumin and mustard seeds, tamarind paste, parsley, ginger, and salt. Stir, cover, and let boil over medium heat for 4 minutes. Add ghee, cover, and simmer on low heat for 10 minutes more. Serve at once.

CURRY POWDER ♡
1 teaspoon chana dhal (yellow split peas)

1 teaspoon urad dhal (Indian black lentils)

1/2 teaspoon fenugreek seeds

1/2 teaspoon cumin seeds

1/2 teaspoon coriander seeds

8 dried whole red chilis, or to taste

7 whole black peppercorns, or to taste

1 teaspoon mustard seeds

1 teaspoon ground turmeric

2 pinches asafetida powder

Combine the chana and urad dhals, fenugreek seeds, cumin seeds, coriander seeds, red chilis, black peppercorns, and mustard seeds in a small cast-iron skillet over medium heat. Stir with a wooden ladle until lightly browned, for about 5 minutes. Remove from heat and allow to cool. Mix in the turmeric and asafetida powders and transfer the mixture into a hand grinder or spice mill. Grind into a fine powder and store in an airtight jar.

GARLIC BROCCOLI SOUP ♡

Serves: 6

1 1/4 gallons water

1/2 cup split mung beans

1 bunch broccoli

1 tablespoon olive oil

4 cloves garlic, crushed

1 tablespoon coriander seeds, crushed

1 teaspoon black pepper, coarsely ground

3 tablespoons barley miso

1/4 cup warm water

Bitter spring greens, for garnish

Bring water to a boil in a large heavy-bottomed soup pot. Wash mung beans and add to the boiling water. Wash broccoli, trim the stems, and cut into bite-size pieces. Add to the soup water. Heat olive oil in a small skillet and lightly roast the crushed garlic, coriander, and black pepper for 15 seconds over medium heat. Add garlic-spice mixture to the soup by stirring it with the small skillet until the spices have combined with the liquid (if possible). Cover and simmer for 30 minutes on medium heat. Dilute miso in warm water, and stir into the soup. Continue simmering for 5 minutes more. Garnish with bitter spring greens of your choice and serve at once.

SWEET MUNG BEAN SOUP ♡

Serves: 6

1 gallon water

2 cups mung beans, split

1 tablespoon rock salt

1 teaspoon turmeric powder

1 teaspoon cardamom powder

1 tablespoon sunflower oil

1 tablespoon cumin seeds

2 tablespoons unrefined brown sugar

1 small bunch fresh cilantro, for garnish

Bring water to a boil in a large soup pot. Wash mung beans, and add to the water, along with salt, turmeric, and cardamom powder. Cover and let simmer on medium heat for 20 minutes. Heat sunflower oil in a small skillet and roast the cumin seeds for about 1 minute over medium heat until golden brown. Then add the spice mixture to the soup pot by stirring the soup with the small skillet (if possible). Add the brown sugar, stir, and simmer for 5 minutes more. Garnish with fresh cilantro and serve at once.

TOFU & PEA SOUP

Serves: 6

1 1/4 gallons water

1 tablespoon corn oil

2 pounds soft tofu

1 tablespoon fresh ginger, minced

1/2 teaspoon cayenne pepper

1 cup fresh peas

1 cup carrots, finely cubed

3 tablespoons barley miso

1/4 cup warm water

4 scallions, chopped

Soft-cooked brown rice, for garnish

Bring water to a boil in a large heavy-bottomed soup pot. Heat corn oil in a large skillet over medium heat. Crumble the tofu and lightly sauté it for about 3 minutes, seasoning it with the ginger and cayenne pepper. Add to boiling water, along with the peas and carrots. Cover and simmer on medium heat for 20 minutes until carrots are very tender. Dilute the miso in warm water and stir into the soup. Cover and simmer for 10 minutes more. Garnish with scallions and serve at once with a dollop of soft-cooked brown rice.

DELICATE DESSERTS

VEDIC ROSE PUDDING CAKE

Serves: 8

1 tablespoon sunflower oil

1 1/2 cups Cream of Wheat

1/2 cup spelt flour

1 cup cow's milk (organic)

1/2 cup rosewater

1/4 cup dates

1/4 cup dried cherries

1/4 cup raisins

1/4 cup Sucanat

1 teaspoon cardamom powder

1/2 teaspoon ground nutmeg

1/2 teaspoon turmeric powder

1 handful dried, organic rose petals for garnish

Preheat oven to 350 degrees. Oil a shallow baking dish using sunflower oil and set aside. Sift Cream of Wheat and flour into a mixing bowl, and add the milk and rosewater. Mix into a smooth batter. Remove pits from dates and cherries, then cut into tiny pieces and add to the batter, along with raisins. Stir in Sucanat and spice powders, and pour batter into prepared baking dish. Bake for 15 minutes until the pudding cake is barely set and the top is golden brown. Spoon out the pudding cake into dessert bowls, and garnish with a few rose petals.

COCONUT CUSTARD ♥

Serves: 4

1 pint almond milk

2 tablespoons Sucanat

1 cup fresh coconut, finely shredded (if fresh coconut is unavailable, substitute with dried coconut)

1/2 teaspoon natural almond extract

1 tablespoon kudzu powder

1/4 cup cold water

Bring almond milk to a boil in a small saucepan over medium-high heat. Add Sucanat, fresh coconut, and almond extract. Cover and simmer on low heat for 5-7 minutes. Dilute kudzu powder in the cold water, then add to the coconut mixture. Stir until the custard thickens. Serve warm.

MELON & MANGO SLICES ♥

Serves: 4

1 small honeydew melon

1 large ripe mango

1 lemon, freshly juiced

1 pinch unrefined brown sugar

Cut melon in half, core, and peel. Cut evenly into 1/2-inch slices, and set aside. Slice mango in half, avoiding its large seed. Peel halves and slice them. Arrange the melon and mango slices on a dessert platter, sprinkle with lemon juice and sugar, then serve.

ALMOND LIME SQUARES

Serves: 4

2 cups barley flour

1/4 cup unrefined brown sugar

2 tablespoons organic ghee (recipe on pages 150-151

1/2 teaspoon rock salt

1/4 cup warm water

1/4 cup toasted almonds, finely crushed

2 limes, freshly juiced

2 tablespoons lime zest

1 tablespoon sunflower oil

Preheat oven to 350 degrees. In a large bowl, combine flour, sugar, ghee, and salt. Add the warm water, crushed almonds, lime juice and zest, then mix into a thick batter. Lightly oil a small square baking dish with sunflower oil and pour batter into it. Bake for 20 minutes, or until a fork inserted comes out clean. Serve warm.

GLAZED STRAWBERRIES ♥

Serves: 4

1 pint strawberries

3 tablespoons sugarless strawberry jam

1 orange, freshly juiced

1 tablespoon orange zest

1 tablespoon honey

Wash strawberries, cut into halves, and set aside. Combine jam, orange juice, orange zest, and honey in a small bowl. Whip together and pour over strawberries. Serve at once.

LIVELY LIBATIONS

SWEET LASSI ♡

Serves: 4

Lassi is a traditional North Indian spiced yogurt drink used as a digestive aid after meals.

I pint organic yogurt

I cup almond milk

2 cups warm water

1/4 cup unrefined brown sugar

I teaspoon cardamom powder

1/2 teaspoon clove powder

1/2 teaspoon rock salt

Fresh mint, for garnish

Blend all ingredients except mint in a large bowl, and whisk with an egg beater until the lassi becomes smooth and frothy. Garnish with mint and serve in large cups.

VIOLET TEA ♡

Serves: 4

I quart water

2 tablespoons dried organic violet leaves

I tablespoon Sucanat

Bring water to a boil in a medium size saucepan. Add violet leaves, then remove from heat. Cover and let steep for 7 minutes. Strain the infusion, retaining the roughage to use in your bath water. Add sugar and serve at once.

HEALING BARLEY BREW

Serves: 8

I gallon water

I cup pearled barley

I teaspoon cinnamon powder

1/2 teaspoon clove powder

1/2 teaspoon black pepper, finely ground

I teaspoon bala powder

2 tablespoons unrefined brown sugar

Bring water to a boil in a large saucepan. Wash barley and add to the boiling water, along with the spice powders, pepper, bala, and brown sugar. Cover and simmer on medium heat for 45 minutes until the barley is very soft and the water is thick. Strain the decoction, retaining barley for other use. Serve at once. (To make a tea-porridge, puree the cooked barley in a hand grinder and combine with the liquid.)

LICORICE SPICED TEA ♡

Serves: 4

1 quart water
1 tablespoon dried licorice roots
7 whole cloves
1 teaspoon cinnamon powder
2 tablespoons honey

Bring water to a boil in a medium-size saucepan. Add licorice roots, cloves, and cinnamon powder. Cover and simmer on low heat for 5 minutes. Strain the decoction, and retain the roughage to use in your bath water. Add honey and serve at once.

JAYADEVI'S SPICED TEA ♡

Serves: 4

1 pint water
1 pint soy milk
1/2 teaspoon black pepper
1/2 teaspoon turmeric powder
1 tablespoon orange zest

Bring water and soy milk to a boil in a medium-size saucepan. Add black pepper, turmeric powder, and orange zest. Cover and simmer on low heat for 5 minutes. Strain the decoction and retain the roughage to use in your bath water. Serve at once.

CINNAMON MINT TEA ♡

Serves: 4

4 cups water
2 cinnamon sticks
12 fresh mint leaves
1/2 teaspoon cinnamon powder
1 tablespoon Sucanat

Bring water to a boil in a medium-size saucepan. Add cinnamon sticks and boil for 10 minutes. Remove from heat; add mint leaves, cinnamon powder, and Sucanat. Cover and steep for 5 minutes before serving. Cinnamon sticks may be removed from tea before serving and retained for other use.

GINGER & RED CLOVER TEA ♡
Serves: 4

1 quart water
1 tablespoon fresh ginger, minced
1 tablespoon dried red clover buds
1/2 lemon, freshly juiced

Bring water to a boil in a medium-size saucepan. Add ginger and red clover. Remove from heat. Cover and let steep for 5 minutes. Strain the infusion, retaining the roughage for your bath water. Add lemon juice and serve at once.

HONEY NUT TEA ♡
Serves: 4

1 pint water
1 pint almond milk
1/4 cup walnuts, pureed
1/2 teaspoon cardamom powder
2 tablespoons honey

Bring water and almond milk to a boil in a medium-size saucepan. Add pureed walnuts and cardamom powder, and simmer on low heat for 3 minutes. Remove from heat, add honey, and serve.

FROTHY CHICORY TEA ♡
Serves: 4

1 pint soy milk
1 pint water
2 tablespoons chicory powder
1 teaspoon cardamom powder
1 teaspoon dried orange peel
5 drops of natural walnut extract

Bring soy milk and water to a boil in a medium-size saucepan. Add the chicory powder, cardamom powder, and orange peel. Cover and simmer on low heat for 7 minutes. Add the walnut extract, and remove from heat. Using a whisk, whip the milky mixture until it is frothy. Serve at once, retaining the orange peel.

ALLSPICE & ALMOND TEA ♡

Serves: 4

1 quart water

1 teaspoon allspice powder

8 drops natural almond extract

1 tablespoon honey

Bring water to a boil in a medium-size saucepan. Add the powder and extract. Remove from heat, cover and let steep for 5 minutes. Stir in honey and serve.

Part Three

SUMMER

I take The Vow of Ahimsa

In my thoughts, speech, and actions

Chapter Ten

SUMMER AHIMSA PRACTICES FOR CELEBRATING SPIRIT

Pitiless heat from heaven pours
By day, but nights are cool;
Continuous bathing gently lowers
The water in the pool;
The evening brings a charming peace:
For summer time is here.
When love that never knows surcease,
Is less imperious, dear.

— Kalidasa

In the Vedic Calendar, the summer months occur in May-July, *Jyeshtha-Shravana* (in the Northern Hemisphere). Summer is a time for happiness, abundance, and celebration. Trees are laden with fruits, nature's bountiful sustenance. Vegetables and herbs are filling out the garden. Tall grasses grace the meadows, and animals take smart reprieve out of the midday sun. Children can be found playing outdoors in bare feet. Naturally, we experience fullness, fulfillment, and leisure. Considered a drying and heating season, energy can be quick to desist unless we follow the rhythms of this prolific and energy-bearing time. Cultures throughout the world celebrate summer by venerating the solar deities, celebrating the bountiful crops, feasting outdoors, and generally honoring their spiritual reunion with the earth.

Summer is a season of fire. The fire element is honored at summer's solstice, the day that marks the point at which the earth has moved halfway around the sun in her annual voyage. Days will now begin to get shorter, and the weather grows milder. Mid-summer, as this time of year is called, is the most prolific time to harvest herbs. In England, the Druids gathered on this day for a sunrise ceremony to pay homage to the solstice. Many cultures throughout the world celebrate the summer season in veneration to the sun. Hindus worship Surya (deity of the sun) and perform fire rituals with pine kindling, dried cow dung, camphor, and ghee to honor the deities. Taking place throughout the summer months, ritual and festival fires blaze the countryside. Native American people use the smudge stick, made with dried summer flowers and herbs such as sage, lavender, basil, and rosemary, to nourish the fire. Summer is also the season of merriment. June marks the month of marriage in many European cultures. The Greeks shower the couple with nuts

and sweets for prosperity and fertility. The Romans decorate the couple with garlands of roses, elderflowers, and magnolias for love and fidelity.

BALANCING THE ENERGY OF SUMMER

To achieve a sense of balance, cooling activities are sought to lessen the heat of the
season. Bathing festivals are a prominent part of the Vedic culture. For example,
Snanam Yatra is an auspicious bathing festival occurring in the summer. On the first
full moon of summer, millions of Hindus join this grand celebration in Crissag with
the recitation of Vedic mantras. One hundred and eight pots of consecrated water
are poured on the forms of the deities that preside over this occasion. After the bath,
the deities are dressed in ceremonial cloth and are retired in seclusion for 15 days.

This season is active, mobile, and mostly lived outdoors. It provides you with
endless chances to cultivate a life of inner harmony—ahimsa—and to ward off
heated emotions and anxieties inherent with living in overdrive. When we take
care to cross over this season's rhythms with mindfulness, we find plentiful energy
to celebrate the abundance and richness of summer that surrounds us. On the other
hand, when we are out of balance with seasonal rhythms, we may find ourselves
listless, lethargic, and exhausted from the heat of summer. To prevent dehydra-
tion, drink plenty of water. If your fire humor, Pitta, is not well cared for during the
spring season, it will manifest through a variety of heat related conditions causing
general Pitta symptoms such as weak digestion, fevers, skin disorders, bile accumulation, sunstroke, irritability, and listlessness.

Cooling reprieve is the mantra for the summer. This is a wonderful time for
rejuvenating baths, swimming and wading, and taking "moon baths" by sitting in
the moonlight to assuage mind and spirit with Goddess Lalita's cooling rays. Surround yourself with fragrant scents from flowers and pure essential oils, and wear
light, natural fibers and light comfortable clothing. Observe the two days of fasting
or semi-fasting each month on the Ekadashi days. To strengthen digestion take
light meals with fresh salads; eat chapati with light grains such as cracked wheat,
bulgur, and basmati rice; and have sprouted beans and *dhals* (bean dishes) made
with mung, kidney, lentil, and soybeans. Eat plenty of fruits: figs, grapes, mangoes,
melons, peaches, and pomegranates. Steam or lightly cook your vegetables. Beets,
broccoli, cauliflower, celery, kohlrabi, okra, radishes, snow peas, string beans,
sugar snap peas, summer squash, sweet corn, sweet peppers, and Swiss chard
are a few of the prolific variety of garden fresh foods available to you during the
summer. Avoid heavy meals, pungent or excessively spiced meals, and intoxicants
during this season. Lessen cohabitation, and instead, increase the innocent play of
kindness, romance, and flirtation with your partner. Take the occasional afternoon
siesta during hot days. Follow the rhythms of summer and you will recover your
feelings of playfulness, joy, and abundance.

THE ENERGY OF SUMMER				
PRIMARY ACTIVITY	PREDOMINANT TASTE	PREDOMINANT ELEMENTS	TIME OF YEAR	DOSHIC NATURE
Celebration	Pungent	Air and Fire	Mid to late-May through mid to late-July (Northern Hemisphere)	Pitta and Vata
			Mid to late-November through mid to late-January (Southern Hemisphere)	

Table 10.1

CELEBRATING SPIRIT

Sacred Water—Sacred Bath

Make a cooling bath a daily activity for rejuvenating the body, mind, and spirit. Approach your summer bath as an act of ahimsa for the well-being of you and your family. Follow in the wise ways of my tradition by regarding every drop of water as a sacred means to evoke nourishment and nurturance. Note on your calendar the tenth day of the first waxing moon of summer occurring around mid-May in the Northern Hemisphere, or mid-November in the Southern Hemisphere. This is an auspicious time of the summer when millions of Hindu people celebrate the festival of *Ganga Dusshera* by taking early morning dips in the sacred Ganges River. They do so to wash away despair, tiredness, negative emotions and experiences, disease, and misfortune. They recognize that the sacred river is everywhere, in every continent and culture, in your streams, rivers, lakes, and in your bath. Indeed, this sublime energy lies within you waiting to be invoked through the act of informed practice.

In Vedic history, the river Ganges is said to have descended on earth on this lunar day. High up in the snow-clad Himalayas, the river emerges at Gangotri, cascading down massive boulders to grace the plains of Northern India until she finally meets the sea in the Bay of Bengal. At Allahabad, the Ganga merges with the river Yamuna and the mythical river Saraswati. The confluence of these rivers, known as Prayag, is considered one of the most powerful sacred junctures on earth.

As the lore goes, to transform its cosmic force and make it gentle for the nourishment of humanity, the god Brahma (the Creator) and the god Vishnu (the Sustainer) asked Shiva (the Cosmic Dissolver) to contain and tame the force of the Mother River within his matted locks. He did so by transforming her wild powers for the benefit of humanity. Henceforth, on the tenth day of the first waxing moon of summer, the festival of Ganga Dusshera is observed. For 10 days, people bathe, pray, and make offerings to the sacred river. They take a handful of river clay to remember her, or take her sacred water sealed in brass containers for use in ceremonies to bless the home and family and to use in the final sacrament of life. At twilight every day in Haridwar, thousands of ghee lamps can be seen floating downstream in the Mother River, placed there by eager devotees who meditate on the goddess to manifest her great power. The Mother River holds a significant place in the consciousness of our humanity.

As you endeavor to make your summer dip into a sacred bath, hold this Living Ahimsa affirmation in your mind:

- I recognize the sanctity of water.
- I bathe not only the physical body, but also the mind and spirit.
- I honor my ancestors.
- May the water element within me be strong and stable.

THE PRACTICE: FULL MOON BATH

OPTIMUM TIMING: Early morning or early evening, or on the full moon day.
- **Northern Hemisphere:** On the 10th day of the waxing moon cycle in mid-May.
- **Southern Hemisphere:** On the 10th day of the waxing moon cycle in mid-November.

Full Moon Herbs & Essential Oils:
Use only organic, soothing dried herbs and essential oils for your Full Moon Bath: elderflowers, hops, lavender, lemon balm, lemon verbena, passionflower, raspberry leaves, rose petals, and violet flowers. If available, you may use fresh seasonal herbs as well. If using loose herbs without a bolus, be certain to use a drain strainer to collect the roughage at the end of your bath. This may be placed on the earth or in your compost. Do not throw these herbs into the garbage.

Sample Recipe:
1 cotton handkerchief
1/2 palmful of rose petals
1/2 palmful of raspberry leaves
12 drops of lavender essential oil

INSTRUCTIONS:

1. First, prepare your herbal bolus by taking a palmful of herbs sprinkled with a few drops of essential oil and wrapping them into a bolus in a cotton handkerchief. To make your herbal ball, tie 2 of the opposite ends of the cloth and then overlap the other 2 ends into a firm knot incorporating all 4 ends into a secure knot on the top of the bolus.

2. Fill your bath with warm water and place the bolus of herbs directly in the bath.

3. Allow it to sit for 5 minutes or so in the water before offering your prayers and entering the bath.

4. After the tub is filled and you have placed the sacred herbs and ingredients into the water, make an offering to the Ganga—the river goddess—before you enter the bath. While facing east or north, scoop a palmful of water with your right hand and ritually wash both of your hands with the water, letting it fall back into the tub. Take another palmful of water in your right hand and this time offer it to the goddess by slowly opening your hand and allowing the water to drip from the tips of your fingers back into the tub.

5. Recite the following mantra 3 times as you pour the water from your hand:

    Om Apah Upa Sprishya Ganga Mata
    (Pronounced: OOM AAPAH UPAH SPRISH-YA GANGA MAA-TAA)

    Onto You, Goddess of the River, I sprinkle water

6. Once this offering has been completed, take your bath. It is important that you complete the bath without interruption once you have offered the water sacrament to Ganga. The act of preparing your tub, ritual washing of the hands, offering of water to the goddess, and finishing your bath must be done in one fluid and complete act for your offering to be received by the goddess and for her water blessings to be returned to you.

SUMMER'S LIGHT FOOD PRACTICES

As the summer sun casts its brilliant glow across the universal plain to feed, nourish, and make abundant life's sustenance and happiness, you can emulate its light by invoking the serene light of awareness within—a sense of inner harmony that can only be illumined by the fire of consciousness. You will discover that in Living Ahimsa, all activities you perform—particularly food practices—evoke personal awareness. This inspired awareness occurs once you enter the sanctuary of the heart. In the *Sama Veda* it is said, "The self resides in the lotus of the heart. Knowing this, consecrated to the self, the seer enters daily that sacred sanctuary. Absorbed in the self, the seer is freed from identification with the body and emerges in pure consciousness."

The following meditative Living Ahimsa practice of making ghee from organic sweet butter is more than a metaphor for harvesting the golden light of peace within. Ayurveda considers milk to be the first and most complete food on earth. Milk was traditionally collected well after the delivery of the cow's calf so that it could be properly digested by the human system. From this peace-generating food comes buttermilk, butter, yogurt, and ghee. Milk is part of a peaceful repast only when its quality remains pure and unadulterated. In the practice that follows we seek to remember our spirit of kindness and bring greater awareness to the harm inflicted on the innocent animals, the cows. We look to enhance our personal understanding of what it means to subsist within the rule of the Mother Consciousness. As a response, you will find Mother's generous blessing awaiting you at the end of the practice—a full jar of ghee—golden elixir for the betterment of health. The ancient *vaidyas* perfected the making of medicinal ghee for use in Ayurveda medicine.

Prepare your ghee on the full moon day or the day following the full moon. The cow is primarily guided by the energies of the moon, and its milk reflects this luminous, calming energy. The guru would often instruct his disciples to "gather a herd of cows." This was a figurative expression meaning "go and gather your wisdom." The making of ghee will help you acquire a sense of sadhana—the egoless sense of awareness you bring to each practice you endeavor.

THE PRACTICE: FULL MOON GHEE RITUAL

This practice can be done each month during the full moon, the day following the full moon, or if necessary during the waxing moon phase. Engage your ghee-making practice in a healthful way as you bear witness to the awesome revelation of the play of light, aroma, sound, and presence of the Mother's gift of food.

OPTIMUM TIMING:
- Full moon day, the day after the full moon, or during the waxing moon phase.
- On Mother's Day (occurring on the 2nd Sunday in May, almost midway in the first waxing moon cycle of the month).

Ingredients:
- 1 pound organic sweet butter
- Heavy stainless-steel saucepan
- Stainless-steel spoon
- Clean glass jar with lid
- Tea strainer

Prepare the ghee in silence minding its progress by listening to its sounds as it matures through various stages of evolution through the fire. In its earliest stage, the ghee is quiet. Then suddenly, as it begins to foam, it awakens with the gentle sound of sunrays glowing across the kitchen. As the foam descends to the bottom of the pot, you hear the sounds of a gurgling stream rushing to meet the reflections of the sun. At once, enhanced by the energy of the melting gold, you are immersed in a deep sense of quietude. The air is filled with its rich, fragrant aroma. When the golden liquid of the ghee begins to bubble, you can almost hear the rhythmic sound of a water drum as each bubble disappears with an occasional "plop" and dissolves into a lasting silence.

COOKING INSTRUCTIONS:

- Sterilize the saucepan, spoon, and storage jar by immersing them in boiling water.
- Melt the butter in the saucepan over a low flame. Continue to heat until it boils gently and a buff-colored foam rises to the surface. Do not stir or remove the foam.
- Allow the ghee to cook gently until the foam thickens and settles to the bottom of the pan as sediment.
- When the ghee turns a golden color and begins to boil silently, with only a trace of air bubbles on the surface, it is done.
- Once it is cool, pour the liquid into a clean glass jar, making sure that the sediment remains on the bottom of the pan.
- The sediment may be eaten as a delicious snack!

THE PRACTICE: OFFERING LIGHT TO THE DIVINE MOTHER

Every day is sacred and every day is Mother's Day. For thousands of years, Hindus have been celebrating a 10-day festival honoring the Mother Consciousness in the lunar cycles of spring and autumn, as well as on numerous auspicious days in between. The festival of Mother's Day, where you venerate your earthly mother, is an extension of the greater reverence to the Divine Mother; each and every mother thrives on the lightness of being.

OPTIMUM TIMING:

- On Mother's Day (occurring on the 2nd Sunday in May, almost midway in the first waxing moon cycle of the month).
- Full moon day, the day after the full moon, or during the waxing moon phase.

INSTRUCTIONS:

- Having completed the practice of ghee-making, offer it in the form of light to the goddess, in whichever cultural form you perceive her.

- Pour a tablespoon of ghee into a dipa (traditional ghee lamp) before imbibing the ghee.
- Light the ghee lamp and offer it to the Divine Mother by placing it on a dedicated kitchen shelf intended to be your food offering altar (see *The Ahimsa Kitchen* section in chapter six for a description of my own food offering altar) or on a kitchen table facing east.
- Using your right hand, light the ghee-lamp and offer it to the goddess by circling it three times in the eastward direction (intended for the goddess).
- Recite the following affirmation:
O Great Goddess, accept this light which is lit with pure ghee and which reflects the purity of my offering to you.

THE PRACTICE: FULL MOON SUMMER FEAST

The Summer's full moons are wonderful opportunities to invite your friends to join you in making fresh summer ghee and then enjoy the fruits of your labors in a delectable Full Moon Summer Feast. On the full moon day, or the day after, prepare a scrumptious feast for your family and friends. You can create your celebratory carte du jour from the abundant recipes in the next chapter, "Summer's Splendid Bounty."

OPTIMUM TIMING: On the full moon day, or the day after.

Sample Full Moon Summer Feast Menu:
- Summer Cress Salad (p 164)
- Wild Strawberry Soup (p 168)
- Tagliatelle in Cream Sauce (p 166)
- Apple & Blueberry Crumble (p 180)

OFFERING LIGHT TO THE MOTHER:
Prior to imbibing any meal, it is a customary practice to offer the first "taste" of your meal preparations to the Divine Mother.
- Choose a beautiful small bowl dedicated for this purpose.
- Place a few morsels of food in your bowl and offer the food with your right hand while chanting this mantra:

Om Amritamastu Amritopastaranamasi Svaha
(Pronounced: OOM AM-RE-TAH ASTU AM-RE-TOW-PAAS-TARA-NAM-ASI SWAH-HA)

O Goddess Mother, let this food I offer before you be transformed into ambrosia.

THE PRACTICE: SUMMER MOON FAST

Although the summer heralds a time of celebration and ease, we must remember to take advantage of the powerful healing opportunities of this season by observing the Summer Moon Fast on the 4 appropriate Ekadashi days. In the summer season, and particularly when fasting, it is beneficial to start each day with a cooling bath and offer prayers of gratitude to the sun.

OPTIMUM TIMING:*
Northern Hemisphere:
- 11 days following the new moon in May (counting the new moon day).
- 12 days following the full moon in May (not counting the full moon day).
- 11 days following the new moon in June (counting the new moon day).
- 12 days following the full moon in June (not counting the full moon day).

Southern Hemisphere:
- 11 days following the new moon in November (counting the new moon day).
- 12 days following the full moon in November (not counting the full moon day).
- 11 days following the new moon December (counting the new moon day).
- 12 days following the full moon in December (not counting the full moon day).

*I highly recommend purchasing a Vedic Calendar to calculate the exact timing of the new and full moons for Ekadashi calculations.

Contra-indications: Do not fast during severe illness, menstruation, or while bleeding. The elderly and young children should also avoid fasting.

INSTRUCTIONS:
- On the optimum Ekadashi days noted above, begin a 4-day Summer Moon Fast. Ekadashi generally occurs twice monthly and you must seize each and every opportunity to observe at least one Ekadashi fasting day in each month.
- Refer to instructions in The Practice: Observing a Fast on Ekadashi on pages 70-73.

This sacred lunar observance is practiced to reclaim your state of inner balance with cyclical rhythms, reclaiming your grace with nature, and thereby healing and nullifying personal health and familial challenges. This fortnight of practice is aligned with the waxing and waning tempo of the moon. (Remember, if you are unable to complete a full fast try to observe a modified Semi-Fast, detailed on pages 73-77.)

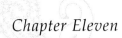

Chapter Eleven

SUMMER'S SPLENDID BOUNTY

Summer is a wonderful time for enjoying nature's abundant foods and harnessing their cooling energies to maintain balance during the solar activities of this season. Your summer menu has plenty of colorful provisions for your nourishment: from light and cooling reprieves to scrumptious and titillating Living Ahimsa feasts with grapes, melons, peaches, mangoes, figs, pomegranates, squashes, snow peas, sweet corn, couscous, and bulgur! Summer is your chance to learn the exquisite art of rolling out Indian flatbreads and dunking them into the blissfully golden nourishment of summer dhals. Divine meals like Mango & Fennel Soup or Barley & Mint Salad, topped off with a Raspberry, Rose Petal & Saffron Cream, will thrill your taste buds while strengthening your deepest sense of nurturance.

SUMMER MENU PLANNING

The Summer Season:
- Northern Hemisphere: Mid-to-late May through mid-to-late July.
- Southern Hemisphere: Mid-to-late November through mid-to-late January.

Vulnerable Time: For Pitta Types*
- Avoid excessively pungent foods like hot peppers, garlic, oily or fatty foods, complex food combinations, and intoxicants.
- * To learn your body type, see appendix one, "Wise Earth Ayurveda Body Types."

SUMMER MENU: DO's & DON'T's	
APPROPRIATE FOODS FOR SUMMER	**FOODS TO AVOID IN SUMMER**
Cool, light, fresh, moist, and fragrant foods	Hot, heavy, stale, oily, and dry foods; intoxicants
Seasonal fruits, vegetables, herbs, beans; and light grains such as bulgur, cracked wheat, chapati, basmati rice, arborio rice, and whole grain pasta	Animal flesh products: meats, fowl, fish, and eggs

Table 11.1

SAMPLE SUMMER MENU

Summer Breakfast:
- Kapha: Breakfast is not recommended.
- Pitta and Vata: See appendix three, "Breakfast of Champions," for a wide array of breakfast choices that can be enjoyed throughout the year.

Summer Lunch:
- Cucumber Raita with Yogurt & Dill (p 161)
- Summer Squash & Couscous Salad (below)
- Mango Lime Decadence (p 180)

Summer Dinner:
- Lentil & Coconut Dhal (p 173)
- Dill & Scallion Chapati (p 177)
- Savory Mango Chutney (p 179)
- Raspberry, Rose Petal & Saffron Cream (p 182)

Gluten-free recipes are indicated by ♥

AMAZING GRAINS

SUMMER SQUASH & COUSCOUS SALAD
Serves: 4

2 cups water
1 cup couscous
1/2 teaspoon rock salt
4 summer squash
3 sun-dried tomatoes
1 tablespoon sunflower oil
1 teaspoon coriander powder
1/2 teaspoon turmeric powder
4 sprigs fresh rosemary, bruised

Bring water to a boil in a large saucepan. Carefully introduce the couscous, stirring frequently to keep it from getting lumpy. Add salt, cover, and simmer over medium heat for 10 minutes until cooked through. Immediately remove the cooked couscous, pour into a colander, and run cold water through it to keep grain from sticking. Wash the squash, then thinly slice on a slant. Slice the sun-dried tomatoes into thin strips. Heat the sunflower oil in a large skillet over medium heat and sauté the squash and tomatoes. Add the spice powders along with a sprinkle of water. Cover and cook for 3 minutes until the tomatoes are flexible. Fold couscous into the vegetables and remove from heat. Allow to cool completely, then garnish with rosemary and serve.

ZUCCHINI POLENTA SALAD ♡

Serves: 4

3 cups water
1 cup polenta
1 pinch rock salt
3 zucchini
1 tablespoon sunflower oil
2 tablespoons fresh parsley, minced

Bring water to a boil in a large saucepan. Carefully introduce polenta, stirring frequently to prevent it from getting lumpy. Add salt and cook over low heat for 20 minutes. Pour cooked polenta into a rectangular pan and allow to cool, then cut into 1-inch squares. Wash and thinly slice zucchini, cutting it on a slant. Heat sunflower oil to medium-high heat in a large skillet and quickly pan fry zucchini for a few minutes until browned on each side. Combine polenta squares and fried zucchini. Garnish with parsley and serve immediately.

BARLEY MINT SALAD

Serves: 4

3 1/2 cups water
1 cup pearled barley
1 ear fresh corn
1 tablespoon walnut oil
1 teaspoon cumin seeds
1/2 teaspoon ajwain seeds
1 teaspoon coriander powder
1 teaspoon rock salt
1/2 lemon, freshly juiced
1/4 cup fresh mint, coarsely chopped
1/4 cup fresh dill, coarsely chopped
1 tablespoon organic yogurt
1 cucumber
1 head of oak leaf lettuce

Bring water to a boil in a medium-size saucepan. Wash barley and add to boiling water. Cover and boil over medium heat for 30 minutes. Strain barley, but retain the cooking water. Bring this water to a boil in a separate saucepan. Husk corn and use a paring knife to remove corn from the cob. Blanch the corn in boiling water for 3 minutes; strain and retain the corn water. Heat walnut oil in a large skillet and lightly roast the cumin and ajwain seeds over medium heat until they turn a dark golden color. Stir in coriander powder and salt, then add the lemon juice. Turn off heat and blend in fresh mint and dill. Pour the corn water into skillet, add yogurt, and whisk mixture gently to mix the dressing.

CILANTRO & LIME BULGUR
Serves: 4

4 cups water
I cup bulgur
I cup fresh peas
I cup carrots, diced
I cup radicchio, finely chopped
1/4 cup cilantro, finely minced
I teaspoon dried tarragon
I tablespoon sunflower oil
1/2 lime, freshly juiced
10 strands saffron
1/2 teaspoon rock salt

Bring 3 cups of water to a boil. Add bulgur, cover, and cook over medium heat for 10 minutes until bulgur is firmly cooked. Remove from heat and pour into a colander. Pour cold water over bulgur to keep the grains from sticking. Blanch the peas and carrots in the remaining water for 5 minutes. Strain and put into a large bowl. Fold in the bulgur, along with radicchio, cilantro, and tarragon. Combine sunflower oil, lime juice, saffron, and salt, then pour over mixture. Toss and serve at once.

CRISPY SNOW PEA & BASMATI SALAD ♡
Serves: 4

3 cups water
I cup basmati white rice
I pound snow peas
I small head red leaf lettuce
I scallion, minced

Bring 2 cups of water to a boil in a medium-size saucepan. Wash basmati rice and add to boiling water. Cover and simmer over low heat for 12 minutes until rice is swelled and fluffy. Use remaining water to blanch snow peas for 3 minutes. Drain snow peas and combine with rice. Tear lettuce apart into whole pieces and arrange on a platter. Fold rice and snow peas over the lettuce. Garnish with scallions. Serve with a poppy seed dressing.

Peel the cucumber and remove seeds by cutting it in half lengthwise and scoring it with a small spoon. Finely dice the cucumber, add the barley, corn, and dressing, then toss the salad. Gently tear the head of lettuce apart, and decorate a large bowl with it. Add the salad to your lettuce-lined bowl. You may drink the healthy, cooling barley water after your meal.

GARDEN POTATO SALAD
Serves: 4

6 cups water
8 new red potatoes, diced
1 pound snow peas
2 medium carrots
1 small daikon radish
3 stalks celery, thinly sliced
1/4 cup fresh parsley, minced
1 tablespoon fresh dill, minced
1 tablespoon sunflower oil
1 orange, freshly juiced
1 tablespoon maple syrup
10 strands saffron
1/2 teaspoon rock salt
1/2 head curly endive, shredded
2 pounds cooked bulgur

Bring water to a boil in a large saucepan and cook potatoes over medium heat for 10 minutes until tender but firm. Strain and allow to cool, retaining the cooking water. Blanch snow peas in the potato water for 3 minutes. Combine potatoes and snow peas in a large bowl. Scrub the carrots and daikon radish. Using a hand grater, coarsely grate them into the bowl with the potatoes and snow peas. Add celery, fresh herbs, and sunflower oil, and use your clean hands to combine the salad. Blend in the orange juice, maple syrup, saffron, and salt. Garnish with endive and serve immediately over the cooked bulgur.

CILANTRO CORN SALAD WITH MILLET BALLS ♡
Serves: 4

5 cups water
1 cup millet
3 ears fresh corn, husked
2 tablespoons corn oil
1 red onion, chopped
1/2 lemon, freshly juiced

I teaspoon maple syrup

1/4 cup fresh cilantro, minced

I tablespoon fresh rosemary, bruised

1/2 teaspoon white pepper, finely ground

1/2 teaspoon rock salt

I head radicchio, shredded

Bring 3 cups of water to a boil in a medium-size saucepan. Wash millet and add to boiling water. Cover and simmer on medium heat for 25 minutes until cooked. Remove from heat and let cool. Wash your hands and rub a small amount of corn oil on your palms. Roll the millet into golf ball-size balls between your palms. In a large saucepan, heat the remaining water and blanch the ears of corn for 5 minutes. Do not discard the water after cooking. Then use a sharp paring knife to remove the kernels off the cob of corn. Heat the corn oil in a large cast-iron skillet. Lightly brown the millet balls over medium heat. In a large bowl, combine the corn with the millet balls. Using the same skillet used for the millet balls, sauté the onions for a few minutes until they turn translucent, then add the corn water, fresh herbs, white pepper, and salt. Whisk the mixture for a few seconds and pour over the millet and corn salad. Garnish with radicchio and serve at once.

SPLENDID SUMMER GREENS

Use of Seasonal Flowers: Whenever possible, make an offering of gratitude to the gods and add more color and vivacity to your salads by decorating them with seasonal flowers from your garden. There is a boundless selection of nature's beautiful flowers throughout the spring, summer, early fall, and autumn. Among the flowers growing during these times are violets, rose petals, yellow mustard and dandelion flowers, white or pink buckwheat flowers, white, red, or lilac clovers, tiny chamomile flowers, apple blossoms, chive blossoms, summer squash blossoms, and nasturtiums.

SUMMER SLAW ♡
Serves: 6

I small white cabbage

I small red cabbage

3 large carrots

2 tablespoons organic ghee (recipe on pages 150-151)

1/4 cup raisins

I tablespoon fennel seeds

I tablespoon fresh orange zest

1/4 cup fresh orange juice

I tablespoon maple syrup

1/2 teaspoon rock salt
1/2 teaspoon white pepper, finely ground
1/2 cup sunflower seeds, roasted

Wash the cabbages, cut in quarters lengthwise, remove cores with a paring knife, and set aside. Finely shred the cabbages lengthwise. Scrub the carrots and nip off and discard the ends. Coarsely grate the carrots and cabbage cores. Combine the cabbage and carrot salad in a large bowl. Melt the ghee in a medium-size cast-iron skillet and sauté the raisins for a minute or so over medium heat until they begin to swell. Add the orange zest and fennel seeds and roast for 30 seconds. Pour the ghee mixture into the salad. Use the same skillet to heat the orange juice for 2 minutes before adding the maple syrup, salt, and pepper. Stir and pour directly over the salad. Toss the salad, sprinkle the roasted seeds over it, and serve at once.

CUCUMBER RAITA WITH YOGURT & DILL ♥
Serves: 4
2 cucumbers
1/2 cup organic yogurt
1 teaspoon fresh lemon juice
2 tablespoons fresh dill, minced
1 pinch black pepper
1 pinch salt

Wash and peel the cucumbers and slice them lengthwise. Remove the seeds by running a teaspoon along the center of the cucumbers. Slice them crosswise, very thinly. In a bowl, combine the yogurt, lemon juice, dill, black pepper, and salt. Add the cucumbers, toss, and serve immediately.

SNAPPY BEAN SALAD ♥
Serves: 4
2 handfuls sugar snap beans
1 handful green beans
3 shallots or spring onions, minced
1 teaspoon fresh oregano, minced
1 teaspoon dried tarragon
1 teaspoon fresh dill, minced
1/2 teaspoon tamarind paste
3 tablespoons warm water
1 tablespoon walnut oil

1 teaspoon Sucanat or brown sugar

1/2 teaspoon rock salt

Blanch all the beans in 2 quarts of boiling water for 3 minutes. Drain them and immediately immerse in a bowl of cold water for 10 minutes before straining them. In a large bowl, combine the beans, shallots, oregano, tarragon, and dill. Wash your hands and use your fingers to dilute the tamarind paste in 3 tablespoons of warm water. Combine tamarind water, walnut oil, Sucanat, and salt, and pour over the salad. Serve immediately.

ROASTED BELL PEPPERS ♡
Serves: 4

4 fresh green bell peppers

1 fresh red bell pepper

2 tablespoons almond oil

1/2 teaspoon rock salt

a few black olives, pitted

Spear the peppers with a long serving fork and scorch the skins over an open flame until they turn black. Immerse them in a bowl of cold water and use your hands to scrape off the charred skin. Carefully cut the peppers in half, lengthwise. Scoop the seeds out with a small spoon. Cut peppers in fine, lengthwise strips, and arrange on a platter. Add salt to the oil and pour over the pepper salad. Garnish with olives. Serve immediately as a side dish.

TOFU SALAD NIÇOISE ♡
Serves: 6

1 pound semi-firm tofu, marinated

1 teaspoon tamari

1 tablespoon sunflower oil

1/2 teaspoon turmeric powder

1 teaspoon coriander powder

1/2 teaspoon rock salt

1/2 cup warm water

1 large head of Bibb lettuce

1/2 pound yellow wax beans

1/2 pound green beans

1/2 pound fresh asparagus

1/4 cup Niçoise olives (available in gourmet markets)

3 tablespoons tiny capers

Slice the tofu into 1-inch square pieces. In a small saucepan, combine the tamari, sunflower oil, turmeric, coriander, and salt with the warm water and heat over low heat for 3 minutes. Pour the dressing in a large, flat-bottomed bowl. Arrange the tofu pieces in the bowl so that each piece is completely immersed in the tamari sauce. Cover with a thin cotton towel and marinate overnight. Wash and tear the lettuce apart, keeping the leaves whole. Nip the hard ends of the asparagus, and along with the beans, blanch in 3 quarts boiling water for 5 minutes. Drain them and immediately immerse in a bowl of cold water for 10 minutes before straining them. Drain the marinated tofu, retaining the sauce and arranging along with the lettuce, asparagus, and beans on a flat-bottomed platter. Decorate with olives and capers. Spoon dressing over the salad and serve at once.

WISE EARTH WALNUT SALAD ♥

Serves: 4

1 large celeriac
2 ounces walnuts, coarsely chopped
1 pound organic green grapes, seeded
1 small red apple
1/4 cup organic cream
1 lemon, freshly juiced
1/2 teaspoon black pepper, finely ground
1/2 teaspoon rock salt

Boil the celeriac in 2 quarts of water for 35 minutes until tender. Remove from water and allow to cool before peeling off the skin. Cut into small cubes and place in a large bowl. Add the walnuts and grapes. Core the apple and cut into bite-size pieces directly before serving the salad (to prevent discoloring). Warm the cream in a small saucepan for 2 minutes and add the lemon juice, salt, and pepper, curdling the cream. Pour into the salad. Toss and serve immediately.

SATTVIC SALAD ♥

Serves: 6

4 heads endive
1 small bunch dandelion leaves
1 small fresh lotus root
1 teaspoon sunflower oil
2 ounces pecans, coarsely chopped
2 firm peaches
1 teaspoon basil vinegar
1 tablespoon fresh fennel, minced

Wash the endive and nip off the root ends to release their petals. Leave the petals whole. Wash the dandelion leaves, nip off the stems, and keep the leaves whole. Combine petals and leaves in a large bowl. Wash, towel dry, and thinly slice the fresh lotus root. Heat the sunflower oil in a small cast-iron skillet and pan fry the lotus slices for a few minutes over medium-high heat until they turn crispy and brown. Add cooked lotus pieces to the salad, wiping the skillet off with a few of the dandelion leaves. Using the unwashed skillet, dry roast the pecans for 2 minutes over medium heat. Core peaches, cut into bite-size pieces, and toss into the salad, along with the roasted pecans and basil vinegar. Garnish with fresh fennel and serve at once.

SUMMER CRESS SALAD ♥

Serves: 4

1 small bunch watercress
1 small bunch land cress
1 cucumber
1 teaspoon sunflower oil
1 teaspoon organic ghee (recpe on pages 150-151)
1 tablespoon coriander seeds
1/2 teaspoon rock salt
1 tablespoon fresh licorice-mint, minced

Wash the cresses thoroughly, leaving their stems on. Peel the cucumber, cut in half lengthwise, and use a small spoon to remove the seeds. Thinly slice the cucumber and combine with the cresses in a large bowl. Combine the sunflower oil and ghee, and warm them in a small skillet. Dry roast the coriander seeds for a few minutes in a separate skillet over medium heat, and then coarsely grind them with a mortar and pestle. Add the crushed seeds to the oil-ghee mixture and roast for 1 minute or so until the ghee begins to foam. Blend mixture into the salad, add the salt and licorice-mint, and toss the salad. Serve at once.

AVOCADO & CHERRY SALAD

Serves: 4

4 new potatoes
1 head chicory
1 ripe avocado
3 stalks celery
1/2 cup oat bran
1 teaspoon sunflower oil
1 lemon, freshly juiced
1/2 teaspoon coriander powder

1 pinch paprika powder
1/2 teaspoon rock salt
1/2 cup Bing cherries, pitted

Scrub the potatoes, cut into quarters, and boil in 2 quarts of water for 10 minutes until tender. Remove from boiling water and immerse in cold water for 10 minutes before straining. Wash chicory and tear the leaves into large pieces. Cut the avocado in half, remove the seed, and carefully release it from its skin. Cut into bite-size pieces. Wash celery and cut thinly, slicing the stalks crosswise. Combine the salad ingredients in a large bowl. Dry roast the oat bran in a skillet over medium heat for 3 minutes, stirring frequently; sprinkle over salad. Combine the sunflower oil, lemon juice, spice powders, and salt and pour into the salad. Toss the salad, making sure the oats are blended in. Garnish with the whole cherries and serve at once.

JICAMA & MANGO SLAW ♥
Serves: 4
1 pound jicama
1 firm, ripe mango
1 lemon, freshly juiced
1 pinch cayenne pepper
1 tablespoon cilantro, minced

Peel the jicama and cut into fine matchsticks. Carefully peel the mango and cut into lengthwise strips, removing the seed. In a bowl, combine jicama and mango, adding the lemon juice and pepper. Garnish with cilantro and serve at once.

PEACEFUL PASTA REPASTS

LINGUINI IN PESTO SAUCE
Serves: 6
1 pound linguini
1 small head rapini or flowering broccoli
1 lemon, freshly juiced
1/4 cup fresh basil
1/4 cup fresh Italian parsley
1/4 cup pine nuts
2 large cloves garlic, peeled
2 tablespoons sunflower oil
1/2 teaspoon black pepper, finely ground
1 teaspoon rock salt

Bring a large, heavy-bottomed pot of water to a boil. Add the linguini and raise the heat to high. Allow the linguini to cook for 7 or 8 minutes until al dente. Strain, retaining a small portion of the cooking water, and pour cold water over the pasta to prevent it from sticking together. Cut the hard ends off the stems of rapini and discard, then blanch rapini in the retained cooking water for 3 minutes, being careful to maintain the vivid green and yellow colors of the leaves and flowers by not over-blanching. Set the rapini aside. In a large hand grater, combine the basil, parsley, pine nuts, and garlic and coarsely grind. Then blend the sunflower oil into the ground ingredients adding the pepper and salt. You may add a palmful of cooking water to make the sauce more fluid. Put pasta in a large bowl and blend in the fresh herbal sauce with clean hands. Garnish with rapini and serve at once.

TAGLIATELLE IN CREAM SAUCE

Serves: 6

1 pound tagliatelle
1 tablespoon sunflower oil
1 small white onion
1/4 cup fresh basil, bruised
1 tablespoon fresh rosemary, bruised
1/4 cup organic cow's cream or soy milk
1 teaspoon coriander powder
1/2 teaspoon white pepper, finely ground
1/2 teaspoon rock salt
1 teaspoon organic ghee (recipe on pages 150-151)
1 handful fresh chives, chopped

Bring a large, heavy-bottomed pot of water to a boil. Add the tagliatelle and cook over high heat for 7 to 8 minutes until al dente. Rinse with cold water to prevent it from sticking together and put into a large bowl. Heat sunflower oil in a medium-size skillet and sauté the onions and rosemary for 2 minutes over medium heat until the onions turn translucent. Stir in the cream or soy milk, along with coriander powder, pepper, and salt, then lower the heat and simmer for 1 minute until the cream begins to bubble. Add the ghee. Garnish with fresh chives and serve at once.

PEPPERY PENNE & ARUGULA

Serves: 6

1 pound penne
2 tablespoons sunflower oil
1 medium red onion, chopped

2 teaspoons fennel seeds

1/2 teaspoon cumin seeds

1 tablespoon fresh oregano, minced

1 tablespoon fresh parsley, minced

1 lemon, freshly juiced

1 handful arugula

1/2 teaspoon rock salt

Bring a large, heavy-bottomed pot of water to a boil. Add penne and cook over high heat for 7 to 8 minutes until al dente. Strain the pasta, running cold water over it to prevent it from sticking together. In a large skillet, heat the sunflower oil and roast the spice seeds for 2 minutes over medium heat until golden brown. Remove from heat and blend in the fresh herbs, along with the lemon juice and salt. Add pasta to the spice and herb mixture. Garnish with arugula or pieces of fresh fennel bulb and serve at once.

SOOTHING SUMMER SOUPS

MANGO & FENNEL SOUP

Serves: 4

1 whole fennel bulb, with tops

1 medium-size ripe mango

1 teaspoon fresh ginger, finely minced

1 tablespoon organic ghee (recipe on pages 150-151)

1 teaspoon coriander powder

1/2 teaspoon cumin powder

1/2 teaspoon white pepper, finely ground

1 teaspoon rock salt

1 cup soy milk

3 cups water

1/4 cup oat bran

Wash and peel fennel bulb under cold water. Cut whole bulb into matchstick pieces, mincing the fresh fennel tops. Set aside the minced fennel for garnish. Wash and peel mango and cut into lengthwise strips. Melt ghee in a large saucepan and sauté the fennel bulb, mango, and ginger for 3 minutes on medium heat. Add the spice powders, pepper and salt, then stir for an additional 30 seconds. Pour in the soy milk, stir, cover, and simmer for 5 minutes over medium heat. Add the water and continue simmering for another 5 minutes. To add body to the soup, introduce the oat bran, stir, cover, and simmer for an additional 3 minutes. Garnish with fresh fennel leaves and serve warm or cool.

WILD STRAWBERRY SOUP ♥
Serves: 4

4 cups water
6 small golden potatoes
I quart ripe, fresh strawberries (organic)
I small bunch fresh cilantro
I tablespoon sunflower oil
I tablespoon cumin seeds
I teaspoon brown mustard seeds
I teaspoon cumin powder
I teaspoon rock salt
I small bunch fresh dill, for garnish

Bring water to a boil in a medium-size soup pot. Scrub the potatoes until all of the skin is almost peeled off. Cut in quarters and add to the boiling water. Cover and simmer on medium heat for 10 minutes until the potatoes are tender. Clean the strawberries, removing the stems, and add to the boiling potatoes. Use a flat-bottomed ladle to puree the potatoes and strawberries while still in the boiling water. Continue cooking this mixture for another 5 minutes. Wash and finely mince the dill and cilantro, reserving sufficient dill for garnish, and add the rest to the soup. Heat the sunflower oil in a small skillet over medium heat and roast the spice seeds for I minute until the mustard seeds begin to pop. Add cumin powder and salt and remove from heat. Add the spice mixture to the soup by stirring the soup pot with the small skillet (if possible). Garnish with fresh chopped dill and serve cool.

CREAMY SPINACH SOUP ♥
Serves: 4

4 cups water
2 handfuls spinach
I teaspoon organic ghee (recipe on pages 150-151)
1/2 white onion, chopped
1/2 teaspoon black pepper, finely ground
1/2 teaspoon rock salt
I small bunch fresh parsley, minced
1/2 lemon, freshly juiced
I cup soy milk

Bring water to a boil in a medium-size soup pot. Thoroughly wash the spinach and add to the boiling water. Cover and simmer on medium heat for 3 minutes. Heat the ghee in a medium-size skillet and sauté the onions over medium heat until they are translucent. Add the pepper, salt, and half of the fresh parsley, and sauté for an additional 2 minutes before adding the lemon juice and soy milk. Simmer over medium heat until the sauce begins to bubble. Then add this mixture to the soup by stirring the soup pot with the small skillet (if possible). Allow to cool, garnish with the remaining parsley, and serve at once.

COSMIC CORN CHOWDER ♥
Serves: 4

4 cups water

1/2 cup pearled barley

3 ears fresh corn, husked

2 medium carrots, diced

1 teaspoon organic ghee (recipe on pages 150-151)

1/2 red onion, chopped

1 teaspoon brown mustard seeds

2 tablespoons organic cashew butter

1/2 cup fresh peas

1 teaspoon rock salt

1/2 teaspoon black pepper, coarsely ground

1 shallot, coarsely chopped

Bring water to a boil in a medium-size soup pot. Wash the barley and add to the boiling water. Use a sharp paring knife to remove the kernels of corn from the cob. Set the kernels aside, and add the bare cobs to the boiling water, along with the diced carrots. Cover and cook over medium heat for 30 minutes until the barley is soft. Remove the corn cobs from the soup and discard them in your compost. Melt the ghee in a small skillet and sauté the onions over medium heat until they are translucent. Add the mustard seeds, cashew butter, and 1/4 cup of the soup water to help dissolve the cashew butter into the sauce. Then add the peas and stir. Simmer for 1 minute before pouring into the soup. Add salt and pepper to the soup pot; stir, cover, and simmer on low heat for 5 minutes. Remove from heat and allow to cool. Garnish with shallots and serve at once.

ZUCCHINI & CHIVE SOUP ♥
Serves: 4

4 cups water

4 medium zucchini

1 large bunch chives

2 scallions

1 tablespoon corn oil

1 teaspoon ajwain seeds

I teaspoon dried marjoram

I teaspoon coriander powder

1/2 teaspoon cayenne powder

I teaspoon rock salt

1/2 lemon, freshly juiced

1/4 cup quinoa

Bring water to a boil in a medium-size soup pot. Wash the zucchini and dice into small pieces. Wash and coarsely chop the chives and scallions. Heat the corn oil in a large skillet and sauté the ajwain seeds and marjoram leaves for I minute over medium heat before adding the spice powders and salt. Immediately add the zucchini, chives, and scallions to the skillet. Stir and cook over high heat for 2 minutes before pouring the mixture into the boiling water. Use some soup water to rinse the oil from the skillet into the soup pot. Add the lemon juice and quinoa. Cover and simmer on medium heat for 7 minutes. Serve warm.

REJUVENATING ROOT SOUP ♡
Serves: 4

4 cups water

2 medium carrots

2 small golden potatoes

I small whole fennel bulb

I medium golden beet

1/2 teaspoon black pepper, finely ground

1/2 teaspoon cardamom powder

I teaspoon rock salt

1/2 cup soy milk

I small bunch fresh licorice mint, minced

Bring water to a boil in a medium-size soup pot. Scrub carrots and potatoes and peel the fennel bulb and beets. Using a hand grater, coarsely grate the roots and bulb, and add to the boiling water. Add the spice powders and salt. Cook for 10 minutes before adding the soy milk. Stir, cover, and simmer over low heat for an additional 3 minutes. Allow to cool, then garnish with fresh mint and serve at once.

YOGURT & MELON SOUP ♡
Serves: 4

4 cups water

3 cups fresh honeydew melon, cubed

1 teaspoon fresh ginger, minced

1 teaspoon cumin seeds

1 teaspoon coriander seeds

1/2 teaspoon black mustard seeds

1/2 teaspoon dill seeds

1 teaspoon sunflower oil

1/2 teaspoon cardamom powder

1 teaspoon rock salt

1 pint organic yogurt

1 small bunch fresh dill, chopped

Bring water to a boil in a medium-size soup pot. Add the melon and ginger, and simmer for 5 minutes over medium heat. Dry roast the seeds together in a medium-size skillet for 2 minutes over medium heat until they turn golden brown. Coarsely crush them in a suribachi. Use the same skillet to heat the sunflower oil. Using a small brush to collect the crushed seeds from the suribachi, add them to the oil, along with the cardamom powder and salt. Stir and blend for 30 seconds before adding to the soup water by stirring the soup pot with the small skillet (if possible). Then allow the soup to cook for an additional 3 minutes. Remove from heat, let cool for a few minutes, and then fold in the yogurt, stirring frequently to prevent it from curdling. Garnish with fresh dill and serve at once.

CAULIFLOWER & TAMARIND SOUP ♥
Serves: 4

4 cups water

1 small head cauliflower

1 tablespoon tamarind paste

1 teaspoon organic ghee (recipe on pages 150-151)

1 teaspoon ajwain seeds

2 scallions, chopped

1 small bunch fresh cilantro, minced

1/2 teaspoon rock salt

1 small bunch celery leaves, chopped

Bring water to a boil in a medium-size soup pot. Wash the cauliflower and carefully cut into tiny florets. Peel the stems and finely dice them. Add florets and stems to the boiling water. Dilute the tamarind paste in a small amount of warm water and add to the soup. Melt the ghee in a small skillet and roast the ajwain seeds for 1 minute over medium heat. Add to the soup, along with the scallions, cilantro, and salt. Cover and simmer on medium heat for 15 minutes. Garnish with fresh celery leaves and serve at once.

COOLING COCONUT & CARROT SOUP ♡
Serves: 4

4 cups water

2 medium carrots

1 teaspoon coriander seeds

1 teaspoon cumin seeds

1 teaspoon organic ghee (recipe on pages 150-151)

3 bay leaves

1/4 cup fresh coconut, grated (if fresh coconut is unavailable,

substitute with dried coconut)

1/2 cup coconut milk

1/2 teaspoon white pepper, finely ground

1/2 teaspoon rock salt

1 small bunch arugula

Bring water to a boil in a medium-size saucepan. Scrub the carrots, dice them into 1/2-inch pieces, and add them to the boiling water. Dry roast the spice seeds in a small skillet for 1 minute over medium heat. Then coarsely crush them in a suribachi. Using the same skillet, melt the ghee and roast the crushed seeds for 1 minute over medium heat. Use a small brush to collect the crushed spice seeds from the suribachi and add them to the soup. Add the bay leaves, shredded coconut and coconut milk, along with the pepper and salt. Cover and simmer over medium heat for 8 minutes. Remove from heat and allow to cool. Tear the arugula in large pieces, garnish the soup, and serve at once.

PINEAPPLE & TOFU SOUP ♡
Serves: 4

4 cups water

1 small pineapple

1 tablespoon coconut oil

1 pound semi-firm tofu, cubed

1 small bunch fresh parsley, chopped

1 teaspoon cumin powder

1/2 teaspoon turmeric powder

1/2 teaspoon cayenne powder

1 tablespoon maple syrup

1/2 teaspoon rock salt

1 handful fresh snow peas

Bring water to a boil in a medium-size soup pot. Peel, core, and cube the pineapple in a large basin to collect the juice, cutting it into bite-size pieces. Add the pineapple pieces, along with the juice, to the boiling water. Heat the coconut oil in a large skillet over medium-high heat and lightly pan fry the tofu for 4 minutes. Add the cooked tofu to the soup, along with the fresh parsley and spice powders. Then add the maple syrup and salt. Stir, cover, and simmer the soup for 5 minutes over medium heat. Garnish with fresh snow peas and serve either warm or cool.

DIVINE DHALS

Dhal is an Indian term for peas, beans, or lentils that have been split and skinned, and also for dishes that have been made with them. It is a rich, savory dish that is traditionally served with flatbread.

MUNG BEAN & SUN-DRIED TOMATO DHAL ♡
Serves: 4

4 cups water

1 cup split mung beans

2 sun-dried tomatoes

1 teaspoon coriander powder

1/2 teaspoon turmeric powder

1/2 teaspoon cardamom powder

1 teaspoon organic ghee (recipe on pages 150-151)

1/2 teaspoon black mustard seeds

1/2 teaspoon ajwain seeds

1 handful curly endive leaves

Bring water to a boil in a medium-size saucepan. Wash and strain the split mung beans and add to the boiling water. Cut the sun-dried tomatoes into thin strips and add to the dhal pot, along with the spice powders. Melt the ghee in a small skillet and roast the spice seeds over medium heat until the mustard seeds begin to pop. Add the roasted seeds to the dhal by submerging the skillet in the dhal pot. Cover and simmer over medium heat for 15 minutes. Tear the endive leaves into large pieces and garnish the dhal. Serve warm with flatbread or over cooked basmati white rice.

LENTIL & COCONUT DHAL ♡
Serves: 4

4 cups water

3/4 cup green lentils

4 bay leaves

1/2 teaspoon turmeric powder

1/2 teaspoon rock salt

I teaspoon coconut oil

I/2 teaspoon cumin seeds

I/2 clove garlic, grated

I fresh green chili pepper (mild)

I/4 cup fresh coconut, grated

(if fresh coconut is unavailable, substitute with dried coconut)

I small bunch fresh cilantro, chopped

Bring water to a boil in a medium-size saucepan. Wash and strain the lentils and add to the boiling water, along with the bay leaves, turmeric, and salt. Cover and simmer over medium heat for I5 minutes. Heat the coconut oil in a small skillet and roast the cumin seeds and garlic for I minute over medium heat until the seeds turn golden brown. Add the cumin seed and garlic mixture to the dhal pot by submerging the small skillet in it (if possible). Add the pepper and shredded coconut, then continue to simmer for an additional I0 minutes. Toward the end of the I0 minutes, introduce the cilantro to the dhal pot. Remove from heat, cover, and allow dhal to sit for 5 minutes before serving. Steamed couscous or flatbread is a delicious complement to this dish.

SPICY SPLIT PEA DHAL ♡
Serves: 4

4 cups water

3/4 cup yellow split peas

I/2 teaspoon ginger powder

I/2 teaspoon mustard powder

I/2 teaspoon turmeric powder

I/2 teaspoon cayenne powder

I/2 teaspoon rock salt

2 scallions, chopped

I clove garlic, grated

2 tablespoons chickpea flour

I teaspoon organic ghee (recipe on pages I50-I5I)

I small bunch fresh dill, chopped

Bring water to a boil in a medium-size saucepan. Wash and strain the split peas and add them to the boiling water, along with the spice powders and salt. Add the scallions and garlic. Cover and simmer over medium heat for I5 minutes. Dry roast the flour in a small skillet for 2 minutes over medium heat until it turns golden brown. Stir into the dhal pot, along with the ghee. Cover and let simmer for an additional 4 minutes. Garnish with fresh dill and serve warm with cooked cracked wheat or flatbread.

RED LENTIL & YELLOW SQUASH DHAL ♥

Serves: 4

4 cups water

3/4 cup red lentils

3 yellow summer squash

I teaspoon cumin seeds

I teaspoon coriander seeds

1/2 teaspoon black peppercorns

I teaspoon walnut oil

I pinch asafetida

1/2 teaspoon rock salt

1/2 pint organic yogurt, for garnish

Bring water to a boil in a medium-size saucepan. Wash and strain the red lentils, then add them to the boiling water. Wash the squash, cut into 1-inch bite-size pieces, and add to the dhal pot. Dry roast the cumin seeds, coriander seeds, and peppercorns in a small skillet for 1 minute over medium heat. Pour into a suribachi and coarsely grind the seeds. Using the same skillet, heat the walnut oil and roast the crushed seeds once more, for 1 minute. Add them to the dhal pot by submerging the small skillet in the dhal water. Then add the asafetida and rock salt. Cover and simmer over medium heat for 20 minutes. Garnish with a dollop of yogurt and serve warm with flatbread.

MUNG BEAN & CILANTRO DHAL ♥

Serves: 4

4 cups water

I cup split mung beans, with skin

I teaspoon fresh ginger, grated

1/2 teaspoon turmeric powder

I teaspoon rock salt

1/2 lemon, freshly juiced

I teaspoon sunflower oil

I tablespoon cumin seeds

I small bunch fresh cilantro, chopped

Bring water to a boil in a medium-size saucepan. Wash and strain the split mung beans and add to boiling water, along with the ginger, turmeric powder, salt, and lemon juice. Cover and simmer over medium heat for 20 minutes. Heat the sunflower oil in a small skillet and roast the cumin seeds over medium heat until golden brown. Add to the dhal (mung bean mixture) by stirring the soup with the small skillet (if possible). Add the cilantro, cover, and allow the dhal to simmer for another 3 minutes. Serve warm with flatbread. (Flatbread recipes follow.)

FLAVORFUL FLATBREADS & INDIAN CHAPATIS

Chapatis are the original unleavened bread made from the flour of stone-ground whole wheat. From ancient times, bread has been an important part of humanity's daily sustenance. From the "breaking of bread" to the "daily bread," this food is the living symbol of communal reaping, harvesting, and sharing the land's bountiful yields. The original chapati was made into dough from whole wheat flour, and then buried under coals in a baking hole dug into the earth. Over the centuries, a multitude of cooking variations developed. Whole wheat is still the dominant form of grain used at the dinner tables of North India.

CLASSIC SPELT CHAPATI
Serves: 4

2 cups spelt flour
1 pinch rock salt
3/4 cup warm water

Combine the flour and salt in a large bowl with your hands by introducing the water gradually, as needed. Knead for about 5 minutes. Cover with a thin, damp cotton towel and allow dough to sit for 2 hours. Set aside a small bowl of spelt flour to use for rolling the chapatis. After 2 hours, uncover the dough, punch it, and knead it briefly before dividing it into 10 balls, each approximately the size of a plum. Using a flat, clean rolling surface and a rolling pin, roll each ball into a thin 6-inch circle. Heat a flat, ungreased griddle on medium heat. Carefully pick up the rolled-out dough, resting it on your open hand, then place it on the heated griddle. When the dough begins to swell, turn it over to cook the other side. Remove the chapati with a pair of tongs and place it over a direct flame for a few seconds. When it begins to puff, remove from heat and serve immediately.

BASIL & ONION CHAPATI
Serves: 4

2 cups whole wheat flour
2 tablespoons fresh basil, minced
1 tablespoon pine nuts, ground
1/2 red onion, minced
1/4 clove garlic, grated
1 teaspoon sunflower oil
1/2 teaspoon coriander powder
1/2 teaspoon rock salt
3/4 cup warm water

Combine all the ingredients. Knead into pliable dough, introducing the water gradually. Knead for about 5 minutes, then cover the bowl with a thin, damp cotton towel and let dough sit for 2 hours. Set aside a small bowl of flour to use for rolling out the flatbread. Follow instructions for making chapati in the Classic Spelt Chapati recipe on page 176. Serve immediately after cooking.

DILL & SCALLION CHAPATI
Serves: 4
2 cups spelt flour
2 tablespoons fresh dill, minced
1 scallion, chopped
1/2 teaspoon black pepper, finely ground
1 pinch rock salt
3/4 cup warm water
1 teaspoon organic ghee (recipe on pages 150-151)

In a large bowl, combine the flour, dill, scallion, pepper, and salt. Introduce the warm water, a bit at a time, and knead into pliable dough for about 5 minutes. Allow dough to sit for 2 hours, covering the bowl with a thin, damp cotton towel. Set aside a small bowl of spelt flour to use for rolling the chapati. Follow instructions from the Classic Spelt Chapati for cooking instructions. Immediately after cooking the chapati, daub one side with the ghee and serve directly.

POTATO FLATBREAD
Serves: 4
Dough:
2 cups barley flour
3/4 cup warm water
1/2 teaspoon rock salt

Potato Filling:
2 small golden potatoes, peeled, boiled, and mashed
1 small white onion, finely chopped
1 tablespoon fresh cilantro, minced
1 teaspoon cumin powder
1 teaspoon coriander powder
1/2 teaspoon rock salt
1 tablespoon warm water

To make the dough, mix all the ingredients in a large bowl, introducing the water gradually. Knead thoroughly for about 5 minutes. Cover with a thin, damp cotton towel and let dough sit for 2 hours. To make the potato filling, combine the ingredients in a large bowl and mix until nicely melded. After 2 hours, uncover the dough, punch it, and then knead it briefly. Divide the dough into 6 balls, each the size of a small orange. Dust each ball with a small quantity of flour and roll them out into 4-inch circles. Place 2 heaping spoonfuls of potato filling in the center of each circle. Gently stretch the perimeters of the dough and fold over the filling, like an envelope. Carefully roll out the potato-filled flatbread, dusting it with sufficient flour to prevent it from sticking on the rolling surface or from spilling its filling. Roll out each flatbread to a 6-inch square piece. Heat a flat griddle over medium heat and lightly oil the surface (sunflower oil preferred). Place the flatbread on the griddle and allow each to cook for about 30 seconds before turning over. Continue to flip the flatbread, pressing it down with a spatula until both sides are lightly browned. Serve immediately.

CLASSIC SWEET FLATBREAD
Serves: 4
2 cups spelt flour
1/4 cup currants
1/2 teaspoon cardamom powder
1/2 teaspoon cinnamon powder
1 tablespoon unrefined brown sugar
5 drops vanilla extract
1/2 teaspoon rock salt
3/4 cup organic cow's milk or soy milk
1 teaspoon organic ghee (recipe on pages 150-151)
1 tablespoon sunflower oil

In a large bowl, combine all the ingredients, except for the milk and ghee. Knead into pliable dough for about 5 minutes, gradually introducing the milk as needed. Cover the bowl and let dough sit for 2 hours. Set aside a small bowl of flour to use for rolling the flatbread. After 2 hours, uncover the dough, punch it, and then knead it briefly. Divide the dough into 6 balls, each the size of a small orange. Dust each ball with a small quantity of flour and roll them out into 6-inch circles. Heat a flat griddle over medium heat and lightly oil the surface (sunflower oil preferred). Place the flatbread on the griddle and allow each to cook for about 30 seconds before turning over. Continue to flip the flatbread, pressing it down with a spatula until both sides are lightly browned. Serve flatbread directly after cooking, daubing a bit of ghee on one side of each flatbread.

SOY & CHIVE FLATBREAD ♡

Serves: 4

1 cup soy flour

1 cup chickpea flour

1 small bunch fresh chives, chopped

1 teaspoon coriander powder

1/2 teaspoon turmeric powder

1/2 teaspoon black pepper, finely ground

1/2 teaspoon rock salt

3/4 cup warm water

1 tablespoon sunflower oil

In a large bowl, combine all the ingredients, gradually introducing the water as needed. Knead for 5 minutes until the dough is pliable. Cover the bowl with a thin, damp cotton towel and let dough sit for 2 hours. Set aside a small bowl of flour to use for rolling the flatbread. After 2 hours, uncover the dough, punch it, and then knead it briefly. Divide the dough into 6 balls, each the size of a small orange. Dust each ball with a small quantity of flour and roll them out into 6-inch circles. Heat a flat griddle over medium heat and lightly oil the surface (sunflower oil preferred). Place the flatbread on the griddle and allow each to cook for about 30 seconds before turning over. Continue to flip the flatbread, pressing it down with a spatula until both sides are lightly browned. Serve immediately after cooking.

SAVORY MANGO CHUTNEY ♡

Serves: 4

1 cup semi-ripe mango, peeled and finely chopped

1/2 coconut, freshly grated

1 cup coconut milk

1 teaspoon lemon juice, fresh

1/2 teaspoon sea salt

1/2 teaspoon black pepper, coarsely grounded

1/2 teaspoon black mustard seeds

1/2 teaspoon sunflower oil

Using a small hand grinder, grind the mango, coconut milk, lemon juice, salt, and black pepper into a thick paste. Sauté the mustard seeds in hot sunflower oil until they pop, then mix into the paste.

MELLOW DESSERTS

MANGO LIME DECADENCE ♥

Serves: 4

2 large ripe mangoes

1 lime, freshly juiced

1 teaspoon organic ghee (recipe on pages 150-151)

1 teaspoon fennel seeds

Using a sharp paring knife, slice each mango lengthwise into 2 pieces, avoiding the large pit in the center. Pare the flesh off each pit and reserve for other use. (Discard the pit in your compost.) Score the flesh of each half, making a fine crisscross pattern, being careful not to cut through the skin. Turn each mango half inside out and pour lime juice over both. Set aside. Melt the ghee in a small skillet and roast the fennel seeds over medium heat until golden brown. Pour equal amounts of the fennel and ghee mixture into the center of each mango half. Serve at once.

TROPICAL FRUIT BOWL ♥

Serves: 4

1 small pineapple, peeled and chunked

1/4 cup fresh coconut, grated (if fresh coconut is unavailable,

substitute with dried coconut)

1/4 cup fresh licorice mint, minced

1/4 cup maple syrup

1/2 cup crushed ice

Combine the pineapple, coconut, and mint in a large fruit bowl. Pour maple syrup over the fruit mixture and garnish with crushed ice. Serve at once.

APPLE & BLUEBERRY CRUMBLE ♥

Serves: 4

3 Gala apples

1 lime, freshly juiced

1/2 pound fresh blueberries

1 cup chickpea flour

1/4 cup unrefined brown sugar

1 tablespoon sunflower oil

1/2 teaspoon rock salt

1/4 teaspoon ground nutmeg

1/4 teaspoon cardamom powder

Preheat the oven to 350 degrees. Peel and core apples, then cut each into 8 slices. Arrange slices in a shallow, oiled baking dish. Sprinkle lime juice over the apple slices. Wash blueberries and evenly lay them over the apple slices. Combine flour, sugar, oil, and salt in a bowl. Cover the fruit with flour mixture. Sprinkle with nutmeg and cardamom, then bake for 20 minutes until the crumble is lightly brown on top.

FRESH WATERMELON & LIME ♡
Serves: 4

1/2 small, ripe watermelon
1 teaspoon rock salt
1 large lime cut into wedges

Use a large, sharp knife to cut the watermelon into wedges. Sprinkle the salt and lime juice on the wedges and serve at once.

APRICOT & VANILLA YOGURT ♡
Serves: 4

1 tablespoon organic ghee (recipe on pages 150-151)
8 fresh apricots, halved and pitted
8 drops vanilla extract
1/4 cup Sucanat
1/2 orange, freshly juiced
1 pint plain yogurt

Melt ghee in a large skillet and arrange the apricot halves on the ghee. Sprinkle apricots with vanilla extract and Sucanat. Pour in orange juice, cover, and simmer over low heat for 20 minutes. Allow to cool, and serve with a dollop of yogurt.

PLUM & CHERRY ASPIC ♡
Serves: 4

6 plums, halved and pitted
1/2 pound Bing cherries, halved and pitted
1 tablespoon fresh orange zest
2 cups water
2 tablespoons agar-agar flakes
2 tablespoons maple syrup
12 strands saffron
Fresh mint leaves, for garnish

Combine the fruits and orange zest in a medium bowl. Bring water and agar-agar to a boil in a small saucepan for 5 minutes, stirring frequently to prevent the agar-agar from lumping. Add the maple syrup and saffron, and remove from heat. Pour directly into the fruit bowl and refrigerate until mixture gels. Garnish with mint leaves and serve at once.

PEACHES & CREAM ♡
Serves: 4

4 large ripe peaches
1/2 cup almond milk
1 tablespoon kudzu powder
3 tablespoons cold water
1 teaspoon cardamom powder
8 drops natural orange extract
1 tablespoon maple syrup

Using a sharp paring knife, slice each peach lengthwise into 2 pieces along the center line, avoiding the pit in the center. (Discard the pit in your compost.) Score the flesh of each half, making a fine crisscross pattern, being careful not to cut through the skin. Turn each half inside out and set aside. Heat the almond milk in a small saucepan. Dilute the kudzu powder in cold water and add to the almond milk, stirring frequently until smooth. Stir in cardamom powder, orange extract, and maple syrup. Remove from heat and whisk briskly into a thick cream. Garnish the peach halves with a dollop of almond cream and serve warm or cool.

RASPBERRY, ROSE PETAL & SAFFRON CREAM ♡
Serves: 4

1/2 pound fresh raspberries
1/2 cup fresh red rose petals (organic)
1 cup almond milk
1 teaspoon arrowroot powder
2 tablespoons cold water
6 drops natural almond extract
2 tablespoons unsweetened raspberry jam
12 strands saffron

Arrange the raspberries and rose petals in a shallow bowl. Heat the almond milk in a small saucepan on medium heat for 3 minutes until milk begins to boil. Dilute arrowroot powder in cold water and add to the almond milk. Lower heat and simmer until mixture is smooth and thick, stirring frequently. Add almond extract, jam, and saffron and blend into a cream. Pour the cream directly over the raspberries and rose petals. Cover and set aside at room temperature for 30 minutes before serving.

MELON & MANGO SLICES ♡

Serves: 4

1 small honeydew melon

1 large ripe mango

1 lemon, freshly juiced

1 pinch unrefined brown sugar

Cut the melon in half, core, and peel. Cut evenly into 1/2-inch slices, and set aside. Slice the mango in half, avoiding its large seed. Peel the halves and slice them. Arrange the melon and mango slices on a dessert platter, sprinkle with lemon juice and sugar and serve.

SUMPTUOUS FRUIT SALAD ♡

Serves: 4

1/2 pound Bing cherries, halved and pitted

2 large peaches, chunked

1 large mango, peeled and chunked

1/4 cup fresh coconut, grated (if fresh coconut is unavailable, substitute with dried coconut)

1/4 cup raisins, poached in 1/4 cup warm water

1 teaspoon fennel seeds, roasted

1 lemon, freshly juiced

1/4 cup maple syrup

Combine all ingredients in a large fruit bowl, toss, and serve.

TANTALIZING TEAS

ROSE & RASPBERRY RAPTURE ♡

Serves: 4

8 cups water

2 tablespoons dried raspberry leaves

1 small handful dried rose petals (organic)

6 wedges of fresh lime

Bring water to a boil in a medium saucepan. Add the leaves and petals, then remove from heat. Cover and let steep for 8 minutes. Strain the infusion, retaining the roughage for your bath water. Serve warm or cold, with wedges of fresh lime on the side.

ORANGE & MAPLE TEA ♡
Serves: 6

6 cups water

2 cups fresh orange juice

1 tablespoon fresh orange peel

3 tablespoons maple syrup

A few fresh mint leaves, for garnish

Bring water and orange juice to a boil in a medium saucepan. Add orange peel and maple syrup and then remove from heat. Stir, cover, and let steep for 8 minutes. Strain the tea, reserving the roughage for your bath water. Garnish with fresh mint leaves and serve warm or cold.

CORIANDER & FENNEL TEA ♡
Serves: 4

8 cups water

1 tablespoon coriander seeds

1 teaspoon fennel seeds

1 tablespoon Sucanat

1 tablespoon fresh fennel, minced

Bring water to a boil in a medium-size saucepan. With a pestle, crush the coriander seeds slightly in a mortar. Add to the boiling water, along with the fennel seeds and Sucanat. Remove from heat, cover and let steep for 8 minutes. Strain the tea, reserving the roughage for your bath water. Garnish with fresh fennel leaves and serve warm or cold.

SWEET "CHOCOLATE" MINT TEA ♡
Serves: 6

8 cups water

16 fresh "chocolate" mint leaves

2 tablespoons unrefined brown sugar

1 tablespoon aloe vera gel

Bring water to a boil in a medium saucepan. Slightly bruise the leaves and add to the boiling water. Stir in the brown sugar. Remove from heat, cover, and let steep for 8 minutes. Strain the infusion, reserving the leaves for your bath water. Stir in the aloe vera gel and serve warm or cool.

LEMON TEA ♥

Serves: 6

8 cups water

1 tablespoon fresh lemon balm, minced

1/2 teaspoon fresh lemon peel

2 tablespoons honey

Bring water to a boil in a medium saucepan. Add fresh lemon balm and lemon peel. Remove from heat, cover, and let steep for 8 minutes. Strain the tea, reserving the roughage for your bath water. Stir in the honey and serve warm or cool.

Part Four

RAINY SEASON

I take The Vow of Ahimsa

To protect Mother Nature and my food source

Chapter Twelve

RAINY SEASON AHIMSA PRACTICES FOR ORGANIZING THE INNER SPACE

Water is greater than food. Where there are no rains,
there will be a deficiency of food. When the great rains
appear, all beings are happy, knowing food will follow.
It is water in different forms that appear as God, earth,
atmosphere, heaven, mountain, men, animals, birds,
grass, trees, flies and ants. All these forms are only
water. Meditate on water.

—The Chandogya Upanishad

The entire universe expresses the energy of reform and reorganization during *Varsha,* the rainy season or early fall, which occurs in the months of July and August in the Northern Hemisphere. The atmosphere during this time of year is ideal for reassessing our inner worlds as we find ourselves naturally drifting inward. The mind is gently nudged to tune-in, take stock, and reorganize its inner space. Cloudy and rainy days have their own special qualities that invoke a desire to create a warm and safe space around us—a Living Ahimsa haven. Instinctually, animals and birds create shelters to retreat to during the rainy season. Lack of sunshine is accompanied by rain drenched days that tend to dampen the mood and lessen the spirit of enthusiasm and invigoration.

At this time, the digestive fire, which is naturally at its height during the summer months, can be adversely affected. By paying careful attention to your daily foods and activities, you can strengthen both digestion and emotional stamina. Ginger, garlic, pippali, black pepper, and lemon juice naturally kindle the digestive fire.

Early fall—called monsoon season in some parts of the world—brings much needed rains to the tropical regions. In Vedic tradition, *Guru Purnima* is celebrated on the full moon day in July, a festival in which the guru or enlightened Vedic spiritual teacher is venerated with an outpouring of love, devotion, and gratitude. This tradition dates back to ancient times with the introduction of the first guru—Veda Vyasa—the supreme saint who edited the four Vedas, wrote the 18 *Puranas*, the

the *Mahabharata*, and the *Srimad Bhagavata*. This time is considered most auspicious for disciples to reinitiate spiritual practices and lessons gleaned from their guru. The day is also widely celebrated by farmers and other stewards of nature as the advent of the monsoon season, which brings the life-generating showers that nourish the earth and preserve life.

When the monsoon season ends, sailors and fishermen in South India continue the ritual of gratitude by observing the festival of *Narali Purnima*. Coconuts are offered to appease the sea god Varuna and to show gratitude to him for the benevolent rains. In my tradition, the coconut fruit, which is used prolifically in Hindu ceremonies, is symbolic of the cosmic womb that produces prosperity and fertility.

The grand celebration of the rainy season continues unabated with the opulent veneration of Lord Ganesha. The birth of Ganesha—the beloved elephant-headed deity with his curving trunk, potbelly, and huge ears—is celebrated on the fourth day of the waxing moon of *Bhadrapada* (August-September), and generally lasts for 10 days. The transcendent Ganesha is beloved by millions around the world. In India, villagers sculpt clay figurines in Ganesha's image, and after two or more days of worshipping these figurines with oblations, they offer them to the holy rivers and streams—the Hindu way of completing a sacred intention by offering it into the water of life. Known for his power to remove obstacles from his disciples' paths, Ganesha is venerated at the onset of virtually every activity in Hindu life.

On the first full moon falling in August, the spirit of love and devotion culminates with the ceremony of *Raksha Bandhana*. This event is a means of strengthening family bonds, and a time when men and boys renew their traditional vows to safeguard their sisters. Young girls and women tie an amulet around the right wrists of their brothers as a token of affection and protection against negative forces. The amulet is called *rakhi* and is made from colorful threads of cotton or silk.

The season of the blessed rains are commemorated throughout the world. Native American Hopis show reverence and gratitude to nature at the end of the Kachina dances. Kachinas are supernatural beings that help to safeguard and protect the tribes. Young men who are considered to be pure of heart perform these dances in order to bring rain and healing energies to the whole community. And in Celtic tradition the *lammas*, the first loaf of bread to be baked from the harvest, is placed on the altar as an offering of gratitude to Mother Nature.

AWAKENING TO THE RAINY SEASON'S RHYTHMS

Aligning with the rhythms of the rainy season will help you achieve inner cleansing and physical and emotional realignment. Use the reforming energy heralded by this season to go indoors and reorganize not only your thoughts, but your physical living and working spaces. Clean out your files and closets, catch up on neglected paperwork, reorganize your home, (especially the kitchen and office areas) and as you do, reevaluate the choices you've made since the last rainy season, redirecting them as necessary. This is a great opportunity to reinvoke your intention to living a life of inner harmony and ahimsa. Since the entire universe is experiencing this vibration of reform, it helps your mind immensely to attune to and be in balance with the greater energies of the cosmos.

During the rainy season the earth releases more gases into the atmosphere, and this tends to aggravate Vata, the bodily air humor. Further aggravation is created by the dampness of the rains and the higher acidity in the water at this time. The rainy season comes at a time when the body is at its point of lowest vitality. Even though the rainy season marks the beginning of a period of strengthening, the body becomes vulnerable, and its resistance to the onslaught of the rains diminishes.

Vata-nourishing foods and activities are the magic balm to relieve typical rainy season symptoms such as: anxiety, arthritis, constipation, distension, emaciation, fearfulness, insomnia, memory loss, and nervous disorders. Vata may be nourished at this time by light, warm, sweet, and semi-unctuous foods. Brown rice, wheat, and barley are excellent grains for this season. Ayurveda recommends warm cow's milk with ghee and honey as the season's elixir (recipe on page 218).

Pitta, the body's fire humor, and Kapha, the body's water humor, are also moderately affected by excessive wetness. To remedy this, lessen your intake of fluids but drink warm stimulating teas such as mint, licorice, vetiver, and ginger. Seasonal vegetables such as beets, carrots, fresh sweet corn, daikon, and squashes should be well-cooked. Eat sautéed greens in moderation and reduce the consumption of beans during this season.

THE ENERGY OF THE RAINY SEASON				
PRIMARY ACTIVITY	PREDOMINANT TASTE	PREDOMINANT ELEMENTS	TIME OF YEAR	DOSHIC NATURE
Reorganization	Sour	Earth and Fire	Mid-to-late July through Mid-to-late September (Northern Hemisphere)	Kapha and Pitta
			Mid-to-late January through Mid-to-late March (Southern Hemisphere)	

Table 12.1

ORGANIZING THE INNER SPACE

As I mentioned earlier, the rainy season brings with it pelting down rains that force us indoors. Sitting inside listening to the hypnotic rhythm of the raindrops naturally cajoles the mind inward and can promote a spirit of comfort when we engage in the appropriate activities. Organizing your living and working spaces helps you gently transition into a calm and sheltered space within yourself where you can experience Living Ahimsa, the profound power of peace. When you apply yourself to clearing out the accumulated glut of old files, drawers, cabinets, and closets—and catching up on neglected paperwork—you will be surprised to feel an abundance of vital energy surging up from within. This vital energy helps you create the mental and emotional inner space to reevaluate your choices and redirect them as necessary; a great opportunity to make a solid investment in your future inner harmony. Your retooling activities at this time will garner potent harmonic support from the cosmos.

Bhastrika Breath~The Fire Power of Peace
The following Bhastrika Breath Practice is a perfect practice to do in the early morning before setting out to the reorganizational tasks at hand. *Bhastrika* is a Sanskrit word for "the bellows" used in a furnace, inferring that the prana, the universal life force, is to be vigorously drawn in and out of the bellows of the lungs in the same way that air is forcibly blasted into a furnace by a pair of bellows to increase the potency of the fire. This practice will energize your entire being and bring warmth and vigor to balance out the chill of the rainy season.

THE PRACTICE: FIRING UP THE BHASTRIKA BREATH

OPTIMUM TIMING: On the full moon day (generally 14-15 days from the new moon), in the early morning.
- **Northern Hemisphere:** On the 10th day of the waxing moon cycles, starting in mid-July and mid-August.
- **Southern Hemisphere:** On the 10th day of the waxing moon cycles, starting in mid-January and mid-February.

INSTRUCTIONS:
1. Sit in a comfortable posture facing east.
2. Deeply exhale the air from the lungs.
3. Take a quick and short in-breath, followed by immediately releasing a blast of air with the out-breath, or exhalation, through the nostrils.
4. For the 1st round of Bhastrika Breathing, release 8 successive short blasts of air with the out-breath, while making a sharp hissing sound.

5. Concentrate on the exhalation (out-blasting) of the breath. (Short intakes of breath will automatically occur in this process.)
6. For the 2nd round, place both hands overlapping on your belly, and this time out-blast the exhalation 12 times with successive rapidity.
7. Afterward, take pause and do alternate nostril breathing at a gentle and leisurely pace for two minutes.
8. Complete the exercise by doing a third round of Bhastrika Breathing by out-blasting the exhalation in successive rapidity 12 times.
9. End the practice with a few minutes of gentle alternate nostril breathing.

RAINY SEASON MOON FEAST

You will discover that in the swell of Living Ahimsa, everything you do counts, and every aspect of your life can be nourished by the foods you choose to eat. As you refine your breath force, your food preferences will change to meet your new awareness. The *Taittiriya Upanishad* states, "May the universe never abuse food, breath is food; the body eats food, this body rests on breath. Breath rests on the body; food is resting on food. The one who knows this becomes rich in food and great in fame."

The Magic of Masala

As you clear your spaces—both external and internal—celebrate the completion of your many long-neglected tasks with the superb sadhana of creating your own masala, or spice blend. Symbolic of the melding of peaceful spirit with body and mind, making masalas has been practiced as a Living Ahimsa art form of sadhana at the Wise Earth School for more than a quarter century. There we chant Vedic mantras and recite sacred intentions while grinding and pounding the spice seeds into aromatic and flavorful blends.

The making of masala is a metaphor for harvesting the spirit of ahimsa and maturing intelligence. The myriad aromas, sounds, tastes, and textures of the cracked spice seeds enliven each and every cell, tissue, and memory of being. In short, when you create a masala you are building the cosmic pillars for primal nourishment through food, breath, and sound. You are honing the vibration of the mind and resuscitating the spirit, bringing them into a state of heightened awareness. The nose becomes a direct route to consciousness; the eyes, the gateway to light; the ears, a pathway to peace. The tongue receives the blessings of flavors, and the sense of touch leads the way to reforming your experience. The more adept you become at this grand practice, the more you will be able to experience peace directly.

These Living Ahimsa food practices not only impart rasa, the pure taste of life, but also nourish and influence your life force. Every bite we eat and every motion and sound we make in the spirit of ahimsa invokes the Mother Consciousness— her vibration, energy, and memory. As you continue to make masalas, your self-expression will blossom. Soon you will want to create your own masala combinations from the vast variety of spice seeds available to you. Inquire into the spices of your own ancestry and use those spices to make magical masalas that will help you heal and reorder your ancestral memories. Invite your family and friends to share in this harmonious practice and together awaken the mother essence of healing—rasa.

THE PRACTICE: MASALA FOR A RAINY DAY— A CONTEMPLATIVE FOOD PRACTICE

OPTIMUM TIMING: On full moon day, or the day after the full moon.
- **Northern Hemisphere:** Mid-to-late July through mid-to-late September, or specifically on Guru Purnima day, the full moon day in July occurring at the mid-to-end of the month.
- **Southern Hemisphere:** Mid-to-late January through mid-to-late March.

Rainy Day Masala Ingredients:
2 tablespoons cumin seeds
1 tablespoon ajwain seeds
1 tablespoon yellow mustard seeds
1 tablespoon white peppercorns
1/2 teaspoon ginger powder
1/2 teaspoon grated nutmeg
1/2 teaspoon cinnamon powder
1/2 teaspoon clove powder

COOKING INSTRUCTIONS:

Begin by roasting the fresh seeds. Use a cast-iron skillet to roast one type of seed at a time for 2-3 minutes over moderate flame until they begin to crackle or pop. Roasting helps renew the energy and memory of the seeds. (Be careful not to burn the seeds.) Keep the roasted seeds in separate bowls, ready to be ground into spice powders.

Spread a large, colorful, natural linen cloth or mat on the center of your floor. Set out your paraphernalia: roasted seeds, a mortar and pestle, suribachi or grinding stones, and sit family-style in a circle. Grind the seeds (one kind at a time) in a clockwise motion. Allow yourself to become immersed in the circular movement of your arm. Be mindful of the heavenly aroma and sonorous resonance of each spice as it is ground. Also be mindful of the inner tranquillity you feel as you grind away the cares and fears of the day. Be aware of the rich taste this sadhana practice gives to your food.

Roast and grind the spice seeds before adding the ginger powder, grated nutmeg, cinnamon powder, and clove powder. Store in a sealed ceramic jar or glass bottle and use within a fortnight. The quantities provided in this recipe will last a family of 4 people about 1 week. See the wonderful masala recipes in the following chapter to create a rainy day feast for your family and friends. (Also see appendix three, "Seasonal Masalas," for additional delectable masala blends.)

Herbert's Story

By age 69, Herbert, a former politician, had developed Alzheimer's disease. Soon after, he also gradually developed an aversion to food. Sarah, his devoted wife of 35 years, was distraught to see her partner physically disappearing before her eyes. He had lost more than 100 pounds by the time Sarah came to see me about her husband's health. Determined not to allow Herbert to die of malnutrition, Sarah attended a Wise Earth Ayurveda & Living Ahimsa food workshop in New York produced by one of our instructors.

Our instructor advised Sarah not to force Herbert to eat, but rather to introduce the daily practice of grinding spices into their home. Like most individuals who first learn about Living Ahimsa practices, Sarah was clearly dubious. What our instructor suggested seemed a ridiculously simple regimen for healing such a complex condition as Herbert's. But the instructor cajoled Sarah into giving it a try. At this point she was willing to do anything to nourish her husband's health. So she went to the Indian grocer and purchased a mortar and pestle along with a variety of spice seeds including fennel, cumin, coriander, mustard, and cardamom.

She decided to perform her daily practice at about 4:30 each afternoon, a time she and Herbert would usually enjoy what was once his favorite tea—Darjeeling. After serving Herbert his cup of tea, she would dry roast a variety of seeds: coriander, cumin, fennel, and cardamom, then grind and mix them in a mortar. Usually, Herbert would be bent over in his armchair while aimlessly changing the TV remote from one station to the next. With a dejected spirit, he would remain inattentive to whatever Sarah was doing in the kitchen. However, by the fifth day of her routine masala practice, Herbert asked Sarah if he could help her with grinding the spice seeds. Sarah was shocked since Herbert was never interested in anything that had to do with cooking or being in the kitchen. She enthusiastically helped set up a grinding station so Herbert could grind away. He remarked on how much he loved the smell of fennel and coriander as he was grinding the seeds.

The next morning, Sarah seized the day by making an oat porridge with milk, maple syrup, and raisins, and served it for breakfast to Herbert. She skillfully placed a bowl of the freshly ground fennel and coriander on the table next to his porridge and sprinkled a few pinches on it. She was literally astounded when Herbert asked her to please sprinkle more of the aromatic condiment on his porridge. Herbert ate the porridge ravenously and continued to request the same breakfast each morning for about three months before asking for a change in the menu. Herbert told Sarah that the porridge reminded him of the scent of his grandmother who had migrated from Russia.

Herbert's story, like the stories of so many before him—Sita, Mary, Shelli, Jaya, Amy, to name a few—is a tribute to the powerful effects of Living Ahimsa studies. These individuals are among the thousands who have survived challenging health crises by leading a life of ahimsa. The magnificent simplicity of these awareness-building practices awakened in Herbert a sense of ancestral well-being, and therefore his memory of taste and desire for food was restored to some degree.

A LIVING AHIMSA MANTRA FOR GRATITUDE

As the benevolent protector of dharma—the cosmic laws of life—Lord Ganesha guides the devotee and the innocent onto the path of harmony. The elephant-headed cosmic force, also known as *Ganapati*, meaning "the one who many follow," rides a mouse as his vehicle. Ganesha's popularity is celebrated by millions of people from faith traditions around the world. Many interesting legends about the birth and the greatness of Lord Ganesha are found in the Vedas. He is known as the god of wisdom, prudence, and prosperity. Every activity in Hindu life begins with an invocation to Lord Ganesha who brings the spirit of gratitude to life within us and renders new beginnings auspicious.

One of the most powerful intentions we can maintain is the spirit of gratitude: for Mother Nature's rains, for the ancestors, for your guru, for the things that please you and the things that do not, for the gifts you recognize, and for those that you can neither see nor fathom. You can secure the impenetrable protection of Lord Ganesha and convert your sacred intention to foster gratitude into an immediate blessing by remembering to be grateful for *everything* in your life. The following is a mantra that serves to keep this intention alive. The ideal time for honoring Lord Ganesha is on his birthday (on the fourth day of the waxing moon cycle in August); however, this mantra can be practiced at any time and is effective at all times.

THE PRACTICE: MANTRA TO INVOKE LORD GANESHA

OPTIMUM TIMING:
- Early morning is the most auspicious time, although this mantra can be practiced at any time.
- For 10 days starting on the 4th day of the waxing cycle in August, not counting the new moon day. (Lord Ganesha's birthday occurs on the 4th day of the waxing moon cycle in August.)

INSTRUCTIONS:
- Facing east in the early morning, sit comfortably in a meditative pose and repeat the following mantra 108 times.
- To maintain the count without distraction, you are advised to get a Vedic Japa Mala, prayer beads, strung with 108 beads. (See instructions on how to use your Vedic Japa Mala on page 32.)
- Recite the following mantra:

Om Ganeshaya Namah
(Pronounced: OOM GAH-NAY-SHAH-YA NAH-MAH-HA)

Reverence onto Lord Ganesha

THE PRACTICE: RAINY SEASON MOON FAST

Ekadashi generally occurs twice monthly. It is imperative that you seize at least one opportunity to observe an Ekadashi fasting day in each month, and it is best if you can work up to observing 4 fasting days during each Ekadashi Fast.

OPTIMUM TIMING:*
Northern Hemisphere:
- 12 days following the new moon in July (not counting the new moon day).
- 11 days following the full moon day in July (not counting the full moon day); this brings you into August.
- 12 days following the new moon in August (not counting the new moon day).
- 11 days following the full moon day in August, Raksha Bandha (counting the full moon day); this brings you into September.

Southern Hemisphere:
- 12 days following the new moon in January (not counting the new moon day).

- 11 days following the full moon day in January (not counting the full moon day); this brings you into February.
- 12 days following the new moon in February (not counting the new moon day).
- 11 days following the full moon day in February, Raksha Bandha (counting the full moon day); this brings you into March.

*I highly recommend purchasing a Vedic Calendar to calculate the exact timing of the new and full moons for Ekadashi calculations.

Contra-indications: Do not fast during severe illness, menstruation, or while bleeding. The elderly and young children should also avoid fasting.

INSTRUCTIONS:

- On the optimum Ekadashi days noted above, begin a 4-day Rainy Season Moon Fast.
- Ekadashi generally occurs twice monthly and you must seize each and every opportunity to observe at least one Ekadashi fasting day in each month.
- Refer to instructions in The Practice: Observing a Fast on Ekadashi on pages 70-73.

This sacred lunar observance is practiced to reclaim your state of inner balance with cyclical rhythms, and thereby heal and nullify personal health and familial challenges. This fortnight of practice is aligned with the waxing and waning tempo of the moon. (Remember, if you are unable to complete a full fast try to observe a modified Semi-Fast, detailed on pages 73-77.)

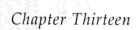

Chapter Thirteen

STIMULATING FEASTS FOR THE RAINY SEASON/EARLY FALL

Your Living Ahimsa feast for early fall is a magic balm of the season's best foods to invigorate the body, mind, and spirit into a solid sense of security and wellness. Stimulating curries, dhals, and a medley of moisture-replenishing cooked grains like: wild rice, millet, and buckwheat seasoned with ginger, scallions, rosemary, and thyme, are accented with warming, exotic teas, spiced tarts and nut cakes, and milk with ghee and honey—the elixir of the season. This pivotal season of the year invites you to take the necessary pause to strengthen your sense of security, confidence, and valor.

RAINY SEASON/EARLY FALL MENU PLANNING

Rainy Season/Early Fall:
• Northern Hemisphere: Mid-to-late July through mid-to-late September.
• Southern Hemisphere: Mid-to-late January through mid-to-late March.

Vulnerable Time: For Vata, Pitta, and Kapha Types*
• Vata: Avoid excess cold, dry foods, and astringent, bitter tastes.
• Pitta: Avoid excess pungent, salty, oily, and fatty foods, and intoxicants.
• Kapha: Avoid excess sweet, salty, cold, oily, and fatty foods.

* To learn your body type, see appendix one, "Wise Earth Ayurveda Body Types."

RAINY SEASON MENU: DO's & DON'T's	
APPROPRIATE FOODS FOR RAINY SEASON	FOODS TO AVOID IN RAINY SEASON
Sweet, moderately salty, and moderately pungent tastes	Sour, bitter, and astringent tastes

Warm, light, moist, moderately unctuous foods	Cold, dry, fermented, heavy foods, and foods in excess
Seasonal fruits and cooked vegetables; grains such as rice, wheat, and barley	Animal flesh products: meats, fowl, fish, and eggs
	Minimize consumption of cow's milk, honey, and ghee

Table 13.1

SAMPLE RAINY SEASON/EARLY FALL MENU

Rainy Season/Early Fall Breakfast:
- Kapha: Breakfast is not recommended.
- Pitta and Vata: See appendix three, "Breakfast of Champions," for a wide array of breakfast choices that can be enjoyed throughout the year.

Rainy Season/Early Fall Lunch:
- Wise Earth Fettuccini Primavera (p 206)
- Cardamom & Ginger Tea (p 217)

Rainy Season/Early Fall Dinner:
- Buckwheat Biryani (below)
- Early Fall Potato Curry (p 208)
- Ginger & Pear Chutney (p 209)
- Berry Heaven Tart (p 214)

*Gluten-free recipes are indicated by ♥

RAINY DAY GRAINS

BUCKWHEAT BIRYANI
Serves: 4
Biryani is a classic North Indian dish, generally made from rice, vegetables, nuts, and dried fruits.

1 cup cracked buckwheat
1 1/2 cups water
1 tablespoon sunflower oil
1 teaspoon cumin seeds

I teaspoon mustard seeds

I teaspoon Early Fall Masala (recipe on page 374)

I teaspoon coriander powder

1/2 teaspoon rock salt

I small russet potato, finely diced

I cup cauliflower florets, finely chopped

1/2 red bell pepper, finely chopped

2 tablespoons cilantro, minced

I teaspoon fresh ginger, minced

2 medium onions, finely chopped

Rinse buckwheat and drain. Bring water to a boil in medium-size saucepan. Add buckwheat, cover saucepan securely, and simmer on low heat for 10 minutes until all the water is absorbed. Heat sunflower oil in a large skillet or wok over medium heat and roast all the seeds for I minute until the mustard seeds pop. Quickly add the masala, coriander powder, and salt; lower heat and stir roasted spices for a few seconds. Add the potato, cauliflower, bell pepper, cilantro, and ginger, stirring frequently. Sprinkle in a palmful of water as you stir the mixture. Cover securely and continue to simmer on low heat for 5 minutes until the potato is cooked. Gently fold in buckwheat and serve warm.

BROWN RICE, SNOW PEA & RAISIN BIRYANI ♡

Serves: 4

I cup long-grain brown rice

2 cups water

I tablespoon olive oil

I handful rapini, finely chopped

I handful snow peas

I medium shallot, chopped

I tablespoon organic ghee (recipe on pages 150-151)

1/2 teaspoon black pepper, finely ground

I teaspoon cumin seeds

1/2 handful raisins

1/2 handful of raw almonds, slivered

12 strands of saffron

A few sprigs cilantro

Rinse the rice well and drain. Bring the water to a boil in a heavy pot. Put in the rice, cover tightly with a lid, and simmer over low heat for 35 minutes until the rice is firmly cooked. Be careful not to allow your rice to become sticky by overcooking. Heat the olive oil in a wok or large skillet, sauté rapini and snow peas over medium heat for a minute before adding the shallots. Cover the wok and steam cook on low heat for another minute or so. Heat the ghee in a small cast-iron skillet. When it starts to bubble, add the almonds, raisins, cumin seeds, and black pepper. Once the almonds turn light brown and the raisins begin to plump, remove from heat and let stand. Stir the saffron into the warm ghee mixture. Remove the wok lid, turn off heat, and carefully fold in the cooked rice with a large wooden spoon. Stir in the ghee mixture and garnish the biryani with a few sprigs of cilantro. Add rock salt or sea salt, if desired. Serve warm.

ROSEMARY WILD RICE ♥

Serves: 6

3 1/2 cups water
1 1/2 cups wild rice
1/2 teaspoon rock salt
1 tablespoon organic ghee (recipe on pages 150-151)
1 tablespoon olive oil
2 sprigs of fresh rosemary

Bring water to a boil in a medium-size saucepan. Wash the wild rice and add to the boiling water, along with the salt. Cover and simmer on medium-low heat for 35 minutes until the rice is tender. Drain excess water. Add the ghee, olive oil, and rosemary. Cover and let stand for 5 minutes. Mix well, and serve.

SOFT MILLET WITH GHEE ♥

Serves: 4

4 cups water
1 1/2 cups millet
1 tablespoon organic ghee (recipe on pages 150-151)
1/2 teaspoon rock salt

Bring water to a boil in a medium-size saucepan. Wash the millet thoroughly and add to the boiling water. Use a chopstick to keep the cover slightly ajar allowing steam to escape. Simmer over low heat for 20 minutes. Stir in the ghee and salt, and add water as necessary to prevent the millet from sticking to the pot. Remove from heat, cover securely, and let sit for 5 minutes before serving.

NUTTY BUCKWHEAT

Serves: 4

3 1/2 cups water
2 cups buckwheat groats

I teaspoon rock salt

I/2 teaspoon black pepper, finely ground

I tablespoon sesame butter

I/4 cup roasted pine nuts

I/4 cup parsley, minced

Bring water to a boil in a medium-size saucepan. Wash the buckwheat and add to the boiling water, along with the salt and pepper. Cover and simmer on medium heat for 15 minutes. Stir in the sesame butter, and continue cooking for 10 minutes. Remove from heat and let sit for 5 minutes. Garnish with roasted pine nuts and fresh minced parsley. Serve warm.

RAINY DAY KICHADI ♥

Serves: 4

3 I/2 cups water

I cup basmati white rice

I/4 cup split yellow mung beans

I cup quinoa

I teaspoon rock salt

2 tablespoons olive oil

I teaspoon grated ginger

I teaspoon cumin seeds

I/4 cup sesame seeds

Endive for garnish, finely chopped

Bring water to a boil in a medium-size saucepan. Wash rice and yellow mung and add to the water, along with the salt. Cover and simmer over medium-low heat for 5 minutes, before adding the quinoa. Simmer over low heat for an additional 7 or 8 minutes, or until the kichadi turns fluffy. Remove from heat, keep covered, and set aside. Heat the olive oil in a small skillet. Roast the ginger, cumin, and sesame seeds for a few minutes until they are golden brown. Gently stir the roasted seeds and ginger into the kichadi. Serve at once.

QUINOA WITH SPROUTED MUNG BEANS ♥

Serves: 4

2 cups water

I I/4 cup quinoa

I cup freshly Sprouted Mung Beans (recipe on page 118)

I tablespoon olive oil

I teaspoon coriander powder

1/2 teaspoon turmeric powder
1/2 teaspoon rock salt
1 tablespoon orange zest

Bring water to a boil in a medium-size saucepan. Wash quinoa in a fine sieve, then add
to the boiling water. Cover and simmer over medium heat for 7 minutes until quinoa is
translucent and cooked. In a large bowl, combine quinoa and sprouts. Over medium heat,
pour the olive oil into a skillet and add coriander, turmeric, and salt. Stir for a minute or so
before adding the orange zest. Fold the grain into the spice mixture. Stir and serve immediately. Garnish with finely chopped endive.

BLESSED BEAN FEASTS
RED LENTILS & QUINOA ♥
Serves: 4
1 cup red lentils
4 cups water
2 dried bay leaves
1/2 teaspoon salt
1 cup quinoa
1 teaspoon organic ghee (recipe on pages 150-151)
1 teaspoon cumin seeds
1/2 teaspoon fresh ginger, minced
1/2 teaspoon garlic, minced
1/4 cup fresh parsley, minced

Thoroughly wash the lentils. Bring water to a boil in a heavy-bottomed soup pot. Add the
beans, bay leaves and salt, and simmer over medium heat for 10 minutes. Wash the quinoa
in a fine sieve and add to the dhal (lentil mixture). Continue to simmer for an additional
5 minutes. Heat the ghee in a small cast-iron skillet, and roast the cumin seeds, ginger,
and garlic for a few minutes over medium heat until they turn golden brown. Remove from
heat and combine the ghee-roasted spices with the dhal by immersing the small skillet in
the soup pot (if possible). Cover and simmer for 3 more minutes. Garnish with parsley and
serve warm.

VADA WITH CILANTRO YOGURT SAUCE ♥
Serves: 2
Vada and amavada are made from ground dhal, spiced, and deep fried into golden patties.
Traditional to South India, the vada are made with urad dhal and the amavada are made
with toor or chana dhal. They are marinated in yogurt and served at religious ceremonies
and wedding festivities.

Vada:

1 cup urad dhal (Indian black lentils)

2 tablespoon shallots, minced

1/4 teaspoon black pepper, coarsely ground

1/4 teaspoon turmeric powder

1/4 teaspoon sea salt

1/2 cup sunflower oil

Soak the dhal for 1 hour. Drain and grind into a coarse paste. Add shallots, black pepper, turmeric, and salt. Shape into 1-inch balls and set aside. Pour the sunflower oil in a wok or frying pan, and heat over medium heat. When the oil begins to bubble, immerse the balls into the oil and deep fry them for about 3 minutes until they are brown on both sides.

Cilantro Yogurt Sauce:

1 cup plain yogurt

1/4 cup water

2 tablespoons cilantro, finely minced

2 tablespoons cherry juice

1 pinch asafetida

1/2 teaspoon of rock salt

Pour yogurt into a bowl and whip with an eggbeater. Slowly add water, cilantro, cherry juice, asafetida, and salt. Continue to beat the mixture until smooth and fluid. Place the fried vadas into the cool yogurt mixture, cover with a clean cotton cloth, and allow them to sit for 30 minutes. Serve with basmati rice.

CARDAMOM & SPELT UPPAMA

Serves: 2

Uppama is a South Indian savory dish made with cracked wheat, or farina (called rava or suji), combined with a variety of finely cut fresh vegetables and fragrant spices such as poppy seeds, coriander seeds, cloves, cumin seeds, cinnamon, and ginger. Finely chopped cashews or coconut may also be added to make a rich and nourishing uppama. This dish is a mainstay in the South Indian breakfast, although it may also be served for lunch and dinner.

1 cup cracked wheat, or farina

1 teaspoon olive oil

1/2 teaspoon mustard seeds

1 teaspoon urad dhal (Indian black lentils)

6 cardamom pods

6 curry leaves

1/4 teaspoon coriander powder

2 tablespoons fresh cilantro, minced

2 cups boiling water

Dry roast the cracked spelt in a cast-iron skillet and set aside. Pour olive oil in a separate medium-size saucepan, and brown the mustard seeds, urad dhal, and cardamom pods for a minute or so over medium heat until the seeds begin to pop. Add curry leaves, coriander powder, and cilantro, and sauté for 30 seconds. Add roasted spelt and stir. Pour in the boiling water, cover, and simmer on low heat for 25 minutes. Serve warm.

CARROT & PARSLEY UPPAMA ♡
Serves: 2

1 cup short-grain brown rice

2 tablespoons sesame oil

2 tablespoons urad dhal (black lentils)

1 red chili

1 minced onion

1/4 cup diced carrots

1/2 teaspoon brown mustard seeds

2 tablespoons fresh Italian parsley, minced

1/2 teaspoon ginger, minced

2 pinches asafetida

1/2 teaspoon rock salt

2 cups boiling water

Roast the rice in a large cast-iron skillet, and then coarsely crack the grain in a mortar and pestle. In the same skillet, add sesame oil and roast the dhal, chili, and mustard seeds over medium heat until the seeds begin to pop. Remove the mixture from the skillet and set aside. Place onions, carrots, parsley, ginger, asafetida, and salt in the same skillet, cover, and sauté the vegetables on low heat for 3 minutes. Then layer the roasted cracked rice over vegetables, add the boiling water, and do not stir. Cover and simmer on low heat for 30 minutes. Serve hot.

NOURISHING NOODLES

WISE EARTH FETTUCCINI PRIMAVERA
Serves: 6

1 pound thin spelt pasta

1 small bunch broccoli

1 small bunch spinach

2 small zucchini

2 medium carrots

1 tablespoon sunflower oil

1 lemon, freshly juiced

1/4 cup fresh parsley, minced

1/2 teaspoon coriander powder

1/2 teaspoon black pepper, finely ground

1/2 teaspoon rock salt

Bring a large heavy-bottomed pot of water to a boil. Add pasta and let it cook over high heat for 7 to 8 minutes until al dente. Strain and retain a small portion of the cooking water. Wash the broccoli and cut the flowers into tiny florets. Peel the usable portion of the stems and cut into matchstick pieces. Thoroughly wash the spinach, nip off a small piece from the ends, and discard. Scrub the carrots and cut them into matchstick pieces. Wash the zucchini and cut into 1/4-inch thick half-moon pieces. Blanch all the vegetables, except for the spinach, in the retained cooking water for 3 minutes. In a large bowl, combine the pasta, blanched vegetables, spinach, oil, lemon juice, parsley, coriander powder, pepper, and salt. Combine the pasta and vegetables, adding a palmful of the cooking water from the vegetables. Serve at once.

FARFALLE WITH RED BELL PEPPER

Serves: 6

1 pound farfalle (bow-tie pasta)

1 tablespoon sunflower oil

1 red bell pepper

1 small bunch chives, chopped

1 head radicchio, shredded

2 shallots, chopped

1/2 grapefruit, freshly juiced

1 teaspoon rock salt

1/4 cup roasted dried coconut

Bring a large heavy-bottomed pot of water to a boil. Add farfalle and cook over high heat for 7 to 8 minutes until al dente. Strain the pasta, running cold water over it to prevent it from sticking together, and put into a large bowl. Coat the pasta with the sunflower oil. Spear the pepper on a fork and scorch it over an open flame until it turns completely black. Run cold water over the pepper and then carefully peel off the charred skin. Cut the pepper in half to remove the seeds and then cut it into lengthwise strips. Add the peppers to the pasta. Introduce the chives, radicchio, shallots, grapefruit juice, and salt. Mix it together, garnish with roasted coconut, and serve at once.

SPELT NOODLES WITH MUSTARD GREENS

Serves: 6

1 pound spelt noodles

2 large handfuls mustard leaves and flowers

1 tablespoon walnut oil

1/4 cup fresh Mexican basil, minced

1/2 lime, freshly juiced

1 teaspoon dried lemon balm leaves

1/2 teaspoon black pepper, finely ground

1 teaspoon rock salt

1 teaspoon brown sugar

Bring a large heavy-bottomed pot of water to a boil. Add the noodles and raise the heat to maximum. Allow noodles to cook for 7 or 8 minutes until al dente. Strain the noodles, retaining a small portion of the cooking water. Wash and cut the mustard leaves in wide diagonal strips, chop the stems finely, and leave the flower shoots whole, if available. Blanch the leaves, stems, and flowers for 2 minutes in the retained cooking water. Strain and retain 1/2 cup of this water. Combine with noodles in a large bowl. Heat walnut oil over medium heat in a skillet and add the basil, lime juice, lemon balm, pepper, salt, and brown sugar. Mix for 1 minute before adding 1/2 cup of retained cooking water. When the sauce begins to bubble, remove from heat, and blend in with the noodles and greens. Serve at once.

CONTEMPLATIVE CURRIES & DHALS

EARLY FALL POTATO CURRY ♡

Serves: 4

12 English potatoes (small, yellow potatoes)

1 tablespoon coriander seeds

1 tablespoon ajwain seeds

1 tablespoon coconut oil

1 teaspoon turmeric powder

1/2 teaspoon cardamom powder

1 teaspoon cumin powder

2 dried red chilis

1 teaspoon rock salt

1/2 cup water

1/2 cup organic yogurt

Scrub the potatoes and cut into quarters. Dry roast the coriander and ajwain seeds for 2 minutes in a large cast-iron skillet until golden brown. Remove from heat and crush the seeds with a mortar and pestle. Heat the coconut oil in the same skillet, and add the seeds, along with the potatoes. Then add turmeric, cumin and cardamom powders, along with the chilis and salt. Stir and simmer for 3 minutes, before adding the water. Cover the pot and let simmer on medium heat for 15 minutes until the potatoes are very soft. Remove from heat and immediately fold in the yogurt. Serve at once over the Buckwheat Biryani with Ginger Pear Chutney (recipe follows).

GINGER & PEAR CHUTNEY ♡
Serves: 4
1 teaspoon black mustard seeds
1 tablespoon organic ghee (recipe on pages 150-151)
1/4 cup grated fresh ginger
1 cup firm Bartlett pears, peeled and thinly sliced
1/4 cup currants
1/2 teaspoon sea salt

Sauté mustard seeds in ghee over medium heat until they pop. Stir in ginger, pear slices, currants, and salt. Stir gently and cook over medium heat for 3 minutes or so until the currants swell.

SPICY CURRIED LENTILS ♡
Serves: 6
1 bunch broccoli florets
1 tablespoon organic ghee (recipe on pages 150-151)
1 tablespoon curry powder (recipe on page 134)
2 cups French lentils
1 teaspoon garlic, minced
1/2 teaspoon ginger, minced
1 teaspoon rock salt
7 cups warm water

Wash the broccoli florets and set aside. Melt ghee in a large saucepan, and roast the curry powder for 30 seconds until the ghee starts to bubble. Add the lentils. Stir, cover, and let simmer for 3 minutes. Add the minced garlic and ginger, along with the salt. Stir, cover, and simmer for 3 minutes more before adding the water. Allow to simmer on medium heat for 20 minutes until the beans are cooked. Add the broccoli florets to the dhal. Cover the pot and remove from heat. Serve warm over cooked a grain of your choice.

SWEET POTATO & MUNG CURRY ♡

Serves: 6

2 cups whole mung beans

4 medium sweet potatoes, diced

1 tablespoon black mustard seeds

1 tablespoon cumin seeds

1 tablespoon olive oil

1 teaspoon turmeric powder

1/2 teaspoon cardamom powder

1 teaspoon cumin powder

2 dried red chilis

1 teaspoon rock salt

10 cups warm water

1/2 cup yogurt (organic)

Scrub the potatoes, dice with skin on, and set aside. Dry roast the seeds for 2 minutes in a small cast-iron skillet over medium heat until golden brown. Remove from heat and crush the seeds with a mortar and pestle. Heat the olive oil in a large saucepan over medium heat, and add the seeds, along with the diced potatoes. Add turmeric, cumin, and cardamom powders, along with the chilis and salt. Stir and simmer for 3 minutes, before adding the warm water. Put in the mung beans, cover, and simmer on medium heat for 35 minutes until the potatoes and beans are thoroughly cooked. Remove from heat and immediately fold in the yogurt. Serve at once over cooked medium or long-grain brown rice or millet.

SPICY RED LENTIL DHAL ♡

Serves: 4

4 cups water

1 cup red lentils

2 dried bay leaves

1 teaspoon olive oil

1 teaspoon cumin seeds

1 teaspoon mustard seeds

1/2 teaspoon fresh ginger, minced

1 teaspoon green chilis, minced

1/4 cup fresh parsley, minced

Thoroughly wash the beans. Bring water to a boil in a heavy-bottomed soup pot. Add the beans, bay leaves, and salt, and simmer over medium heat for 10 minutes. Heat the olive oil in a small cast-iron skillet over medium heat, and roast the cumin and mustard seeds for a few minutes until golden brown. Add the minced ginger and chilis. Stir, remove from heat, and immediately pour the roasted spices into the dhal. Cover and simmer for 10 more minutes. Garnish with parsley and serve warm over bulgur or soft millet.

CELESTIAL SALADS & DIVINE DRESSINGS

ARUGULA WITH MUNG BEANS ♡
Serves: 4

1 bunch arugula
1 small bunch red leaf lettuce
2 large carrots
1 small red cabbage
1 cup mung beans cooked and warm
1/2 cup sunflower seeds, toasted

Wash and towel dry the arugula and lettuce, and tear into large pieces in a large wooden salad bowl. Scrub and coarsely grate the carrots, adding them to the salad bowl. Wash the cabbage and thinly slice it along the grain, after removing the core. Dice the core and, along with the cabbage, mix into salad. Add the mung beans and toss the salad. Garnish with toasted seeds. Serve with a dressing of your choice. (Dressing recipes follow on pages 213-214.)

CILANTRO & CHICKPEAS ♡
Serves: 4

1 bunch cilantro
1 bunch radicchio
2 cups chickpeas, cooked and warm
1 cup golden beets, finely grated
1 avocado, thinly sliced

Wash the cilantro and tear into bite-size pieces. Wash and towel dry the radicchio. Combine all ingredients, except the avocado, in a wooden salad bowl. Then arrange the avocado pieces in a swirling design over the salad. Serve with a dressing of your choice (pages 213-214).

BLACKBERRY & ADUKI BEANS ♡
Serves: 4

1 bunch curly endive
1 cup jicama, matchstick cut
2 cups aduki beans, cooked and warm
1 cup fresh blackberries

Wash the endive and combine with all other ingredients, except for the blackberries, in a wooden salad bowl. Wash the blackberries and gently place them over the salad. Serve with one of the delicious dressings from the next section.

APPLE & WALNUT LENTILS ♡

Serves: 4

1 large bunch romaine lettuce

1/2 cup currants, soaked in 1/2 cup hot water

3 golden apples, thinly sliced

1 cup carrots, matchstick cut

1/4 cup roasted walnut pieces

Wash and towel dry the lettuce and tear into large pieces. Strain the currants and reserve the soaking water. Combine apples, carrots, and walnut pieces in a wooden salad bowl. Serve with one of the delicious dressings from the next section.

YOGURT CABBAGE SLAW ♡

Serves: 4

1 large white cabbage

1/4 cup fresh chives, minced

1 teaspoon celery seeds

1 teaspoon cumin seeds

1 tablespoon poppy seeds

1 tablespoon fresh lime juice

3 tablespoons yogurt (organic)

1/4 cup soy milk

1 teaspoon kudzu or arrowroot powder

1/2 teaspoon rock salt

1/2 teaspoon white pepper, finely ground

Wash the cabbage and cut in quarters, lengthwise. Remove the core with a paring knife. Finely shred the cabbage lengthwise and then again crosswise. In a large bowl, combine the shredded cabbage and chive salad. Dry roast the celery and cumin seeds in a small saucepan for 3 minutes over medium heat until they turn golden brown. Then add the poppy seeds for 30 seconds or so until they begin to pop. Mix the seeds in the salad. Combine the lime juice, yogurt, and soy milk in the same saucepan and warm over low heat for 3 minutes. Thoroughly dilute the kudzu in 3 tablespoons cold water and pour the kudzu solution into the milk mixture, along with the salt and pepper, stirring it frequently until the sauce begins to thicken. Remove from heat. Toss the salad, coating it with the sauce. Cover the bowl and allow it to sit in a quarter of a sink full of cold water for 10 minutes before serving.

ALMOND VINAIGRETTE DRESSING ♡

1/2 cup currant water (reserved from soaking the currants)

1/4 cup fresh orange juice

1 tablespoon basil vinegar

2 tablespoons almond oil

1/2 cup toasted almonds, coarsely ground

A sprinkle of dried red pepper flakes

Combine all ingredients in a glass jar with a tight-fitting lid. Vigorously shake for 30 seconds or so until the dressing is mixed. Pour amply over salad and serve immediately.

ORANGE & BASIL DRESSING ♡

1/2 cup fresh Mexican basil leaves

1/2 cup warm bean water (reserved from cooked beans)

2 tablespoons fresh orange juice

1/2 teaspoon sunflower oil

1/2 teaspoon rock salt

Wash and mince the basil leaves and combine with other ingredients in a glass jar, secured with a tight-fitting lid. Vigorously shake the jar for 30 seconds or so until the dressing is combined. Pour onto the salad and serve warm.

TAMARIND DRESSING ♡

1/2 cup warm bean water (reserved from the cooked beans)

1 tablespoon sesame oil

1 teaspoon honey

A sprinkle of cayenne powder and black pepper

1/2 teaspoon tamarind paste, diluted in 2 tablespoons hot water

Combine all ingredients in a glass jar with a tight-fitting lid. Shake the jar vigorously for 30 seconds or so until the dressing is completely combined. Toss the salad with enough dressing to amply coat it.

SAVORY MUSTARD DRESSING ♥

I/2 cup warm bean water (reserved from the cooked beans)

I teaspoon mustard (organic)

I teaspoon sunflower oil

I teaspoon fresh lemon juice

A sprinkle of black pepper, finely ground

Combine all ingredients in a glass jar with a tight-fitting lid. Shake vigorously for 30 seconds or so until the dressing is completely combined. Toss the salad with enough dressing to amply coat it.

DISTINCTIVE DESSERTS

BERRY HEAVEN TART

Serves: 6

Sweet Tart Shell:

I cup unbleached whole wheat flour

I tablespoon unrefined brown sugar

I pinch rock salt

2 tablespoons sunflower oil

I/4 cup warm water

Filling:

2 cups fresh blackberries

I cup fresh raspberries

I/2 cup unrefined brown sugar

2 tablespoons arrowroot starch

I/8 cup cold water

I pinch rock salt

To make the tart shell, combine flour, sugar, and salt, gradually adding the oil. Use sufficient water to knead the dough into a firm ball. Roll out the dough into a circle, large enough to cover an 8-inch tart pan. Chill until the shell is stiff. If filling and crust are to be baked together, dough is now ready to be used. (If using a pre-baked pastry shell continue with the following directions.) Place shell in an oiled rectangular baking dish. Preheat oven to 370 degrees. Wash the berries and mash half of them into a pulp. Set aside the whole berries. Pour the mashed berries and sugar into a medium-size saucepan and bring to a boil on high heat. Dilute the starch in cold water and pour into fruit mixture, along with the salt. Reduce heat, stir frequently until mixture thickens, then remove from heat and set aside. Arrange the whole berries in the unbaked tart shell and pour the fruit mixture over them. Bake for 30 minutes until the edges of the shell turn golden brown. Serve warm with Almond Cream (recipe on page 260)

BANANA CREAM PIE ♡
Serves: 8

2 cups almond milk

1 teaspoon natural vanilla essence

1/4 cup maple syrup

1 teaspoon cardamom powder

10 ripe bananas

1/4 cup dried pineapple, unsweetened

3 tablespoons arrowroot starch

1/4 cup cold water

Prepare an 8-inch pre-baked Short Crust Pastry Shell. (See recipe on page 302.) Combine the almond milk, vanilla extract, maple syrup, and cardamom powder in a medium-size saucepan and bring to a boil on high heat. Peel the bananas and thinly slice them. Cut dried pineapple into tiny cubes and add to the boiling milk mixture, along with the sliced bananas. Dilute starch in cold water and pour into the milk-fruit mixture. Stir frequently until mixture thickens. Lower the heat, cover the saucepan, and allow the creamy mixture to simmer for 15 minutes until the pineapple is tender when pierced. Pour the banana-pineapple cream into the pre-baked pastry shell. Allow pie to cool for 1 hour before serving.

MILLET HALVA ♡
Serves: 4

1 cup millet flour

1 tablespoon walnut oil

2 cups water

1 teaspoon cardamom powder

1/2 teaspoon ginger powder

1 small handful of raisins

1 small handful of cashews, coarsely chopped

3 tablespoons honey

Heat a large skillet over medium heat and lightly parch the flour for 2 minutes until it turns slightly brown. Pour in the oil, water, spice powders, raisins, and cashews. Mix thoroughly, and let simmer on medium-low heat, for about 7 minutes, stirring frequently to avoid burning. When the mixture becomes thick, remove from heat. Blend in honey and serve warm.

WISE EARTH NUT CAKE

Serves: 8

2 cups spelt flour

I cup unbleached whole wheat flour

I teaspoon baking powder

1/4 cup sesame seed butter

3 tablespoons unsalted butter

1/4 cup unrefined brown sugar

I cup cow's milk (organic)

1/2 cup cinnamon tea

I pinch of rock salt

A few fresh mint leaves and slivered almonds, for garnish

Preheat the oven to 350 degrees. Sift the flours and baking powder together into a large mixing bowl. Cut in the butters and sugar and mix thoroughly with your hands. Pour in the milk and cinnamon tea, adding the crushed nuts and salt. Blend into a thick batter and pour into a deep, oiled baking pan. Bake for 35 minutes until a fork inserted in the center of the cake comes out clean. Allow to cool for 30 minutes. Arrange fresh mint leaves and slivered almonds, pressing slightly to dent top of cake. Serve warm with Cinnamon Mint Tea (page 140).

BLUEBERRY YOGURT CAKE ♡

Serves: 6

I cup soy flour

I cup chickpea flour

I teaspoon baking powder

1/2 cup plain yogurt (organic)

I tablespoon almond oil

8 drops natural almond extract

1/4 cup unsweetened blueberry jam

1/4 cup maple syrup

I cup fresh blueberries

Preheat oven to 375 degrees. Sift the soy and chickpea flours and baking powder into a mixing bowl. Pour in yogurt, almond oil and almond extract, and mix well. Add blueberry jam and maple syrup, and thoroughly blend the batter. Pour into a deep, oiled baking pan. Wash blueberries and arrange them on top of batter. Bake for 35 minutes until a fork inserted in the center of the cake comes out clean. Serve warm, with Cardamom & Ginger Tea (page 217).

BLACKBERRY KUCHEN ♥

Serves: 8

Topping:

1 cup fresh blackberries

1/2 cup grape juice

1/4 cup Sucanat

1/2 fresh lemon, juiced

Batter:

1 1/2 cups chickpea flour

1/2 cup soy flour

1 teaspoon baking powder

3 tablespoons unsalted butter (organic)

1/4 cup unrefined brown sugar

3/4 cup soy milk

Preheat oven to 350 degrees. Oil a shallow baking dish and set aside. In a small saucepan, combine all ingredients for the topping. Cover and simmer on medium heat for 5 minutes. Sift the chickpea flour, soy flour, and baking powder into a mixing bowl. Cut in the butter and mix thoroughly with your hands. Add sugar and soy milk, and stir into a batter. Pour batter into prepared baking dish and bake for 10 minutes. Pour blackberry topping over cake and bake for 20 minutes more. Serve warm with Raspberry & Clove Tea (page 218).

TEMPTING TEAS FOR A RAINY DAY

CARDAMOM & GINGER TEA ♥

Serves: 6

8 cups water

1 teaspoon fresh ginger, peeled and grated

10 cardamom pods

1/2 teaspoon cardamom powder

1/2 fresh lemon, juiced

Bring water to a boil in medium-size saucepan. Add ginger and cardamom pods, cover, and simmer for 5 minutes. Strain the tea and reserve roughage to use in your bath water. Add cardamom powder and lemon juice to tea. Cover and steep for 5 minutes before serving.

SAFFRON & ROSE PETAL TEA ♥

Serves: 6

8 cups water

1 small handful dried rose petals (organic)

12 strands saffron

1 tablespoon honey

Bring water to a boil in medium-size saucepan. Remove from heat and add rose petals and saffron. Allow to steep for 10 minutes. Add honey to the warm tea. You may serve with the petals or strain the tea and reserve the petals for your bath water.

RASPBERRY & CLOVE TEA ♥

Serves: 6

4 cups water

2 cups cow's milk (organic)

2 tablespoons dried raspberry leaves

8 whole cloves

1 pinch clove powder

1 pinch cardamom powder

1 pinch cinnamon powder

1 tablespoon unrefined brown sugar

Combine all ingredients in medium-size saucepan and bring to a boil. Reduce heat, cover, and simmer for 8 minutes. Strain the decoction, retaining the roughage for your bath water. Serve the tea hot.

MILK, GHEE & HONEY ELIXIR ♥

Serves: 4

1 cup water

2 cups whole milk

2 tablespoons ghee

1 tablespoon honey

Bring the water and milk to a boil in a medium-size saucepan. Remove from heat, add the ghee, cover, and let sit for 5 minutes. Stir in the honey directly before serving. Serve the elixir warm, an hour or so after dinner.

VANILLA & LICORICE TEA ♡
Serves: 6

6 cups water

2 cups soy milk

1 vanilla bean, split

2 tablespoons dried licorice root

1 tablespoon maple syrup

Combine all ingredients in a medium-size saucepan and bring to a boil. Reduce heat, cover, and simmer for 10 minutes. Strain the decoction, retaining the roughage for your bath water. Serve the tea hot.

INDIAN SPICED TEA ♡
Serves: 6

8 cups water

6 whole cloves

2 cinnamon sticks

1 teaspoon fennel seeds

2 star anise, whole

4 cardamom pods

Bring water to a boil in medium-size saucepan. Add all ingredients and reduce heat. Cover and simmer for 25 minutes.

Part Five

AUTUMN

I take The Vow of Ahimsa
To preserve the heart of peace and love

Chapter Fourteen

AUTUMN AHIMSA PRACTICES FOR HARVESTING NURTURANCE

The autumn comes, a maiden fair
In slenderness and grace,
With nodding rice-stems in her hair
And lilies in her face.
In flowers of grasses she is clad;
And as she moves along,
Birds greet her with their cooing glad
Like bracelets' tinkling song.
—Kalidasa

Autumn is the season of the harvest, reaping the fruits of your labor, and paying homage to Mother Nature by receiving her bountiful foods and honoring the ancestors and the spirit world. As the sun drifts away from the North Pole, the "Night of the Gods" begins. Daylight hours start to shrink, and light and darkness share equal time in the sky, a time we call the Autumn Equinox or "Equal Night."

Autumn, *Sharada*, occurring in the months of August and September in the Northern Hemisphere, is the most resplendent season, as she boasts a kaleidoscope of colors, textures, and sounds. Deep greens, burnt oranges, muted pinks, reds, and purples of the leaves, bark, and fruits are braced by the tinkling sounds of falling leaves or the brisk movement of clear waters in the rivers and streams. In northern climates, the entire landscape comes alive with clarity: The tall grasses hide a family of deer in the meadows, and the wheat and barley fields crisply ripen in the golden sun awaiting their profound sacrifice to the harvest. The earth opens her bosom and offers her bounty of Living Ahimsa food on a richly hued landscape. The frosty months are just around the corner, and a coolness of demeanor sets in. Autumnal browns, rusts, greens, and grays decorate the landscape as we take to safeguarding our health from the dramatic change of environment occurring within and without.

As the rainy season gives way to the glorious autumn, the Vedic culture commemorates the birth of Lord Krishna in the major celebration of *Janmashtami*. Krishna and his consort, Radha, symbolize the eternal and divine lovers. On this day, images of both deities are bathed and adorned with fineries after early morning ablutions. This occurs on the eighth day of the waning moon at the end of August or beginning of September.

Goddess Durga, the ten-armed celestial warrior, is celebrated in India twice a year in the festival of *Navaratri*, a practice I describe in more detail at the end of this chapter. According to Vedic lore, Durga rides a lion, plays the rattle drum, and defeats evil to protect her people. The autumn Navaratri celebration begins on the first lunar day of the waxing moon in *Ashvini*. Sacred grass, flowers, leaves, lamps, incenses, and grains from the autumnal harvest are offered in gratitude to the goddess for her protection. Barley is sprouted in clay pots and its sheaf worn on caps and behind the ears as symbols of the final day of Navaratri.

Harvest festivals celebrating the earth's abundance abound throughout the world in almost all cultures during this time. In rural areas farmers celebrate the harvesting of their crops in time-honored ways. In Lithuania, a community of people dance with the last sheaf of corn reaped. The corn is dressed as an old woman and danced around to bring blessings and good fortune. Among the Greeks, Althea, goddess of abundance, and Dionysus, god of the vine, are worshipped during harvest season. Sati, goddess of abundance, is honored in Egypt. The Basques worship Mari, goddess of the weather, and the Hindus give thanks to Saranya, goddess of the clouds.

The apple trees are laden with majestic fruit in the autumn, and picking apples is a feat celebrated with great fervor throughout the world. In Cornwall, England, it is believed that on October 27th, if unmarried women or men purchase Allan apples, tuck one under their pillow for the night, and eat it first thing the next morning without making a sound, their life partner will manifest shortly thereafter. After having eaten the apple, imbibers go outdoors in their nightgowns in the early autumnal morning light and stand under a tree, and the very first person of the opposite gender that passes by is believed to be his or her future spouse.

In mid-October, the Feast of the Ingathering, also known as the Feast of the Tabernacles, occurs among the Jewish people who honor the land's harvest. The celebration lasts nine days, during which families design a Sukkah (a booth made of leaves and branches) or set out a symbol of the holiday with parts of four different trees (a palm, willow, citron, and myrtle) within the home, reminders of living in accord with universal laws such as studying of the scriptures, doing good deeds, and leading a wholesome life.

AWAKENING TO AUTUMN'S RHYTHMS

The powerful influence of the moon during the southerly phase of the sun's movement is reflected in the moisture of autumn. From the Ayurveda perspective, accumulated Pitta from the rainy season becomes aggravated during the autumn season. This is a time when the digestive fire is already heavily taxed by the long, dry period of the previous phase when the sun has been focusing its attention on the northern hemisphere.

This moist heat of autumn is generally not conducive to good health. Ulcers, high blood pressure, strokes, paralysis, and diabetes are some of the conditions that prevail at this time of year. Special Pitta-reducing foods and activities are necessary during this season in order to maintain optimum health. Seasonal foods with sweet, bitter, and astringent energy that can assuage the Pitta dosha are recommended. Apples, barley, basil, buckwheat, cabbage, cauliflower, cilantro, cucumbers, dates, figs, kale, lentils, melons, mint, mung beans, pears, soybeans, spelt, squash, string beans, sugar snap beans, and thyme are a few Pitta-reducing choices of the season. Avoid hot, pungent, oily, and fermented foods such as yogurt, soy sauce, and alcohol at this time. Foods that are excessively alkaline in nature, such as salt, millet, radish, and ginger, should also be avoided. Avoid going outside where there is early morning dew. Daytime napping is also contraindicated during this season.

Autumn is the sacred season of the harvest. Give yourself permission to reap the benefits of the year's hard work. This is a good season to simplify your living and working spaces in order to provide yourself plenty of room to move, breathe, and practice the nourishing autumnal practices that follow in this chapter.

THE ENERGY OF AUTUMN				
PRIMARY ACTIVITY	PREDOMINANT TASTE	PREDOMINANT ELEMENTS	TIME OF YEAR	DOSHIC NATURE
Harvesting	Salty	Water and Fire	Mid to late-September through mid to late-November (Northern Hemisphere)	Pitta
			Mid to late-March through mid to late-May (Southern Hemisphere)	

Table 14.1

VIRECHANA—AUTUMN MOON CLEANSE

According to the principles of Pancha Karma, autumn is one of the two most vulnerable seasons of the year—spring being the other. Ayurveda recommends the entire body be cleansed of its cumulative ama (harmful toxins caused by dosha aggravation that can occur from season to season). It is essential to cleanse the bodily tissues during this season to prevent the build up of ama in the system. The ideal time for cleansing the body of its toxicity (using a cleansing routine such as fasting or purgation) is at the latter part of the season, when the doshas are in their most fluent form.

Because the human body maintains a delicate homeostasis, the sensible process of eliminating its manifested doshas, or wastes, is a systematic act of tempering, cajoling, and nurturing. Excess doshas are never forcibly removed from the body. In Wise Earth Ayurveda practice, we take into consideration the overall condition of the individual, the seasonal effects on the vital tissues, and the phases of the moon. Purgation therapy, or Virechana, one of the five profound therapies used in Ayurveda, is the process by which bodily wastes are effectively eliminated through the lower pathways of the body. A primary therapy for Pitta disorders relating to digestive issues and disorders of bile and blood, Virechana cleanses Pitta's main site—the stomach and small intestines. This practice is also good for clearing out excess Kapha from the stomach, which also aids the proper performance of Vata's air in that region of the body.

Virechana is an excellent autumnal bodily cleansing and revitalizing program. This purgation therapy helps to alleviate a plethora of conditions: abdominal distention, asthma, burning sensations, constipation, cysts/breast disorders, edema, excessive body heat, fever, gastrointestinal disorders, headaches, inflammation of the eyes, irregular peristalsis, jaundice, nausea, painful hemorrhoids, poisoning, swelling of the spleen or prostate, toxicity in the body, tumors, urinary problems, and worms/parasites in the intestines. Seasonal cleansing of the body in this way increases ojas, or immunological buffers, and therefore, increases stamina, prevents aging, relieves mental stress, and revitalizes the body, mind, and spirit. (For more details on seasonal cleansing and revitalization therapies, refer to my book *Ayurveda: Secrets of Healing*.)

The following autumnal purgation practice has been tailored to allow you to perform your seasonal cleanse at home. For an effective purgation, the minimal time of three days should be observed. However, if you can't take that much time out of your busy life, reduce the number of days and do the cleanse anyway. In order to get the most benefit from this cleanse, it's vital that a Semi-Fast accompany your days of cleansing, as follows.

THE PRACTICE: VIRECHANA HOME THERAPY CLEANSE

OPTIMUM TIMING: Mornings between 7:30–8:30 a.m. (Semi-Fasting required before, during, and after purgation.)

- **Northern Hemisphere:** For 3 consecutive days during the week prior to the first new moon in October.
- **Southern Hemisphere:** For 3 consecutive days during the week prior to the first new moon in March.

Semi-Fasting Contra-indications: Do not fast during severe illness, menstruation, or while bleeding. The elderly and young children should avoid fasting.

SEMI-FAST INSTRUCTIONS:

- For 3 days prior to the Virechana Cleanse, observe a Semi-Fast (see The Practice: Observing a Semi-Fast on pages 73-77).
- For 3 days during the Virechana Cleanse, Semi-Fast on only White Basmati Kichadi (recipe on page 74).
- For 3 days after the Virechana Cleanse, observe a Semi-Fast.
- You will be Semi-Fasting for a total of 9 days.

Virechana Purgation Contra-indications: Do not take this therapy if any of the following conditions exist: bleeding from the lower pathways; menstruation; strong abdominal cramps and pain (especially if it could be appendicitis); exhaustion; spasms or pain in the chest and heart; uncontrollable coughing; spasms in the limbs; or a prolapsed rectum. Do not take purgation after meals. Do not eat any solid foods until you have evacuated the system 3-4 times.

VIRECHANA PREPARATION:

Clear your work schedule for 3 consecutive days, take time to rest, and for 3 days prior to purgation, take a warm bath in the morning, towel dry the body, and do a vigorous rubdown of your body with warm sesame oil. This practice can be used continually during the cold seasons since it helps to cajole the mind and loosen tightness in the muscles while stimulating ama to flow out of the body.

Virechana Purgative Ingredients:

4 cups warm water

3 tablespoons Ayurveda medicated castor oil

I glass orange juice, freshly squeezed

4 lemon wedges, in case of nausea

VIRECHANA INSTRUCTIONS:

Do not take breakfast. Instead, drink 2 of the 4 cups of warm water. Prepare the fresh orange juice and set aside. Wait for a few minutes before taking the castor oil. To warm the castor oil, pour 3 tablespoons in a small bowl and place it in a larger container of hot water. Do not mix the oil in the water. Drink the oil and quickly chase it down with the remaining 2 cups of warm water. Afterward, drink the orange juice to help keep down the oil.

It is important that you lounge around indoors in a comfortable robe and keep a good book as company for the remainder of the day. After drinking the oil, do some mild indoor exercises like gentle walking about the house or light cleaning for about 15 minutes or so, until the oil is digested. Do not eat any solid foods until you have evacuated the system 3-4 times. Depending on your constitution, your timing for evacuation and number of eliminations will vary.

- Pitta types tend to respond faster to the purgative (within the first hour) and can have as many as 5-7 evacuations.
- Kapha types take longer to digest the purgative and may experience signs of nausea. Generally, Kapha types take about 2 hours before elimination begins.
- Vata types take the longest to move the bowels (as many as 3-4 hours) and sometimes experience no elimination whatsoever. They can expect to have 2 or 3 eliminations at the most.

If nausea occurs, drink a cup of warm water with the juice of 1/2 a lemon. Keep lemon or lime wedges handy. If nausea continues, suck on the wedges.

DURING THE VIRECHANA CLEANSE:

You will most likely experience a certain degree of emotional vulnerability:

- Pitta types tend to experience irritability or anger.
- Kapha types may feel sluggish or needy.
- Vata types may feel nervous, anxious, or fearful.

Allow these emotions to simply be what they are. Seek shelter in the privacy of your home or room and dress for the occasion—wear your most comfortable clothes, perhaps your favorite pajamas, robe, nightgown, or yoga outfit. The idea is to wallow in the comfort of being exactly who you are in the present moment. There is no one there to see you; the only witness is yourself. This is a perfect time for you to put your inner witness to practice by observing your emotions, thoughts, and feelings and simply letting them be what they are, where they are, without attempting to renegotiate or repattern them! Make a pact with yourself that this is your time, and let nothing intrude on your moment of being. Put away all gadgets, cell phones, laptops, etc. In between trips to the restroom, kitchen, and your couch, you may play soothing chants or music and songs that inspire you. You can catch up on journaling or simply rest and allow the mind to empty itself with the Cleanse. Drink plenty of warm water.

If you are a Vata type having difficulty eliminating, think of something really scary like a great big anaconda, or fierce lion rearing through the front door; Pitta types should think of something soothing like the serene surface of a lake glimmering in the early morning eastern light. Kapha types can keep down the nausea by reinforcing the idea of having your favorite sweets when this purge is over—keep a good stack of tissues close by and weep to your heart's content. And remember, doing this Virechana Cleanse once (in the autumn) or twice (in the spring and autumn) a year will safeguard your health for years to come!

To relieve stressful or negative emotional states experienced during your Virechana Cleanse, you may also refer to the Warm Teas for Semi-Fasting set out on page 73. Choose the teas that address your specific emotional requirement.

THE PRACTICE: AUTUMN MOON FAST

As you know, Ekadashi generally occurs twice monthly; it is imperative that you seize at least one opportunity to observe an Ekadashi fasting day in each month, and it is best if you can work up to observing 4 fasting days during each Ekadashi Fast.

OPTIMUM TIMING:*
Northern Hemisphere:
- 11 days following the full moon at the end of August, counting the full moon day (this brings you into September).
- 12 days following the new moon in September, not counting the new moon day.
- 11 days following the full moon at the end of September, counting the full moon day (this may bring you into October).

Southern Hemisphere:
- 11 days following the full moon at the end of February, counting the full moon day (this brings you into September).
- 12 days following the new moon in March, not counting the new moon day.
- 11 days following the full moon at the end of March, counting the full moon day (this may bring you into April).

*I highly recommend purchasing a Vedic Calendar to calculate the exact timing of the new and full moons for Ekadashi calculations.

Contra-indications: Do not fast during severe illness, menstruation, or while bleeding. The elderly and young children should avoid fasting.

INSTRUCTIONS:
- On the optimum Ekadashi days noted above, begin a 4-day Summer Moon Fast.
- Ekadashi generally occurs twice monthly and you must seize each and every opportunity to observe at least one Ekadashi fasting day in each month.
- Refer to instructions in The Practice: Observing a Fast on Ekadashi on pages 70-73.

This sacred lunar observance is practiced to reclaim your state of inner balance with cyclical rhythms and reclaim your grace with nature, and thereby heal and nullify personal health and familial challenges. This fortnight of practice is aligned with the waxing and waning tempo of the moon. (Remember, if you are unable to complete a full fast try to observe a modified Semi-Fast, detailed on pages 73-77.)

PITRI PAKSHA—NOURISHING OUR ANCESTORS

Amid the richness of harvest, the Vedic culture takes time to honor the ancestors. Ancestors play a significant role in the affairs of our lives. Although they have passed on, their energy continues to guide and protect our living relations, especially when we remember that we are forever at one with them. The rishis taught that prayers help our ancestors achieve the status of a *Pitri*, or Celestial Being. Once attained, this evolution also benefits us.

In Vedic tradition, every year rites are performed to honor the ancestors during *Pitri Paksha*, which occurs during the waning moon of *Ashvini*, in September and October according to the Western Calendar. Although we should honor the forebears at all times, in Living Ahimsa this ancestral season is the most powerful time to connect with the energy of the ancestors, as nourishment and oblations offered to them are most readily received. This observance, which I will detail in the paragraphs that follow, helps to revive within us the memory of our people and nourish the spirits of our ancestors. The practice involves two weeks of reciting special prayers, as well as offering grain, water, and milk to appease the ancestors. Portions of the food offerings are also given to the cows and crows, animal friends linked to the ancestral spirits. The last and most significant day of Pitri Paksha falls on the new moon, when prayers and offerings are deemed most necessary.

Perhaps there is an ancient link between Pitri Paksha and the Day of the Dead or All Soul's Day. Many cultures have different ancestral beliefs and observances that coincide with the turn of the autumnal moon. The Japanese people also venerate their ancestors at the Autumn Equinox. And among the Buddhists, this is a day to practice oblations to souls. They observe the practice of *Higan*, meaning "other shore," relating to the habitat where souls abide.

Offerings performed during Pitri Paksha are said to directly reach the ancestors because of a special boon granted to humanity by Lord Yama—the cosmic purveyor of death. The genesis of Pitri Paksha may be traced back to Karna, the renowned hero of the *Mahabharata*, who ascended to the celestial world after his death. He was rewarded with gold and silver for the charitable deeds he had done while on earth. Unfortunately, he had not performed any offering of food to the ancestors, or any act of generosity concerning food while on earth, and therefore he was rewarded no food in his celestial abode. Dismayed by this revelation, he prayed to Lord Yama that he may return to earth to recompense for his neglect.

Lord Yama did allow him to return to earth, but only for 14 days. During that short time, known as *Mahalaya Paksha*, he nourished the brahmins and the poor with a great abundance of food. As a result of this penance, Yama granted certain additional boons to all of humanity. By Yama's decree, all Pitri Paksha offerings performed in the world serve to benefit every departed soul.

According to the Hindu tradition, one of the highest universal laws is *Pitri Rina*, repaying our debt to the ancestors, which includes parents, grandparents, and spiritual teachers. Our ancestral lineages are not limited to those with whom we share a genetic heritage. Vedic seers have bequeathed humanity with a vast wellspring of knowledge and ceremony, which, when understood and practiced in rhythm with nature, serves to retain the memory of consciousness on earth.

At early dawn in India, millions of Hindus may be seen offering oblations to their ancestors in the holy rivers. Priests prepare sacred water as an offering to the departed souls with the chanting of specifically energized mantras. Customarily, the sacred water is poured from a spoon-shaped vessel called *kosha* into the Ganges, the sacred conduit through which the offering reaches the souls of the deceased forefathers. This ritual of offering water to the souls of one's predecessor is called *tarpana*. (In Hindu protocol these ancestral rituals are usually performed for the departed relatives by the eldest male in the family going back three generations.) Once you remember to honor your cosmic human obligation, you will discover your ancestral spirit manifesting in your everyday Living Ahimsa practice as grace, success, joy, and harmony.

HONORING OUR ANCESTRAL CONNECTION

The Vedic sages recognized that each of us exists as an interdependent being and that we are all linked to the universe through our ancestry. They predicted that the collective grief of the modern world would be caused by the loss of our ancestral memory; that human memory impairment would be the most crucial cause for the breakdown of dharma, the cosmic and social intelligence that guides and safeguards our Living Ahimsa values and purpose as they relate to the self, family, community, and nature. They understood that honoring the ancestors keeps us living in harmony with our forebears and the whole of humanity.

I believe the present state of chaos and restlessness in the world within and without has its roots in our relationship to the ancestors. As the principles of Living Ahimsa deteriorated in our modern lifestyle, so too did our connection to the energy of the forebears. Vedic tradition–like many native cultures–informs that the ancestors play a significant role in our daily lives. They have a vital connection with the world of the living since their subtle energy intimately presents itself to guide, inspire, and safeguard our progress and well-being on the earth. The *Taittiriya Upanishad* (verse 1.11.2) advises, "Let there be no neglect of the duties to the gods and ancestors. Be one to who mother is god. Be one to who father is god." Ancestors serve as the direct pathway to help us connect our earthly experiences to consciousness.

Honoring Ancestors is a dynamic methodology (part of the Wise Earth Ayurveda Inner Medicine program) based in the Vedas, which Hindu populations have been observing for thousands of years. For almost two decades at the Wise Earth School, we have been invoking this profound work to bring alive the requisite memories and indelible purposes that the ancestors serve in our daily lives. In restoring this significant ancestral work for the global community, I have pared it down to simple sacred intentions that all cultures can use.

I receive scores of letters each month from students and participants who recognize the importance of restoring ancestral memories as well as the necessity for doing these practices. I share one of these compelling notes from Linda, a Wise Earth instructor. One of her community members, Candice, had recently died from breast cancer. Linda held a memorial service for her during Pitri Paksha and invited Candice's husband, David, who knew very little about Vedic rites. Linda's sharing follows:

> Together, as a community, we chose to support our friend Candice's journey of the soul with this work. I thought Mother would like to hear the profound effect Wise Earth's ancestral practice had on David. He is a kind, sweet, and gentle man. He doesn't attend yoga or Ayurveda classes, so I wasn't sure how he would respond to the ancestral mantras or ceremony. I was certain, though, of his depth of love for Candice. We began with Mother's words, then a few words describing the purpose for gathering, and followed it with Wise Earth's meditation practice. Each person shared her beautiful memories about Candice before we recited the Pitris Mantra. You could feel the emotion of oneness, which created a supreme expression of love and support among us.

At first David was visibly uncomfortable, but softened as the evening progressed. He stumbled along with the chants. He watched carefully as each person came up and poured the sesame seed and water mixture into the bowl, and came up last and did it too. He was in tears as he offered the rite of nourishment for the peaceful journeying of Candice's spirit. Afterward, he looked deeply into my eyes. "Thank you so much," he said with such genuine warmth in his eyes. "I feel so much better.... I really feel so much better!" I could see the change in both his body and his energy. He was breathing more freely. His eyes were softer. He continued, "I am so relieved and happy to know I can support Candice's soul to move on and that I will not be holding her back. Every soul should have the support like this to move on! I didn't know there was such a thing I could do but I am so happy I do now. It is a great comfort and relief to me." David took the gift of a jar of black sesame seeds along with keen instructions on how to continue performing the ancestral nourishing rites at home for the duration of the Pitri Paksha season.

Thank you Mother for teaching this work; I am so grateful to serve in this way. I am so happy we are doing the Ancestor Conference again this year.

HEALING ANCESTRAL HURT—RECLAIMING CELESTIAL POWER

As we stand poised this autumn to enter the season of the ancestor, it is the perfect time to take pause, remember, and release memories we have had locked up within us. Release the ancestral patterns that prevent us from claiming our body, mind, and spirit of ahimsa, and reclaim our celestial power to heal and nourish. This is the perfect time to identify and let go of ancestral memories and inured habitual patterns that impede our happiness, health, and well-being.

As noted in my book *Women's Power to Heal through Inner Medicine*: "We are all healed. We heal in life. We heal in death. We heal in rebirth. And ultimately, we heal into consciousness." Remembering the ancestor is one of the most significant Living Ahimsa practices we can do to heal ancestral karmas. Healing is a subtle thing—it is initiated within us through our awareness. Healing has to do with our ongoing relationship to the earth, sun, moon, sky, water, forest, animals, children, and ancestors. In reality, we live in perennial initiation with our ancestors. What we love becomes part of our vital tissues, our immunity, and our destiny. Unfortunately, what we dislike or despise also becomes a part of our karmic anatomy.

In accord with Vedic tradition, we recognize that the profound power of healing must be applied to the spirit as much as it is to the body and mind, as all are intertwined. Through simple rites that honor our ancestors, we will find long-forgotten memories that have the potential to heal ourselves and our lineage. Each one of us has the capacity to utilize our own Inner Medicine, enter the vast cosmos within us, and become infinitely more conscious. Restoring these forgotten lessons of the ancestors immediately increases our awareness. Over the decades I have witnessed the miraculous healing of countless numbers of people; people who had suffered great losses or near-fatal diseases, and through their dedication to this practice, have repatterned and regained abundant blessings and life force.

At the recent Honoring Ancestors Conference that I hold every year, one of the participants—Stephanie, a 62-year-old woman—flatly refused to partake in the ancestral ceremony for nourishing her ancestors. She declared to the entire audience that she hated her parents who had both passed on, found them to be unloving and abusive, and saw no reason to "remember them, far less honor them! Why should I honor people I don't even like?" Stephanie is certainly not alone in this mindset of harboring familial grievances. I assured her that the more she kept the hatred and anger for her ancestors alive, the more space within her they would occupy. As my late father would say, "When we honor the ancestors we stand on their shoulders, and when we don't, we carry them on our backs!"

At first, she was reluctant to let go of the inured hurt which had inadvertently become a tenacious tenant in the inner abode of her heart, yet she consented to let me guide her through the rites of offering food to her ancestors. Afterward, she fell down to the floor in heart-wrenching tears. I picked her up and hugged her for a long time. In her ear I whispered, "I'm giving you 10 hugs for every hug you did not get from your mother and father." Because of her profound healing experience, Stephanie is now free from despair. Three months later, she lost 30 excess pounds without trying to lose weight, found a brand new job that inspires her, and can hardly wait for the next Honoring Ancestor Conference.

One of the most effective ways for us to immediately free ourselves from the devastation of ancestral hurt, illness, and despair is by repatterning hurtful memories into auspicious karmas. On every step of our journey, if we are to recover our ancestral memories, we are obligated to help ourselves and our predecessors heal the devastation that has spanned the centuries! At this significant time of the year when ancestors are energetically open to receiving nourishment, we have an incredible chance to remember them, and in so doing, to free ourselves from ancestral karmas of grief, disease, and despair. Vedic education teaches us rites of passage that transcend the boundaries of all traditions. They are easy to incorporate and use in our daily lives to bring forth healing, health, and spiritual freedom to our families and to ourselves.

Honoring ancestors helps us—through the exquisite practice that follows—to unearth traumas and past hurt that have been carried on through family lines. Like Stephanie, we can also free ourselves from carrying our ancestors on our backs. Because their memory patterns are deeply embedded within our vital tissues and cells, we continually reenact patterns that originated in the history and memories of our ancestors. When we do not recognize ancestral traumas, we are likely to ferry them into every aspect of our lives. Negative emotions, feelings of alienation from the Divine, restlessness, mental hyperactivity, and unhealthy food habits and cravings are all indications that ancestral memories may be blocked. The good news is that we can resolve our karmic history by honoring our ancestors; we can trade in hurt, grief, and illness for celestial guidance.

Open to spirit and learn the time-honored traditions for aligning with our ancestors and they will become our guides to experiencing joy, harmony, and prosperity. Once we reconnect to the memory of our present and past, we accelerate our Living Ahimsa sense of abundance and joy. Indeed, the kind cosmos provides us with many opportunities for healing; a perennial healing coming forth from remembering those who have come before us.

THE PRACTICE: OFFERING FOOD TO THE ANCESTORS

OPTIMUM TIMING: Pitri Paksha, the time of the ancestors.
Northern Hemisphere:
- The Ancestor's Moon begins with the last full moon that occurs either at the end of September or the beginning of October, and lasts for a fortnight ending at the new moon.

Southern Hemisphere:
- During the last full moon that occurs either at the end of March or the beginning of April, ending a fortnight later at the new moon.

In the warm and communal environment of your home, I encourage you to invite like-spirited friends and family to come together and perform this sublime practice to connect to greater joy and abundant healing. By performing this Vedic rite, you will dissolve untoward ancestral karmas and release energy that may be impeding you through angst and hurt. I especially encourage those of you who feel stuck or unhappy in your lives, or who may suffer from repeated illnesses with no apparent cause, to seize the precious opportunity that this time of year offers to reorient your psyche and reorder your life free from ancestral baggage and hurt.

INSTRUCTIONS:
1. Find a serene place outdoors in nature (preferably by a river) and sit facing south, or sit indoors at your altar facing south.
2. Facing south in the early morning light, recite the following Vedic mantra for ancestors at each offering, staying mindful of the welfare of your ancestors—known and unknown.

Om Namo Vah Pitrah Saumyah Svadha
(Pronounced: OOM NAH-MO VAPH PE-TRAS SAUM-YA HA SWA-DHA)
(saum as in "sour")

Obeisance to You, O Gentle Ancestors

3. Place one anjali (2 hands cupped together) of black sesame seeds in a brass or stainless-steel urn or pitcher dedicated for this use. (You may also use black rice, which may be purchased at gourmet or health food stores.)
4. Fill the urn or pitcher with 4 cups of water.
5. Mix the rice or seeds and water in the urn.
6. If making the offering indoors, place the urn in a large bowl into which you will be pouring the food offering. (The food offering takes about 10-15 minutes.)
7. Using your left hand, connect the tips of your thumb and index finger thereby forming a circle.
8. Use your right hand (even if you are left-handed) to pour the rice/seed and water mixture from the vessel through the opening of the circle created in your left hand. Pour the mixture slowly into the large bowl, or onto the earth, keeping in mind that you are feeding and nourishing your ancestors. While you are pouring the offering, recite the Vedic mantra for ancestors, noted above. Continue to repeat the mantra after the offering.
9. Sit in meditation and connect to the powerful energy of the Mother Consciousness.
10. Hold the mantra internally and let it float in your mind without deliberately reciting it.
11. Pray for loved ones who have recently passed on, and for the safe travel of their souls to the celestial sphere.
12. Visualize their entry into the abode of the Pitris, tantamount to heaven.

After the ritual, take the offering to a place where birds and animals can partake of it. Do not discard it in the garbage.

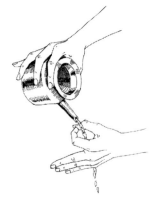

Figure 14.1 Mudra for Ancestral Food Offering

NAVARATRI—AUTUMN MOON FEAST FOR THE GODDESS

Your dedication to the work of the spirit follows with a splendid feast—the heart-fulfilling occasion of Navaratri—nine days of feasting and nights of celebration in honor of the Great Goddess Durga. The exquisite goddess is venerated in the form of the fierce warrior who safeguards her charges with tenacity; boasting 10 heads and mounted on top of her lion. This occasion begins at the end of the Ancestor's Moon, which is the new moon day in *Ashvini* (September-October). The following day, Navaratri begins.

Although during these nine days our attentions are especially attuned to the Great Mother, every day of the year is the goddess's day. For thousands of years Hindus have been honoring the Mother Consciousness in the lunar cycles of spring and autumn, as well as on numerous auspicious days in between. In energizing the body, mind, and spirit during your cosmic reward of the feast, keep in mind the purpose of this feast is to celebrate the immutable spirit of the Mother that nurtures us all at every moment. On each one of the nine days, invite friends, family members, and co-workers to join you in preparing and enjoying the Living Ahimsa feast of autumn. Create your feasts from the abundant Autumn Recipes set out in the following chapter.

THE PRACTICE: AUTUMN MOON FEAST FOR THE GODDESS

OPTIMUM TIMING:

Northern Hemisphere:

- 9 days beginning on the day after the new moon in *Ashvini* (September-October).

Southern Hemisphere:

- 9 days beginning on the day after the new moon in March-April.

INSTRUCTIONS:

- Before imbibing this Autumnal Moon Feast for the goddess made with delicious autumn recipes, gather your friends and family and venerate the Great Mother, asking for her protection by reciting the following mantra 18 times.
- Visualize the goddess Durga on her mount, the lion. (Durga champions the cause of the feminine and protects her charges with invincible strength.)
- Prior to imbibing the meal, it is a customary Vedic practice to offer the first "taste" of your meal preparations to the goddess. Offer the food with your right hand while chanting the mantra that follows:

Om Durgayai Namah

(Pronounced: OOM DUR-GAA-YAI NAH-MAH-HA)

My Reverence onto Goddess Durga

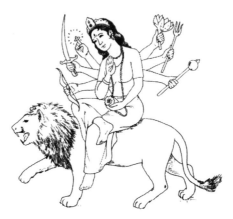

Figure 14.2   Goddess Durga Riding Lion

Chapter Fifteen

AUTUMN'S GOLDEN HARVEST

Autumn heralds the first signs of the frosty months that lie ahead, when nature's muted browns, rusts, and greens canvas the landscape with the rustling sounds of leaves and vivid light streaks down from the heavens. This season offers abundant, fragrant repasts as the warmth of summer days becomes a fleeting memory. Bountiful opportunities present themselves to apply Living Ahimsa practices in nature's garden and kitchen. Autumnal foods help safeguard health: apples, barley, basil, dates, figs, kale, lentils, melons, mint, mung beans, spelt, and thyme are just a few of the ingredients used to create scrumptious recipes such as Honey Mustard Mung Bean Salad, Peppery Purple Kale, Basmati Rice Pullau, and Heavenly Chai.

AUTUMN MENU PLANNING

The Autumn Season:
- Northern Hemisphere: Mid-to-late September through mid-to-late November.
- Southern Hemisphere: Mid-to-late March through mid-to-late May.

Vulnerable Time: For Vata Types*
- Avoid excess cold, dry, astringent, and bitter foods.

*   To learn your body type, see appendix one, "Wise Earth Ayurveda Body Types."

AUTUMN MENU: DO's & DON'T's	
APPROPRIATE FOODS FOR AUTUMN	FOODS TO AVOID IN AUTUMN
Sweet, bitter, and astringent tastes	Salty, sour, and pungent tastes
Sweet, cool, light, and fresh foods	Fermented, salty, excessively oily, and alkaline foods
Seasonal fruits, vegetables, herbs, beans, and grains such as barley, buckwheat, spelt, wheat, corn, and basmati rice	Meats, fowl, fish, eggs, and intoxicants

Table 15.1

SAMPLE AUTUMN MENU

Autumn Breakfast:
- Kapha: Breakfast is not recommended.
- Pitta and Vata: See appendix three, "Breakfast of Champions," for a wide array of breakfast choices that can be enjoyed throughout the year.

Autumn Lunch:
- Creamy Potato Casserole (p 253)
- Wise Earth Mesclun Salad (p 245)
- Wise Earth Fruit & Nut Compote (p 262)

Autumn Dinner:
- Cosmic Kichadi (p 241)
- Garlic Broccoli Goodness (p 246)
- Ganesha's Glorious Pudding (p 259)

Gluten-free recipes are indicated by ♥
Yeast-free recipes are indicated by ❶

HEAVENLY GRAINS

CREAMY RISOTTO WITH PURPLE KALE ♥
Serves: 4

1 small bunch purple kale

1 tablespoon sunflower oil

1 medium onion, sliced in half moons

2 garlic cloves, minced

1 tablespoon fresh oregano, minced

1 tablespoon fresh flat leaf parsley

1 tablespoon fresh rosemary

2 cups arborio rice

5 cups boiling water

1/2 teaspoon black pepper, coarsely ground

1/2 teaspoon rock salt

Wash kale, cut leaves into diagonal strips, and finely dice the tender parts of the stems (discard the hard ends of stems). Heat the sunflower oil in a wok or large skillet. Sauté the onions and garlic on high heat for a few minutes, being careful not to burn the garlic. Slightly bruise the fresh herbs and add them along with dried stems of kale to the onion and garlic mixture. Quickly rinse rice in water, and combine with cooked herbs. Cook the rice for a few minutes, stirring frequently, before putting in the kale leaves. Continue cooking over medium heat for 2 minutes before adding half of the boiling water (2 1/2 cups). Add pepper and salt. Cover and simmer gently over medium heat for 15 minutes or so, until all water is absorbed. Pour in remaining hot water, stir, cover, and continue to cook gently for 15 more minutes until the rice is firmly cooked. Because of the starchy nature of the arborio rice, your risotto will be moist and creamy.

COSMIC KICHADI ♡
Serves: 4

3 1/2 cups water
2 cups basmati white rice
1/4 cup split yellow mung beans
1 teaspoon rock salt
1 teaspoon sesame oil
1 teaspoon cumin seeds
1 head red oak lettuce

Bring water to a boil in a medium-size saucepan. Wash rice and mung beans, and add to the water along with the salt. Cover and simmer on medium-low heat for 12 minutes or until the kichadi turns fluffy. Remove from heat and set aside. Heat the sesame oil in a small skillet over medium heat. Roast the cumin seeds for a few minutes until they are golden brown. Gently stir the roasted seeds into the kichadi. Serve at once over whole lettuce leaves.

BASMATI RICE PULLAU ♡
Serves: 4
Pullau is a traditional rice dish of North India, made with a myriad of aromatic spices.

1 cup basmati white rice
1 1/2 cups water
1/2 teaspoon rock salt
1 tablespoon organic ghee (recipe on pages 150-151)
1 teaspoon cumin seeds
5 whole cloves
8 whole black peppercorns
5 cardamom pods
2 one-inch cinnamon sticks
5 dried curry leaves
2 medium red onions, chopped
12 saffron strands

Rinse rice and drain. Bring water to a boil in a medium-size saucepan. Put in rice and salt, cover tightly, and simmer on low heat for 15 minutes until rice becomes fluffy. In a large cast-iron skillet, dry roast all spice seeds, cardamom pods, cinnamon sticks, and curry leaves for a few minutes over medium heat until the cumin seeds turn golden brown. Add onions, cook, and stir until onions turn translucent. Fold in rice gently with a large wooden spoon. Remove from heat and mix in the saffron. Traditionally, the uncrushed spices are served in pullau—advise your guests to avoid eating them.

PEACEFUL PILAF ♥
Serves: 4

Pilaf is a traditional dish of North India, made from basmati rice, vegetables, and mildly spiced masalas.

1 cup basmati brown rice
2 cups water
1 tablespoon walnut oil
1 handful broccoli florets
2 small golden beets, cubed
1 medium red onion, chopped
3 mustard leaves, thinly sliced
1/2 teaspoon black pepper, finely ground
1/2 teaspoon red chili flakes
A few sprigs fresh parsley, for garnish
A few sprigs fresh burnet, for garnish

Rinse the rice well and drain. Bring the water to a boil in a heavy pot. Add the rice and cover tightly with a lid. Simmer over low heat for 35 minutes until the rice is firmly cooked. (Be careful not to allow your rice to become sticky through overcooking.) Heat the walnut oil in a wok or large skillet and sauté the broccoli and beets for a few minutes over medium heat, then add the onions. When they turn translucent add the mustard leaves, stirring frequently until the leaves turn limp. Cover wok and turn off the heat. Fold in the cooked rice with a large wooden spoon. Tear the parsley and burnet into pieces, and garnish the pilaf. Serve warm.

DELECTABLE DHALS
CLASSIC MUNG BEAN DHAL ♥
Serves: 4

1 cup split mung beans
1 teaspoon sunflower oil

1/2 cup white onions, finely chopped
1/2 teaspoon brown mustard seeds
1/2 teaspoon turmeric powder
1 tablespoon cilantro, minced
2 red dried chilis
1/2 teaspoon rock salt
1/2 teaspoon tamarind powder
4 cups water

Thoroughly wash the split mung beans (dhal) with your hands. Heat sunflower oil in a heavy-bottomed soup pot and sauté the onions over medium-low heat until translucent. Add the mustard seeds and stir for 30 seconds or so. Then add the turmeric powder, cilantro, chilis, and salt, allowing the spices to roast for 1 minute before adding the water. Cover the pot and bring the broth to a boil. Stir in the mung beans, cover and allow to cook over medium heat for 10 minutes. Then dissolve the tamarind paste in the dhal mixture, and continue to cook for an additional 5 minutes. Remove from heat and serve warm over cooked long-grain brown rice.

KARHI—CHICKPEA FLOUR SOUP ♥
Serves: 4
Karhi is a traditional soup of South India made from chickpea flour, yogurt, and aromatic spices.

1 cup chickpea flour
2 cardamom pods
2 one-inch cinnamon sticks
4 whole cloves
1 teaspoon brown mustard seeds
1 teaspoon whole black peppercorns
3 cups water
1 teaspoon coriander powder
4 dried curry leaves
1 teaspoon Sucanat
1 teaspoon rock salt
1 teaspoon fresh lime juice
1/2 pint plain yogurt, for garnish

Roast the flour along with the cardamom pods, cinnamon sticks, cloves, mustard seeds, and peppercorns in a large cast-iron skillet over medium heat for a few minutes until the flour turns light brown. In a heavy-bottomed soup pot, bring water to a boil. Add the flour and spice mixture, stirring frequently until the flour is dissolved and turns into a smooth milky soup. Add the coriander powder, curry leaves, Sucanat, salt, and lime juice to the broth. Cover and simmer on low heat for 20 minutes. Use a sieve to remove the uncrushed spices and discard them in your compost. Serve hot topped with a dollop of yogurt.

ADUKI DHAL ♥
Serves: 4
1 cup aduki beans
6 cups water
1 tablespoon coriander seeds
1 tablespoon sunflower oil
1 teaspoon cumin seeds
1 teaspoon brown mustard seeds
1 teaspoon unrefined brown sugar
1/2 teaspoon rock salt

Soak beans in 3 cups of water for 4 hours. In a heavy-bottomed soup pot, bring the remaining water to a boil. Add the aduki beans and discard the soaking water. Cover and simmer over medium heat for 30 minutes. Dry roast the coriander seeds in a small cast-iron skillet for 1 minute or so over medium heat, then coarsely grind them with a mortar and pestle. Heat sunflower oil in the same skillet and lightly roast the crushed coriander seeds and cumin seeds until golden brown. Add the mustard seeds. When they begin to pop, pour the spice mixture into the dhal by stirring the soup pot with the small skillet, if possible. Add the sugar and salt, cover, and continue simmering the dhal for an additional 20 minutes until it becomes thick. Serve over cooked cracked spelt.

HEARTY HARVEST GREENS
PEPPERY PURPLE KALE ♥
Serves: 4
1 large bunch purple kale
1/2 cup raw sunflower seeds
1/2 teaspoon rock salt
1/4 teaspoon cayenne powder
1/2 lime, freshly squeezed

Wash the kale and cut finely on a bias, using the stems as well. Steam kale for 3-4 minutes. In a separate cast-iron skillet, roast the sunflower seeds over medium heat until they are golden brown. Stir the salt and cayenne into the sunflower seeds and remove from heat. Squeeze the lime juice over the kale and remove lime seeds from kale (if any). Sprinkle the roasted seeds over the kale and serve over medium-grain brown rice.

WISE EARTH MESCLUN SALAD ♥

Serves: 4

Mesclun is a Provencal term for a salad mixture of greens and young, tender lettuces. Mesclun mix has become very popular recently in the big chain supermarkets and health food stores.

1 small head oak leaf lettuce
2 curly endives
2 tablespoons sunflower oil
1 lemon, freshly juiced
1/2 teaspoon black peppercorns, freshly ground

Wash and towel dry the lettuces. Tear them into small pieces and place in a large salad bowl. Pour sunflower oil, lemon juice, and pepper into a jar. Cover with a tight-fitting lid and shake to mix the dressing. Toss the salad with just enough dressing to coat the greens.

SPINACH & ONION SAUTÉ ♥

Serves: 4
2 bunches New Zealand spinach or baby spinach
2 large red onions
1 teaspoon sunflower oil
1/2 teaspoon black pepper, finely ground
1 teaspoon lemon juice, freshly squeezed

Wash spinach thoroughly. Soak the red onions in cold water for 5 minutes and then peel the outer skin. Roast the whole onions on a grill or open flame for a few minutes turning them frequently with a pair of tongs. When the outer layers of the onions become some-what charred remove from heat. Set aside to cool. Heat sunflower oil in a medium-size skillet and sauté the spinach for 2 minutes over medium heat. Cut the onions in half-moon slices, and add to the spinach, along with the black pepper. Cover and simmer on low heat for 3 minutes. Pour the lemon juice over the spinach and onions. Serve warm over cooked cracked wheat or bulgur.

GLORIOUS STEAMED GREENS ♥

Serves: 4
2 leaves of kale
3 leaves of collards
1 small bunch land cress
1 small bunch arugula
2 medium carrots

2 tablespoons sesame seeds

1 teaspoon mustard seeds

1 tablespoon sesame butter

1/2 teaspoon rock salt

1 teaspoon rice vinegar

1/4 cup hot water

Wash greens thoroughly, remove all stems and set aside. Tear the leaves into large pieces and finely chop the stems with a knife. Steam leaves and stems for 5 minutes. Scrub the carrots and coarsely grate them. In a separate cast-iron skillet, dry roast the sesame seeds for a few minutes over medium heat, until they turn golden and can easily be popped between the thumb and index finger. Remove the seeds from the skillet. Dry roast the mustard seeds for 1 minute until they begin to pop. Combine with the sesame seeds and coarsely grind in a hand mortar. Pour hot water into a small bowl and dissolve the sesame butter with the back end of a spoon. Add salt and vinegar. Toss the steamed greens, grated carrots, and partially ground seeds in a large salad bowl. Pour in the sesame butter mixture and serve as a warm salad over couscous.

GARLIC BROCCOLI GOODNESS ♥

Serves: 6

1 bunch white sprouting broccoli, with leaves

1 bunch purple sprouting broccoli, with leaves

1 bunch rapini

1 teaspoon olive oil

4 cloves garlic, finely minced

1/4 cup water

Wash the bunches of broccoli and rapini thoroughly, separating leaves from sprouts. Heat olive oil in a large skillet and brown the minced garlic for 2 minutes over medium heat, being careful not to burn it. Add the leaves and sprouts. Pour in water, stir, cover, and simmer for 3 minutes. Serve hot over mixture of cooked basmati white rice and quinoa.

CURLY GREENS CASSEROLE ♥

Serves: 6

1 bunch curly kale

1 bunch curly mustard

1 bunch curly parsley

2 cups boiling water

1 cup soy milk

1/2 cup chickpea flour

1 tablespoon dried rosemary

1 teaspoon dried thyme

1/2 teaspoon turmeric powder

1/2 teaspoon red chili flakes

1/2 teaspoon white peppercorns, finely ground

1/2 teaspoon rock salt

1/2 teaspoon sunflower oil

Thoroughly wash the greens and finely chop them, using the stems as well. Blanch the greens for 2 minutes in the boiling water. Strain the greens and retain the water. Preheat the oven to 400 degrees. Roast the flour in a separate large cast-iron skillet over low heat for a few minutes until golden. Add the dried herbs, turmeric, chili, white pepper, and salt, stirring frequently for a few minutes, until the aroma of the herbs and spices are released. Pour the soy milk into a large bowl and fold in the flour mixture until it is a smooth batter. Oil a large casserole dish and pour in the batter. Mix in the blanched greens, along with enough water from the greens to completely cover the vegetables. Bake uncovered for 25 minutes until the batter becomes crispy. Remove from oven and allow to cool for 10 minutes. Use a metal spatula to loosen the casserole from the dish and turn it over onto a serving platter. Slice and serve warm.

SAUTÉED PAK CHOI WITH ALMONDS ♡

Serves: 4

8 heads of pak choi (baby choy)

1 tablespoon sesame oil

1/4 cup raw almonds, blanched and slivered

1/2 teaspoon rock salt

Fresh basil, for garnish

Wash the pak choi and leave each head whole. Heat sesame oil in a medium-size skillet over low heat and roast the almonds for 2 minutes until golden brown. Add the pak choi along with a palmful of water and the salt. Stir, cover, and allow to simmer for 3 minutes. Remove from heat and serve warm over spelt pasta. Garnish with minced fresh basil, if desired

CAULIFLOWER CONFETTI ♡

Serves: 6

1 head purple cape cauliflower

1 head early fall ivory cauliflower

1 head alverda (lime green cauliflower)

1 tablespoon sunflower oil
1 tablespoon fresh ginger, minced
1 teaspoon coriander powder
1/2 teaspoon red chili powder
1/2 teaspoon cardamom powder
1/2 teaspoon cumin powder
1 teaspoon brown mustard seeds
1/2 teaspoon rock salt
1/4 cup water
Finely chopped fresh cilantro, for garnish

Wash and firmly break the cauliflower florets apart. Use a sharp paring knife to finely cut the florets and stems into small pieces. Steam the cauliflower pieces for 5 minutes. Heat sunflower oil in a large heavy-bottomed pot, and roast the fresh ginger and spice powders for 1 minute over medium heat, until dark brown. Add the mustard seeds and salt. When the seeds begin to pop, add the steamed cauliflower, stirring frequently. Add water, cover, and simmer on low heat for 5 minutes. Garnish with cilantro and serve hot over long-grain brown rice.

COCONUT & CABBAGE MASALA CURRY ♡

Serves: 6
2 heads Chinese cabbage
1 cup fresh coconut
4 green cardamom pods
1 tablespoon coriander seeds
4 cloves
1 two-inch piece of cinnamon
1/2 teaspoon rock salt
1 teaspoon coconut oil
1 small white onion, thinly sliced
2 green chili peppers, finely minced
1 teaspoon fresh ginger, finely minced
2 tablespoons water

Wash and shred the cabbage. Heat a small cast-iron skillet and dry roast the pods, seeds, and cinnamon stick for 2 minutes over medium heat. Using a hand spice grinder, grind all roasted spices along with the salt into a fine masala powder. Using the same skillet, dry roast the fresh coconut over medium heat for 3 minutes, until it begins to exude a sweet aroma and partially turns golden brown. Heat the coconut oil in a large skillet over medium heat and roast the masala powder in it for 1 minute before adding onions, chilis, and ginger. Stir the masala mixture for 2 minutes until onions turn translucent. Add the cabbage and sauté for 3 minutes, stirring frequently. Then stir in the roasted coconut and a few tablespoons of water. Cover and simmer over medium heat for 5 minutes until cabbage turns limp. Serve warm over cooked millet.

THE JOY OF CHOY ♡

Serves: 4

1 head bok choy

1 head gai choi (Chinese bok choy)

1 teaspoon sesame oil

1/4 cup raw cashew pieces

2 tablespoons currants

1 teaspoon fresh orange rind, grated

1/2 teaspoon coriander powder

1/2 teaspoon cardamom powder

1/2 teaspoon black peppercorns, finely ground

1/2 teaspoon rock salt

Thoroughly wash the greens, breaking them one stem at a time. Cut stems in large diagonal pieces, keeping the leaves whole. Heat sesame oil in a large cast-iron skillet and roast the cashews and currants together for 3 minutes over medium heat until the cashews turn slightly golden and the currants swell. Add orange rind, coriander, cardamom, pepper, and salt. Stir in the greens, leaves first. Sprinkle in a palmful of water, cover, and turn up heat slightly. Cook for 2 minutes before adding the stems. Cover again and simmer over low heat for 2 more minutes. Remove from heat and serve warm over long-grain brown basmati rice.

GRACIOUS GREEN BEANS

HARVEST BEAN MÉLANGE ♡

Serves: 6

1 handful golden beans

1 handful wax beans

1 handful pole beans

1 red bell pepper

2 tablespoons organic ghee (recipe on pages 150-151)

1/2 teaspoon black peppercorns, freshly ground

1/2 teaspoon cardamom powder

1/2 teaspoon cinnamon powder

1 lime, freshly juiced

1/2 teaspoon rock salt

Wash the beans and snap off the stringy ends. Gather a bunch at a time and cut diagonally in 3 pieces. Wash the red bell pepper and remove the stem and the core using a paring knife. Cut in half and then slice lengthwise in 1/2-inch pieces. Melt the ghee in a large skillet. Add pepper, cardamom, and cinnamon powders and roast in the ghee over low heat for 1 minute until the ghee begins to froth or bubble. Add the medley of beans along with the lime juice and salt. Sprinkle in a handful of water. Cover and simmer over medium heat for 7 minutes. Serve warm over medium-grain brown rice.

STRING BEANS ALMONDINE ♡

Serves: 4

4 handfuls young string beans

1 tablespoon sunflower oil

1/2 cup almonds, blanched and slivered

1/2 teaspoon brown mustard seeds

1 teaspoon cumin seeds

1 teaspoon coriander seeds

Wash the string beans and snap off the ends. Heat sunflower oil in large cast-iron skillet and sauté the almonds over medium heat, until they turn slightly brown. In a suribachi, partially grind the cumin, coriander, and mustard seeds to a coarse texture. Combine with the sautéed almonds, stirring frequently for about a minute or so. Add the string beans, sprinkle a palmful of water, then cover and simmer over medium heat for 5 minutes.

MESCLUN SALAD WITH SWEET SUGAR PEAS ♡

Serves: 4

1 small head oak leaf lettuce

1 handful fresh sugar peas

2 curly endives

2 tablespoons sunflower oil

1 lemon, freshly juiced

1/2 teaspoon black peppercorns, freshly ground

Wash and towel dry the lettuces and peas. Tear them into small pieces and place in a large salad bowl. Pour oil, juice, and pepper into a jar. Cover with a tight-fitting lid and shake to mix the dressing. Toss the salad with just enough dressing to coat the greens.

HONEY MUSTARD & MUNG BEAN SALAD ♡

Serves: 4

2 cups fresh Sprouted Mung Beans (recipe on page 118)

1 head bib lettuce

1 handful plantain or purselane leaves*

1/4 cup roasted peanuts, coarsely ground

1 lemon, freshly juiced

1 teaspoon sourwood honey

1 teaspoon yellow mustard seeds, freshly ground

1/2 teaspoon white peppercorns, freshly ground

1/2 teaspoon rock salt

2 tablespoons extra virgin olive oil

*Purselane is a tasty, tangy wild green

Wash and towel dry the sprouted mung beans, lettuce, and plantain or purselane leaves. Combine the peanuts, lemon juice, honey, ground mustard, white pepper, salt, and olive oil in a jar with a tight-fitting lid, and shake to mix the dressing. Toss the salad with just enough dressing to delicately coat the sprouts and leaves.

RESPLENDENT ROOTS

ROSEMARY NEW POTATOES ♡

Serves: 4

2 handfuls small red potatoes

1/2 fresh lemon

2 tablespoons fresh rosemary, finely chopped

1/2 teaspoon black peppercorns, freshly ground

1/2 teaspoon rock salt

1 teaspoon sunflower oil

2 handfuls mizuna greens, washed

Preheat oven to 350 degrees. Scrub new potatoes and cut into halves. Squeeze lemon over potatoes and remove fallen lemon seeds (if any). Toss potatoes with fresh rosemary, pepper, and salt. Amply daub a baking dish with sunflower oil. Pour in mixture and bake for 1 hour. Serve over the invigorating mizuna greens with a mixture of long-grain brown and wild rice.

DILL RUSSET POTATOES WITH GHEE ♡

Serves: 4

2 handfuls small russet potatoes

1 tablespoon organic ghee (recipe on pages 150-151)

2 tablespoons fresh dill, coarsely chopped

1/2 teaspoon fresh white peppercorns, crushed

1/2 teaspoon nutmeg, freshly grated

1/2 teaspoon rock salt

4 Belgian endives, washed

1/4 cup water

Scrub russet potatoes and cut into halves. In a large cast-iron skillet, melt the ghee over medium heat. Lay the potatoes face down in the skillet for a few minutes, until they are browned. Stir in fresh dill, pepper, nutmeg, and salt. Add water, cover, and simmer over low heat for 20 minutes. Pull the endives apart, leaf by leaf, and arrange in the shape of a flower on a serving platter. Pour the potato mixture in the center and serve warm over cooked basmati white rice.

REJUVENATING ROOT MEDLEY ♡

Serves: 4

1 handful red beets

1 handful new potatoes

1 medium parsnip

1 medium carrot

2 tablespoons organic ghee or butter (ghee recipe on pages 150-151)

1/2 teaspoon rock salt

1/4 cup flat leaf parsley, finely minced

Scrub the root vegetables and cut them into 3/4-inch chunks. Bring sufficient water to a boil in a large, heavy-bottomed soup pot to cover the vegetables. Add the vegetables, cover, and boil over medium heat for 10 minutes, until the vegetables are cooked but partially firm. Cook the beets separately in the same manner, to retain the individual colors of the other vegetables. Strain the vegetables and save the water for soup stock. Melt the ghee in a small skillet and pour over the vegetables, then add salt. Toss the parsley into the vegetable mixture and serve warm.

PURPLE POTPOURRI ♡

Serves: 4

2 heads purple cabbage

2 handfuls small purple potatoes

1 tablespoon sesame oil

1/2 teaspoon brown mustard seeds

4 dried bay leaves

1 teaspoon dried tamarind

I small bunch green onions
I/2 teaspoon rock salt
2 tablespoons hot water

Wash the cabbages and cut both in half along the grain. Use a small knife to remove the white stalks, then turn face down. Finely dice the cabbage stalks and scrub and dice the potatoes. Heat sesame oil in a large cast-iron skillet over medium heat. Roast mustard seeds and bay leaves for 30 seconds before adding cabbage and potatoes. Cover and simmer on low heat for 5 minutes. Soak the tamarind in the hot water. Wash and chop the green onions, discarding only the root fibers. Wash hands and pulp the soaked tamarind, discarding the roughage in your compost. Pour the tamarind pulp and water into the vegetable mixture. Add the salt, stir, and cook over high heat for 5 minutes. Garnish with green onions, turn off heat, cover skillet and allow to sit for 5 minutes. Serve over soft cooked millet.

CREAMY POTATO CASSEROLE ♥
Serves: 4
2 handfuls small golden potatoes
2 cups water
2 tablespoons olive oil
2 medium white onions, thinly sliced
I tablespoon fresh sage
I tablespoon fresh thyme
I teaspoon fresh rosemary
I teaspoon coriander powder
I/2 teaspoon black peppercorns, freshly ground
I/2 teaspoon turmeric powder
I/2 teaspoon rock salt
I cup soy milk
Mizuna greens, finely chopped for garnish

Preheat oven to 400 degrees. Scrub the potatoes and slice them into I/2-inch pieces. Steam or boil them in 2 cups of water for 5 minutes only. While they are still firm, drain and set aside while retaining the cooking water. Wash the fresh herbs and slightly bruise them. Heat I tablespoon olive oil in a cast-iron skillet. Sauté onions and herbs over high heat for approximately 3 minutes, stirring frequently. When the onions become translucent, add the spice powders and the salt. After I minute, remove from heat and add potatoes. Use the remaining oil to grease a 2-quart casserole dish. Spread the potato and herb mixture into the dish. Pour the potato water and the soy milk over the mixture. Bake uncovered for 25 minutes or until top of casserole is brown. Serve with mizuna greens over cooked long-grain basmati brown rice.

BLISSFUL BEET STEW

Serves: 4

2 handfuls golden beets, with green tops

4 medium carrots, with green tops

2 small new potatoes

1 teaspoon sunflower oil

1 tablespoon fresh basil, minced

1 small bunch shallots

1 tablespoon dried parsley

1 tablespoon dried oregano

1 teaspoon dried marjoram

1 teaspoon cumin seeds

1 teaspoon cumin powder

1 teaspoon rock salt

1/2 cup oat bran

1/2 cup quinoa

6 cups water

1 cup organic plain yogurt, for garnish

A few sprigs finely chopped fresh parsley, for garnish

Remove the green tops (if any) from the beets and carrots. Scrub them along with the potatoes, then cut into 3/4-inch pieces. Wash the green tops, remove the stems, and finely chop. Heat sunflower oil in a large heavy-bottomed soup pot over medium heat. Wash and coarsely chop the fresh basil and shallots. Sauté them in oil for 3 minutes before adding the dried herbs. When the shallots turn limp, stir in the cumin seeds and powder. Allow the seeds to turn golden before adding the root vegetables, stirring frequently. Cover the pot and cook vegetable mixture for about 3 minutes until it turns slightly brown. Add water and salt, cover, and cook for 15 minutes before adding greens. Continue cooking for 10 minutes, then add oat bran and quinoa. Lower heat, cover, and simmer for 10 minutes. Serve hot in soup bowls garnished with a dollop of yogurt and a sprinkle of fresh parsley.

BOUNTIFUL BREADS & MAJESTIC MUFFINS

WISE EARTH WALNUT DATE BREAD

Serves: 8 (3 loaves)

1 tablespoon unsalted butter

1/4 cup pitted dates, minced

1/4 cup walnuts, finely chopped

2 1/2 cups warm water

4 cups whole wheat flour

1/2 teaspoon rock salt

1 tablespoon natural yeast

1 tablespoon maple syrup

Melt the butter in a heavy skillet and lightly sauté the dates and walnuts for about 2 minutes, then set aside. Combine water, flour, salt, and yeast in a large bowl and stir until yeast dissolves. Stir in the date-walnut mixture then transfer the sticky dough into a large oiled bowl. Cover with a secured lid and let rise in a warm place for 40 minutes until it doubles in size. Punch down the dough and divide equally into 3 oiled loaf pans, brushing the tops amply with maple syrup. Bake at 425 degrees for 10 minutes. Reduce heat to 350 degrees and bake for 20 minutes more.

SCOTTISH OATMEAL BREAD

Serves: 8 (3 loaves)

2 cups boiling water

2 cups rolled oats (plus extra for garnish)

1/4 cup unrefined brown sugar

1/2 cup warm water

1 tablespoon natural yeast

1/2 teaspoon rock salt

1 tablespoon sunflower oil

2 cups spelt flour

2 cups unbleached whole wheat flour

Pour boiling water over the oats and let stand for 30 minutes. Combine the sugar, warm water, yeast, and salt, stirring until the yeast dissolves. Pour into oat mixture. Blend in the sunflower oil and flour and knead until smooth. Place in large oiled bowl, cover securely, and allow to sit in a warm place for 60 minutes. Then punch down the dough, cover, and let rise for an additional 60 minutes. Divide dough into three equal parts and place in oiled loaf pans. Sprinkle with oats and bake at 425 degrees for 10 minutes. Reduce heat to 350 degrees and continue baking for 20 minutes more.

CARAWAY & ONION BREAD

Serves: 8 (3 loaves)

1 tablespoon caraway seeds

2 tablespoons unsalted butter

1 white onion, minced

2 cups warm water

4 cups spelt flour

1/2 teaspoon rock salt

1 tablespoon natural yeast
1 teaspoon sunflower oil

Brown caraway seeds in a heavy dry skillet over medium heat until golden. Add butter. After butter has melted, add onions and sauté for 10 minutes on low heat until translucent. Set aside. Combine water, flour, salt, and yeast in a large bowl and stir until yeast dissolves. Add onion-caraway mixture and fold into the flour, mixing into a sticky dough. Transfer the dough to a large oiled bowl and cover with a secure lid. Let rise in a warm place for about 40 minutes until it doubles in size, then punch down the dough. Oil 3 small bread pans and divide the dough equally among them. Brush the tops of dough with oil, sprinkle with a few caraway seeds, cover, and allow to sit for 40 more minutes until the dough doubles in size. Preheat oven to 425 degrees and bake for 10 minutes. Then reduce heat to 350 degrees and bake for an additional 20 minutes.

YOGURT BUCKWHEAT BREAD
Serves: 8 (3 loaves)

2 cups warm water
1/2 cup organic yogurt
1/2 teaspoon salt
1/2 teaspoon black pepper
4 cups buckwheat flour
1 teaspoon sunflower oil
1 tablespoon cumin seeds

Combine water, flour, yogurt, salt, and pepper in a large bowl. Add the flour and mix into a sticky dough. Transfer dough to a large, oiled bowl and cover with a secure lid. Let rise in a warm place for about 40 minutes until it rises about an inch. Punch down the dough and divide equally into 3 oiled loaf pans. Brush tops of dough with oil, sprinkle with cumin seeds, then cover and let rise for another 30 minutes. Preheat oven to 425 degrees and bake for 10 minutes, then reduce heat to 350 degrees and bake for another 20 minutes.

CELERY SEED LEMON BREAD
Serves: 8 (3 loaves)

1 tablespoon sunflower oil
1 tablespoon ajwain seeds
2 cups warm water
4 cups whole wheat flour
1 tablespoon natural yeast
1/2 teaspoon rock salt

1/2 lemon, freshly juiced

1 teaspoon fresh lemon rind

Heat sunflower oil in a skillet and roast the ajwain seeds for a minute or so over medium heat until golden. Set aside. Combine water, flour, yeast, salt, lemon juice, and rind in a large bowl. Add the reserved ajwain-oil mixture and stir until the yeast dissolves. Transfer the sticky dough to a large oiled bowl. Cover with a secured lid and let rise in a warm place for 40 minutes until it doubles in size. Punch the dough and divide equally into 3 oiled loaf pans. You may sprinkle a few ajwain seeds on top of the dough before baking. Preheat oven to 425 degrees and bake for 10 minutes. Then reduce heat to 375 degrees and bake for 20 minutes more.

TAMARIND SUNFLOWER LOAF ♡

Serves: 8 (3 loaves)

1 tablespoon sunflower oil

1/4 cup sunflower seeds, unsalted

1 teaspoon tamarind paste

1 tablespoon boiling water

1 tablespoon natural yeast

2 cups boiling water

1/2 teaspoon rock salt

4 cups barley flour

Heat sunflower oil in a heavy skillet over medium heat and lightly roast the sunflower seeds until golden. Set aside. Dilute the tamarind paste in 1 tablespoon boiling water and combine with yeast, water, and salt. Stir until the yeast dissolves. Blend in the flour and transfer the sticky dough to a large oiled bowl. Cover securely and let rise for 40 minutes. Punch down the dough and then let rise for another 40 minutes until it doubles in size. Divide the dough equally into 3 oiled loaf pans. Bake at 425 degrees for 10 minutes. Then reduce heat to 350 degrees and continue baking for 20 minutes more.

BLACKBERRY MUFFINS

Serves: 6

1/2 pound unsalted butter

1/2 cup unrefined brown sugar

1 lemon, freshly juiced

1 teaspoon kudzu powder

1 cup cold water

1 1/2 cups spelt flour

1 teaspoon baking powder

1/2 teaspoon rock salt

1/2 cup fresh blackberries

Preheat oven to 350 degrees. Allow butter to soften then whisk with sugar until smooth. Add lemon juice. Dilute the kudzu powder with 1 cup of water and blend into the butter-sugar mixture. Sift flour with baking powder and salt. Gradually mix the flour into the butter-sugar mixture until a smooth batter forms. Carefully fold in the blackberries. Pour batter into an oiled muffin tin and bake for 20 minutes.

RASPBERRY MUFFINS

Serves: 6

1 tablespoon almond oil

1 tablespoon sunflower oil

1/2 cup maple syrup

1 orange, freshly juiced

1/2 cup warm water

1 1/2 cups soy flour

1 teaspoon baking powder

1/2 teaspoon rock salt

1/2 cup fresh raspberries

Preheat oven to 350 degrees. Combine the oils, syrup, juice, and water, then briskly whisk for a few minutes. Sift flour with baking powder and salt, gradually blending into the liquid mixture. Gently fold in the raspberries. Pour batter into oiled muffin tins and bake for 20 minutes.

CARROT ALMOND MUFFINS

Serves: 6

1 tablespoon sunflower oil

1 tablespoon organic ghee, softened (recipe on pages 150-151)

1/2 cup warm almond milk

8 drops natural almond extract

1 teaspoon cinnamon powder

1 teaspoon cardamom powder

1 cup water

1/2 teaspoon rock salt

1/4 cup almonds, crushed

1/2 cup carrots, grated

1/2 cup millet flour

1 teaspoon baking powder

Preheat oven to 350 degrees. Heat sunflower oil in skillet for 1 minute over medium heat. Add ghee, almond milk, and almond extract along with cinnamon and cardamom powders, water, and salt. Stir the mixture until blended and remove from heat. Combine the almonds, carrots, flour, and baking powder then carefully fold into the spiced milk mixture. Blend into a batter. Pour batter into oiled muffin tins and bake for 20 minutes.

VIRTUOUS DESSERTS

ALMOND CREAM ♡

Serves: 6

1 cup raw almonds

1/2 cup almond milk

1/2 cup water

8 drops natural vanilla extract

2 tablespoons maple syrup

1/2 teaspoon cardamom powder

1/2 teaspoon ground nutmeg

1 tablespoon arrowroot powder

3 tablespoons cold water

Soak the raw almonds in hot water for 1 hour until the skin loosens. Wash your hands and slip the almonds out of their skins. Grind almonds to a pulp using a medium-size hand grinder. Combine almond milk and water in a medium-size saucepan and bring to a boil. Blend in the puréed almonds, vanilla extract, maple syrup, cardamom, and nutmeg. Dilute arrowroot powder in the cold water and add to thicken the mixture. Stir frequently to prevent the cream from lumping. Serve over tarts, pies, fresh or cooked fruits.

GANESHA'S GLORIOUS PUDDING ♡

Serves: 4

2 cups chickpea flour

1/4 cup almond oil

1/4 cup warm water

1 tablespoon organic ghee (recipe on pages 150-151)

1/4 cup unrefined brown sugar

1/2 teaspoon natural almond essence

1/2 teaspoon cardamom powder

Mix all the ingredients together in a large bowl. Heat a large cast-iron skillet and pour in the batter. Cook on medium heat for 15 minutes, until the batter is slightly browned. Remove from heat, and let stand for 5 minutes before serving.

RICE DATE PUDDING ♥

Serves: 6

1 cup water

2 cups soy milk

1 cup cooked arborio rice

1/4 cup dates, halved and pitted

1/4 cup currants

1 tablespoon dried orange peel

1 teaspoon cardamom powder

1/2 teaspoon cinnamon powder

1/2 teaspoon ground nutmeg

1/2 teaspoon white pepper, finely ground

2 tablespoons Sucanat

Bring the water and soy milk to a boil in a medium-size saucepan. Add the rice, dates, currants, orange peel, spice powders, and sugar. Stir, cover, and simmer on medium heat for 25 minutes until the pudding is thick and creamy. Serve warm.

MOTHER'S APPLE TART

Serves: 6

Sweet Tart Shell:

1 cup unbleached whole wheat flour

1 tablespoon unrefined brown sugar

1 pinch rock salt

2 tablespoons sunflower oil

1/4 cup warm water

Filling:

2 Granny Smith apples, cored and thinly sliced

1/2 lemon, freshly juiced

10 saffron strands

1/4 cup maple syrup

To make the tart shell, combine flour, sugar, and salt, gradually adding the oil. Use sufficient water to knead the dough into a firm ball. Roll out the dough into a circle large enough to cover an 8-inch tart pan. Chill until the shell is stiff. If filling and crust are to be baked together, dough is now ready to be used. (If using a pre-baked pastry shell continue with the following directions.) Preheat oven to 400 degrees. Take an 8-inch Sweet Tart Shell and prick the bottom every 1/2 inch with a fork. Arrange the apple slices in layers on the crust. Sprinkle lemon juice and saffron over the apple slices and bake at 400 degrees for 8 minutes. Then pour the maple syrup over baked apples, lower oven temperature to 350 degrees, and continue baking for 10 minutes more. Serve warm.

CREAMY WHEAT RAISIN PUDDING
Serves: 4

1 cup Cream of Wheat
1/4 cup unrefined brown sugar
1/4 cup raisins
1/2 teaspoon turmeric powder
1 teaspoon cardamom powder
1/2 teaspoon rock salt
1 vanilla bean, split
1 cup water
12 saffron strands
A few crushed almonds

Preheat oven to 325 degrees. In a large bowl, combine the Cream of Wheat, sugar, raisins, turmeric and cardamom powders, and salt. In a small saucepan, combine the water and milk. Add the vanilla bean and bring to a boil. Remove the bean and pour the liquid into the Cream of Wheat mixture. Blend thoroughly into a fluid batter. Oil a shallow baking dish and pour the batter in. Sprinkle saffron and crushed almonds on top, then bake for 30 minutes until the pudding is golden brown on top.

WISE EARTH TAPIOCA ♥
Serves: 4

2 cups cold water
1/2 cup small bead tapioca
1 cup almond milk
8 drops natural almond extract
1 vanilla bean, split
1/2 teaspoon turmeric powder
2 tablespoons Sucanat
A few saffron strands, for garnish

Preheat oven to 400 degrees. Soak the tapioca in the cold water for 30 minutes. Bring almond milk to a boil in a medium-size saucepan. Add the tapioca and soaking water to the milk. Then add the almond extract, vanilla bean, turmeric powder, and Sucanat, stirring frequently to prevent sticking. Simmer on low heat for 10 minutes until the tapioca beads are completely transparent. Pour tapioca mixture into an oiled shallow baking dish. Bake for 15 minutes until the top of custard is golden brown. Remove the vanilla bean, garnish with saffron, and serve warm.

BLACKBERRY TART

Serves: 6

1 Sweet Tart Shell (recipe on page 260)

1 1/2 pints ripe blackberries

1/2 cup sugarless blackberry jam

Preheat oven to 350 degrees and bake the shell for 15 minutes until the edges are lightly brown. Cool on a rack. Arrange the blackberries on crust and cover with jam. Serve plain or with Almond Cream (recipe on page 259).

WISE EARTH FRUIT & NUT COMPOTE ♡

Serves: 4

2 cups water

1/4 cup apricots, halved and pitted

1/4 cup dried figs, thinly sliced

1/4 cup raisins

2 one-inch cinnamon sticks

6 cardamom pods

1 tablespoon unrefined brown sugar

1/4 cup pecans, coarsely chopped, for garnish

Bring water to a boil in a heavy-bottomed saucepan. Add all ingredients, cover, and simmer on low heat for 30 minutes until all the fruits are tender. Garnish with pecans and serve warm.

WALNUT PEAR CAKE

Serves: 6

2 tablespoons organic ghee (recipe on pages 150-151)

1/4 cup unrefined brown sugar

1/2 teaspoon natural vanilla extract

1 teaspoon cinnamon powder

1/2 teaspoon ginger powder

1/2 teaspoon ground nutmeg

1/2 teaspoon rock salt

1/2 cup spelt flour

1/2 cup water

2 large Bartlett pears, cored and thinly sliced

1/2 cup crushed walnuts

Preheat oven to 350 degrees. Oil and flour baking pan, set aside. Combine ghee, sugar, vanilla extract, spice powders, and salt in a bowl. Add a palmful of water and whisk the mixture until smooth. Gradually fold in the flour, adding the remaining water. Mix in the walnuts and sliced pears. Pour the batter into the prepared pan and bake for 30 minutes at 350 degrees.

RASPBERRY GLAZED APPLES ♡

Serves: 4

4 Red Delicious apples

1/8 cup unsweetened raspberry jam

1 teaspoon cinnamon powder

Preheat oven to 350 degrees. Cut the tops off apples and core them, being careful not to core through the apples. Fill each cavity with 1 tablespoon of jam. Sprinkle the cinnamon on top of the raspberry filled apples and bake for 30 minutes, until the apples are tender. Serve warm.

TRANSCENDENT TEAS & ELIXIRS

LEMON VERBENA & LAVENDER TEA ♡

Serves: 2

2 cups water

1 teaspoon lemon verbena leaves

1 teaspoon lavender flowers

1 teaspoon honey

Steep the leaves in 2 cups of boiling water. Cover and let stand for 5 minutes. Strain the leaves and sweeten with honey. Drink warm.

SUBLIME SPICED TEA ♡

Serves: 2

2 cups water

1 cup milk

6 cardamom pods

2 one-inch cinnamon sticks

1 pinch clove powder

1 pinch cayenne powder

1 pinch saffron strands

Fresh organic cream, for garnish

Combine water and milk and bring to a boil. Add cardamom pods, cinnamon sticks, and all spices then simmer over low heat for 5 minutes. Strain and serve warm with a dollop of cream, if desired.

PEPPERMINT & LEMON BALM TEA ♡

Serves: 2

2 cups water

1 teaspoon peppermint leaves

1 teaspoon lemon balm leaves

1 teaspoon honey

Bring water to a boil and add all the leaves. Lower heat and simmer for 5 minutes. Strain, add honey, and serve warm.

HEAVENLY CHAI ♡

Serves: 2

1 teaspoon black tea

1/2 cup soy milk

1 cup spring water

1/2 teaspoon cardamom powder

1/2 teaspoon cinnamon powder

1 pinch clove powder

1 pinch ginger powder

Add black tea to soy milk and water then boil for 20 minutes. Add cardamom, cinnamon, clove, and ginger. Stir and serve warm.

PEACEFUL PEACH LASSI ♡

Serves: 2

1/4 cup organic plain yogurt

1/2 cup organic cow milk

3 cups water

1 cup fresh peaches, quartered

I teaspoon Sucanat

A few drops almond extract

Place all ingredients in blender and blend for a few minutes until smooth. Serve at room temperature.

ALMOND & SAFFRON MILK ♥

Serves: 2 cups

1/2 cup almond milk

I cup water

I teaspoon orange peel

I pinch saffron strands

I pinch nutmeg

Bring milk and water to a boil. Add orange peel, saffron, and nutmeg. Simmer for 10 minutes on low heat. Strain and serve warm.

LAVENDER & SAFFRON MILK ♥

Serves: 2

2 cups organic cow's milk

1/2 cup water

I teaspoon lavender leaves

I pinch saffron strands

I pinch black pepper

Bring milk and water to a boil and add lavender leaves, saffron, and black pepper. Simmer over low heat for 5 minutes. Remove from heat, strain, and drink warm.

ENLIVENING AUTUMN ELIXIR ♥

Serves: 2

2 cups water

I cup milk

1/8 cup raisins

6 dates

3 figs

I tablespoon aloe vera gel

Bring milk and water to a boil and pour into a blender along with the other ingredients. Blend for a few minutes until the drink is semi-smooth. Use as an energy booster.

Part Six

EARLY WINTER

I take The Vow of Ahimsa

To stengthen my power of personal awareness

Chapter Sixteen

EARLY WINTER AHIMSA PRACTICES FOR STRENGTH & ILLUMINATION

To you each known delight,
Bring all that women count as worth
Pure happiness and bright;
While villages, with bustling cry,
Bring home the ripened corn,
And herons wheel through wintry sky,
Forget sad thoughts forlorn.

—Kalidasa

Hemanta, meaning "golden," is the Sanskrit name for early winter. This golden season when the earth is lit with its myriad hues of leaves, forest, and sky offers ample opportunities for us to gather our gold and store it within for the days ahead in the cozy cocoon of winter. Early winter affords us time to strengthen our inner reserves. Like the squirrels that know precisely when the moment arrives for their active scurrying and collecting of nuts, seeds, and sustenance for the cold winter to come, we humans can emulate this instinct of the little creatures and make a sadhana practice of stocking up on food supplies for the winter months.

Early winter brings with it an air of invigoration as the earth reveals her sweetness. The last leaves scatter on the earth as she is carpeted with colors of gold, bronze, burnt rust, and rich sienna. As the air becomes perceptibly thinner and brisker, a sense of fragmentation sets in as mind and emotion reflect the rapidly changing uncertainty of the season.

After giving thanks to the Mother for the autumnal harvest, we now must give our attention to conserving our resources and making provisions for the coming harsh winter. Our spiritual efforts are accelerated by the rapidly approaching snows, sleet, ice, and cold. Quiet efforts are enhanced as we complete unfinished tasks for the year, asserting a demeanor of frugality and practicality in all we do, while deepening friendships and family ties. Spiritual studies yield great benefits during this golden season, a time that naturally fosters the urge for quieting the thoughts and slowing activities.

Each season offers generous support for strengthening specific sadhanas in our cyclical lives. At this time of year, deepening Living Ahimsa practices such as Shanti Mudra (on page 57) and Living Ahimsa Meditation (on pages 28-31), help re-energize our commitment to harmony. In particular, mindful activities help bolster emotional fortitude and mental clarity. This is the perfect time to increase stamina through nurturing activities such as storing grains and dried beans; stocking root cellars; canning vegetables and fruits; preparing winter masalas; making warm sattvic meals; walking in nature; practicing yoga; sitting in contemplation; listening to the harmonious sounds of nature; and practicing drumming.

In India, the golden season is heralded by the Hindus in the lavish five-day long celebration of *Dipavali*, the festival of lights. Throughout the land, millions of lights are lit on cotton wicks placed in tiny clay bowls filled with ghee or oil. This celebration occurs on the last day of the waning moon in *Kartika* (October-November) in the Northern Hemisphere. The festival commemorates the victory of god Rama over Ravana, the malevolent king, symbolizing the triumph of universal and ethical principles over evil. Dipas, ghee lamps, were lit in the city of Ayodhya to welcome Rama's triumphant return home.

Dipavali is also associated with Lakshmi, goddess of prosperity and wealth. During this time the goddess is said to visit the homes of her devotees. Devotees clean and lavishly decorate their homes with flowers, fruits, colorful *papier mâché*, and earthen lamps to welcome her presence. In the evening she is also worshipped through sacred ceremonies.

Dipavali marks the coming of a new season—a time for family and community to reconcile their differences with each other. In southern climates this is also a season for sowing new crops. The golden light of Dipavali is a metaphor for cultivating personal awareness and consciously moving away from habituated negative behaviors and ignorance. Early winter is a natural time in the cosmic cycle of the seasons to fortify your connection to the Mother Consciousness.

The Dervishes, who belong to the Sufi religious order, use dance as a means to cultivate and accelerate spiritual awareness. In the early winter season, the Turks take in a week-long celebration to honor their Dervish tradition. They practice dance as a form of worship and spirituality to invoke their intuitive and cosmic powers. Dervishes gather in big cities and dance in spiraling groups in huge, circular skirts. The Turkish people honor this time with candy making and have a reputation for producing some of the best-known candies in the world. To quote the prophet Mohammed, "Love of sweetness comes from faith." Divine faith helps us all to cultivate a life of ahimsa—the loving care each and every person and culture requires to grow in consciousness. Sweet is the predominant taste of the early winter.

In this season, the Mayans gather to observe their festival of *Kukulcan*, named after their supreme god. *Kukulcan* means, "feathered serpent," and this god is depicted as a feathered water snake. He originated from Toltec myth, where he taught the

Toltecs fishing, healing, and agriculture, and gave them laws and the calendar. He is considered the god of birth and rebirth and also the god of arts and crafts.

Early winter offers a vast and wider view of the landscape, giving more chances to refresh the eyes with the sheer beauty of nature. The seasons are nature's children, and tree worshipping is a fitting activity to perennially celebrate nature. In Japan, venerations are given to one of the world's oldest trees, planted in 288 BCE during early winter. The Buddha is said to have gained enlightenment under the bower of its direct predecessor. Among the Japanese, the sun is also worshipped at this time with homage to Amaterasu, the goddess who is said to be the sister of the moon. Saffron colored rice and bamboo shoots are offered to the sun in her honor.

According to the Vedic Calendar, the actual winter solstice occurs on the eleventh day of the waning moon of *Margashirsha* (November-December). Popularly celebrated on December 21st of each year around the world, the winter solstice commemorates the awakening of the gods from six months of slumber. On this day, offerings of rice, ghee, milk, and jaggery (raw sugar) are made to the gods. True to the Vedic spirit of love, cows and oxen are anointed with fragrant water and sandalwood paste is applied to their horns. Black cows and oxen are adorned with sacred grasses, fruits, and garlands made of flowers, and then led through the streets of the villages to bestow blessings and good fortune on the villagers. Spiritual aspirants observe fasting and prayers for the day. Brahmins, the spiritual guardians of Hinduism, are offered gold, silver, and other fine gifts so that the giver is ensured a peaceful and prestigious life.

AWAKENING TO EARLY WINTER'S RHYTHMS

Strength, vitality, and appetite are enforced during the early winter season. Our digestive fire is generally fortified because the fire element is strong in the atmosphere, and we are able to eat and digest larger quantities of food. Plenty of wholesome, immunity-building, unctuous foods are required at this time: cooked fruits, soft-cooked whole grains, milk beverages, honey, ghee, butter, and yogurt. Bean soups are also highly recommended for this cool and brisk season. Winter grains such as buckwheat, corn, millet, and wheat are also powerful stabilizers for the body and mind. Eating plenty of beans is necessary to compensate for the diminishing vegetables and greens on the good earth in northern climates. Seasonal root vegetables (carrots, beets, turnips, potatoes, onions, shallots, and leeks) as well as low to the ground vegetables (pumpkins, winter squashes, and parsnips) are the healing foods of the season. Many greens such as beet greens, broccoli, broccoli rabe, cabbage, endive, kale, lettuce, spinach, and turnip greens still avail themselves until the end of early winter. Imbibing small quantities of the Ayurveda rejuvenating tonic *Drakshadi*—a medicinal grape "wine" that stimulates vital tissue function—is recommended at this time.

Warm baths with fragrant essential oils, oil massages, and steam baths are the rejuvenating Living Ahimsa practices that help the body and mind relax into the quietude of the season. Walks in nature, yoga, and other healing exercises are also recommended at this time. Early winter is the time for building the foundation for good health that will last the whole year ahead. This season induces sound sleep, clarity of mind, and bodily strength—all qualities to be savored in this over-driven 21st century of profound stress and modernity. The energy of sweetness during this season makes this a perfect juncture for loving and caring activities like cohabitation, conscious family planning, and intimate sharing that strengthen the marital bond and deepen commitment.

THE ENERGY OF EARLY WINTER				
PRIMARY ACTIVITY	PREDOMINANT TASTE	PREDOMINANT ELEMENTS	TIME OF YEAR	DOSHIC NATURE
Gathering	Sweet	Water and Earth	Mid-to-late November through mid-to-late January (Northern Hemisphere)	Kapha
			Mid-to-late May through mid-to-late July (Southern Hemisphere)	

Table 16.1

EARLY WINTER PRACTICE: GATHERING WISDOM & STRENGTH

Among the months, I am Margashirsha (November-December).
—Lord Krishna

Dipavali–The Season of Light

As I mentioned earlier in this chapter, *Dipavali* or *Diwali*, as it is commonly called, is known as the Festival of Light. It is a five-day celebration that falls on the fifteenth day of the waning moon cycle at the beginning of early winter, which is the new moon in early November in the Northern Hemisphere. We celebrate light during Dipavali as a symbol of the "light of knowledge" we seek to acquire that will free us from personal ignorance and the dark energies of prejudice, hatred, ill will, despair, and poverty. It is a time for embracing our shared sense of humanity when an abundant feeling of lightness and human goodness overtakes us.

Various origins are attributed to this festival: It celebrates the marriage of Goddess Lakshmi and Lord Vishnu; commemorates the auspicious day on which the triumphant Lord Rama returned to Ayodhya after defeating the demon, Ravana; and in Bengal, Dipavali is dedicated to the worship of Kali, the fierce warrior goddess that eradicates evil and restores justice.

Waking up during *Brahmamuhurta*—the 4:00 a.m. time period Hindus deem astrologically most auspicious—is the perfect hour of the day to easily access cosmic energies and receive infinite blessings, and therefore the best way to prepare for the day's festivities. Following the customary purifying oil bath, we don new clothing and offer abundant prayers and meditations for the health, welfare, and harmony of all people. That evening, there are dazzling firework displays which represent the burning of effigies of the demon Narakasura, killed by Lord Krishna on this day. Infinite rows of ghee or oil lamps are lit on the altars and windowsills of every home to invoke the spirit of inner illumination. These Vedic rites and celebrations are metaphors for illuminating the inner self—acquiring greater consciousness and attaining personal wisdom.

ILLUMINATING THE SELF

As you have been learning, meditation–a central practice in Living Ahimsa–reveals the workings of the mind in ways that allow us to guide our thought processes into a state of harmony. The focus of the following practice is to cultivate an awareness of the light of consciousness within. It is the faculty of our awareness that sheds light on all things external. As you begin to foster the knowledge of who you truly are and experience the lightness and intelligence that exist within your primordial core, you will witness your perspectives changing and your attitudes shifting. Your life will transform as you become attuned to your own finer, lighter vibration. The meditation practice that follows will help you explore, develop, and expand your mind's focus on your inner light. In short, you will recognize that you are the primal source of illumination.

The Sanskrit word for meditation is *dhyanam*, meaning "discern, measure, ponder, or contemplate." Ultimately meditation enables us to be free from all the limitations and standards by which we measure ourselves. It is the primary means for cultivating a heightened sense of personal and cosmic awareness and for connecting to the pure reality of our individual purpose. The early winter climate provides a profoundly peaceful time for collecting our thoughts, calming our mind and senses, and striving to bring everything in our lives into perfect communion. Take advantage of this priceless moment in time!

VASTU YANTRA—ILLUMINATING MEDITATION

My recent pilgrimage to Tiruvannamalai on the mountain of Arunachala, where Lord Shiva declared his love to Goddess Parvati, illumined me with great insight. As I paid homage to the Eight Shrines representing the Eight Shaktis, or cosmic directions, I felt my heart awakened and my mind illumined. The layout of the shrines mirrored the cosmic flow of creation. Positioned in the center of the energetic axis of the Vastu Mandala was the deity Brahma who is responsible for issuing the Primordial Desire that creates manifestation and fuels love. What is notable here is that Brahma is not represented by a shrine because the central force of love is invisible, infinite, and immutable. It is forever divinizing the surrounding cosmic forces into the universal state of love, maintaining the space of love within our hearts.

The space of love is the center of our home, the center of our life, and the center of our physical body, which is the heart chakra. At the center of our being is love. It is love that is the absolute source of everything. It is the central wellspring of cosmic memory and the maternal core of universal energy from which all other energies are sourced. As such, it protects and nourishes the foundational intelligence responsible for manifestation and consciousness.

Here are the Eight Shaktis that safeguard the physical world and our human consciousness, holding them together through Love:

- **Indra:** *East Direction*—Lord of the Firmament; oversees the overarching affairs of the world and their successful outcome
- **Agni:** *Southeast Direction*—Lord of Fire; generates energy and bestows health and wellness
- **Yama:** *South Direction*—Lord of Death; recycles and balances individual karmas and debts
- **Nirtti:** *Southwest Direction*—Lord of the Ancestors; resolves negative emotions and actions
- **Varuna:** *West Direction*—Lord of Water; oversees the physical world of sustenance and social development
- **Vayu:** *Northwest Direction*—Lord of the Winds; responsible for movement and disseminating information
- **Kubera:** *North Direction*—Lord of Wealth; responsible for economic, financial, and prosperity wellness
- **Ishana:** *Northeast Direction*—Lord of All Quarters of the Universe; safeguards the meditative mind and individual awareness

THE EIGHT DEITIES & THEIR CORRESPONDING COMPASS DIRECTIONS

DEITY	DIRECTION	DOMAIN
Indra	East	Lord of the Firmament
Agni	Southeast	Lord of Fire
Yama	South	Lord of Death
Nirtti	Southwest	Lord of Ancestral History
Varuna	West	Lord of Water
Vayu	Northwest	Lord of the Winds
Kubera	North	Lord of Wealth
Ishana	Northeast	Lord of All Quarters of the Universe

Table 16.2

THE PRACTICE: VASTU YANTRA–ILLUMINATING MEDITATION

OPTIMUM TIMING: Early morning, before dawn.
- **Northern Hemisphere:** New moon day and evening in early November.
- **Southern Hemisphere:** New moon day and evening in early May.

You are in the process of creating permanent luminosity with love in your heart and home—a serene place in your home for your ongoing meditation practice. In this way, you are broadcasting light and love to the entire universe.

YOU WILL NEED:
- 1 square 2' x 2' slate or marble flat stone tile
- 1 new 6' x 6' square cloth to be positioned as a diamond
- 1 cup of rice flour
- 10 traditional dipas* (1 for your altar, 9 for your Vastu Yantra)
- 2 cups organic, pure ghee or sesame oil* (for the dipas)
- 10 cotton wicks, 2 1/2-inches long* (for the dipas)

    *Small brass, stainless-steel, or earthen bowls used as dipas or ghee lamps, the cotton wicks and pure ghee or sesame oil used to light them are commonly available in most Indian grocery stores and also through the Internet.

CREATING THE VASTU YANTRA:
1. Assemble the 10 dipas half-filled with ghee or sesame oil and cotton wicks.
2. Place and light the first dipa on your altar, and set out to create your Vastu Yantra. The lighting of each sacred lamp is an offering to the goddess and symbolizes

illumination, the awakened heart of love.

3. Spread the diamond-shaped cloth on the clean floor and place the flat stone in the center of the cloth (see illustration that follows this practice.)

4. Use the rice flour to create a graph consisting of 8 equal squares, representing the compass directions. Take about a tablespoon of rice flour between your fingers and slowly release the flour to draw the lines.

5. Place an unlit dipa in the center of the mandala and in each one of the eight squares drawn. Be careful to set each lamp on a flat surface and away from anything flammable.

ILLUMINATING THE UNIVERSE WITH PRAYER:

1. Before you begin, invite your family to join in and help create this wondrous nexus of light in your heart and home.

2. Use a match to first light the dipa in the center, which will invoke the cosmic energy of the creation for greater harmony and tranquillity.

3. Then light the dipas representing the other eight directions, beginning with the east and continuing clockwise until all the outer eight directions have been lit.

4. While lighting the lamps, invoke the light of consciousness within. The Bhagavad Gita informs us that each individual houses Infinite Consciousness—the space of love that neither the sun, moon, nor fire can compete with. All sources of illumination in the universe depend on one light only: the Light of Love, the light by which all other lights are eclipsed.

5. You may recite the following mantra in adulation of Goddess Lalita Maha Tripurasundari, Mother of Love, Mother of the Universe:

Om Prema Rupayai Namah
(Pronounced: OOM PRAY-MAH RUE-PAA-YAI NAH-MAH-HA)

Reverence to Her, who is Pure Love

6. Having lit all the lamps, sit facing the beautiful, flickering mandala of lights while facing east.

7. Assume a meditative posture with your hands in the Shanti Mudra (see illustration on page 57) with your palms resting on your knees, facing toward the ceiling to receive energy, and your index fingers and thumbs pointing upwards and lightly touching.

8. Lightly close your eyes to shut out external distractions. Allow the flames of the dipas to illuminate your inner sight.

9. Fortify your emotional and physical posture with this affirmation:

   I am sitting in Love. I am the Source of Immutable Light.

10. Keep the mantra floating gently in your mind as long as you like; as you do, you are invoking inner harmony and tranquillity.

Figure 16.1   Dipa–Ghee Lamp

THE PRACTICE: EARLY WINTER MOON FAST

OPTIMUM TIMING:*

Northern Hemisphere:
- 11 days following the full moon at the end of November (counting the full moon day), bringing you into December.
- 12 days following the new moon in December (not counting the new moon day).

Southern Hemisphere:
- 11 days following the full moon at the end of May (counting the full moon day), bringing you into June.
- 12 days following the new moon in June (not counting the new moon day).

*I highly recommend purchasing a Vedic Calendar to calculate the exact timing of the new and full moons for Ekadashi calculations.

Contra-indications: Do not fast during severe illness, menstruation, or while bleeding. The elderly and young children should avoid fasting.

INSTRUCTIONS:
- On the optimum Ekadashi days noted above, begin a 3-day Early Winter Fast.

- Ekadashi generally occurs twice monthly and you must seize each and every opportunity to observe at least one Ekadashi fasting day in each month.
- Refer to instructions in The Practice: Observing a Fast on Ekadashi on pages 70-73.

This Living Ahimsa lunar observance is practiced to reclaim your state of inner balance with cyclical rhythms, reclaiming your grace with nature, and thereby healing and nullifying personal health and familial challenges. This fortnight of practice is aligned with the waxing and waning tempo of the moon. If you are unable to complete a full fast try to observe this modified Early Winter Semi-Fast:

SEMI-FAST INSTRUCTIONS:
OPTIMUM TIMING:
Northern Hemisphere:
- Semi-Fast for 7 days prior to the first new moon in November.
- Semi-Fast on only White Basmati Kichadi (see recipe on page 74).

Southern Hemisphere:
- Semi-Fast for 7 days prior to the first new moon in May.
- Semi-Fast on only White Basmati Kichadi (see recipe on page 74).

THE PRACTICE: EARLY WINTER MOON FEAST

OPTIMUM TIMING:
- Mid-to-late November through mid-to-late January.
- On Dipavali, the new moon day in early November, and on the day following the new moon in early November.
- Full moon day in the latter part of November.

PREPARATION:
Prepare your Early Winter Moon Feast for your friends and family from the many lavish recipes provided in the next chapter, "Early Winter's Reprieve." First, take a moment to bring illumination to your precious limbs of action—your hands. To truly appreciate the Living Ahimsa feast you are about to enjoy, bring the palms of your hands together in prayer, or Anjali Mudra, and offer your traditional prayer of gratitude to Mother Earth for her bountiful foods. Nourish yourself, and nurture and heal your family and friends with the creation of a feast made from the mind of lightness.

AN OFFERING TO THE GODDESS:
Before you serve the feast, offer the first bite to the goddess as a token of gratitude. As mentioned earlier, our tradition places food offerings in a small brass pot lit with the help of natural camphor resin as an offering into the fire of consciousness. The offering pot can be kept on a stand or altar in the kitchen. The offering may be accompanied with prayers from your own culture, but no matter what your faith or spiritual tradition, the act of prayer encourages confidence, joy, and fearlessness as it evokes divine protection. In any form of prayer, by bringing the palms of your hands together in the Anjali Mudra, you are stimulating the prana, which circulates through the heart increasing vitality and bringing about a sense of clarity. The act of prayer supported by the Anjali Mudra helps to heal the heart. As a result, the wounds of the present life and hurtful karmas incurred through timeless rebirths can be dissolved. When your hands meet each other at the palm, you are transforming the five elements into their single source of *tejas*—the subtle, sacred fire of consciousness held within. You immediately feel the support of the Mother Consciousness, whether or not the desired result is forthcoming.

INVOKING THE LIGHT WITHIN

Following is a Bija Mantra to the goddess of wisdom, which you may use at any time to help your mind remember to do what is wise, precious, and nurturing. Saraswati is the goddess of wisdom, creativity, and light. Recitation of this mantra will help you to elevate your awareness and intuitive ability. Invoking Saraswati will enable you to access the lightness of self.

Aim Saraswatyai Namaha
(Pronounced: AH-EEM SAH-RAHS-WAT-YI NAH-MAH-HA)

Reverence onto Saraswati

Chapter Seventeen

EARLY WINTER'S REPRIEVE

The golden season of early winter inspires the imagination and rekindles hope and health as you spend quiet days gathering your innermost strength to brace the winter months. This is the perfect time to increase stamina through nurturing activities such as storing grains and dried beans; stocking root cellars; canning vegetables and fruits; preparing winter masalas; and making warm sattvic meals—from comforting curries and casseroles to bountiful baked dishes like Red Pepper Loaf, Potato Dill Scones, and yeast-free Cranberry Cake. Hold a bowl of soft-cooked brown rice or millet in your hands and feel its warmth radiating through you while savoring the rich smell of health and happiness. Bountiful foods such as apples, barley, currants, dates, figs, millet, mung beans, and raisins; and herbs such as lemon balm, lemon verbena, licorice mint, rosemary, and thyme are but a few of the nourishing ingredients of this season that enhance your inner light and support the magic of the early winter.

EARLY WINTER MENU PLANNING

The Early Winter Season:
• Northern Hemisphere: Mid-to-late November through mid-to-late January.
• Southern Hemisphere: Mid-to-late May through mid-to-late July.

Vulnerable Time: For Kapha Types*
• Vata: Avoid excess sweet, cold, oily, or fatty foods.

* To learn your body type, see appendix one, "Wise Earth Ayurveda Body Types."

EARLY WINTER MENU: DO's & DON'T's	
APPROPRIATE FOODS FOR EARLY WINTER	FOODS TO AVOID IN EARLY WINTER
Sweet, moderately salty, and sour tastes	Sour, bitter, and astringent tastes
Unctuous, warm, substantial, and stimulating foods	Pungent, bitter, and astringent tastes

Seasonal vegetables such as arugula, beets, broccoli, cabbage, carrots, endive, kale, mustard greens, parsnips, potatoes, pumpkin, sweet potatoes, turnips, and winter squash	Meats, fowl, fish, and eggs; dry, cold, and light foods
Herbs such as basil, cinnamon, dill, marjoram, mint, oregano, parsley rosemary, sage, and thyme	
Stimulating roots such as garlic, ginger, onions, and shallots	
Fruits such as seasonal winter berries, apricots, baked apples, dates, dried figs, pears, and peaches	
Good quality cow's milk (or almond or soy milk), butter, cream, ghee, honey, raw sugar, and yogurt	

Table 17.1

SAMPLE EARLY WINTER MENU

Early Winter Breakfast:
* Kapha: Breakfast is not recommended.
* Pitta and Vata: See appendix three, "Breakfast of Champions," for a wide array of breakfast choices that can be enjoyed throughout the year.

Early Winter Lunch:
* Fresh Baked Red Pepper Loaf with Melted Ghee (p 289)
* Garlic Basil Scones (p 297)
* Sage Lemon Thyme Tea (p 305)

Early Winter Dinner:
* Shakahari Shepherd's Pie (p 295)
* Millet Supreme (p 294)
* Walnut Pear Cake (p 301)

*Gluten-free recipes are indicated by ♥
*Yeast-free recipes are indicated by ✿

ILLUMINATING GRAINS & BENEFICENT BEANS

SESAME RICE ♡

Serves: 4

1 cup medium-grain brown rice

3 1/2 cups boiling water

1 pinch rock salt

1/8 cup sesame seeds

1 tablespoon sesame oil

1 teaspoon cumin seeds

2 red chilis

Wash rice and add to boiling water with salt. Cover and simmer for 35 minutes on low heat. Wash sesame seeds and dry roast them in a cast-iron skillet over low heat until golden. In a separate skillet, add sesame oil and lightly roast cumin seeds for 2 minutes or so on low heat until evenly brown. Use a mortar and pestle to grind sesame seeds with chilis into a fine powder. Allow rice to stand for 5 minutes before garnishing with roasted cumin seeds and sesame seeds. Serve warm.

WHOLE OATS

Serves: 4

2 cups whole oats

1 small cinnamon stick

1 pinch rock salt

4 cups water

1 tablespoon caraway seeds

Soak oats in water overnight. Strain oats and add them along with water, salt, and cinnamon stick to a pressure cooker. Cover, bring to pressure, and cook for 45 minutes on medium heat. Allow pressure to fall naturally before opening the pot. In a small cast-iron skillet, dry roast the caraway seeds over medium heat until golden, then mix into the cooked oats. Allow mixture to cook on low heat without pressure for an additional 10 minutes. Serve warm.

SOFT BROWN RICE ♡

Serves: 4

1 cup short-grain brown rice

5 cups boiling water

8 cardamom pods

Wash rice and place in a pot of boiling water along with the cardamom pods. Cover and let simmer on low heat for 50 minutes until the rice becomes soft and creamy. Remove from heat and serve warm. Sprinkle with plentiful Tila Namak condiment (recipe below).

TILA NAMAK ♡
1 cup sesame seeds, washed
1 tablespoon sea salt

Place sea salt in a stainless-steel pan over a medium flame. Dry roast for 2 minutes until salt becomes dry. Using a mortar and pestle, grind to a fine powder. Place the washed sesame seeds in the pan over a medium flame. Dry roast for several minutes. Stir constantly with a wooden spoon to avoid burning and shake the pan frequently to brown the seeds evenly. When the seeds begin to pop and are golden, the roasting process is finished. Place the roasted seeds in the mortar and pestle with the ground sea salt and slowly, but firmly, grind to a coarse powder until the seeds are semi-crushed. Allow to cool completely; then place in an airtight glass or ceramic container.

SWEET RICE & ADUKI BEANS ♡
Serves: 4
2 cups short-grain sweet rice
1 cup aduki beans
4 1/2 cups boiling water
1/2 teaspoon cinnamon powder
1/2 teaspoon clove powder
1 pinch rock salt

Soak rice and beans together in water overnight. Drain the rice and beans and place in a pressure cooker with the boiling water. Add spice powders and salt. Bring to pressure, reduce heat to medium, and cook for 40 minutes. Allow pressure to fall naturally before opening the cover. Serve warm and sprinkle with plentiful Tila Namak condiment (recipe above).

MILLET WITH ROASTED PINE NUTS ♡
Serves: 4
2 cups millet
4 1/2 cups boiling water
1 pinch turmeric powder
1 pinch sea salt
1 tablespoon olive oil

1 red onion, diced

1/2 handful pine nuts

Wash the millet thoroughly and add to boiling water. Add turmeric and salt and bring water back to a boil before reducing the heat to low. Cover and let simmer for 25 minutes. In a small cast-iron skillet, heat the olive oil and brown the onion and pine nuts together over medium heat for a few minutes until the onions turn translucent. Fold the mixture into the cooked millet. Serve warm.

CITRUS-SPICED BULGUR BALLS

Serves: 2

1/2 cup roasted bulgur

2 tablespoons walnut oil

1 teaspoon coriander seeds

1 teaspoon cumin seeds

3 dried curry leaves, crushed

2 tablespoons orange juice

1/2 teaspoon orange rind, finely grated

1/2 teaspoon cardamom powder

1/4 teaspoon turmeric powder

1/2 teaspoon sea salt

1 1/2 cups water

1 tablespoon fresh cilantro, minced, for garnish

Grind roasted bulgur to a coarse flour. Heat walnut oil in a skillet over medium heat and roast coriander seeds, cumin seeds, and curry leaves. In a large bowl, mix bulgur flour, orange juice, orange rind, cardamom powder, turmeric, salt, and water thoroughly, then knead into a soft dough. Cover the dough with a cotton cloth and let stand for 15 minutes. With lightly oiled hands, roll into small balls and place a few inches apart in a steamer or on an idli tray. Steam the bulgur balls for 20 minutes. Remove from heat, garnish with cilantro, and serve warm.

TOOR & ASPARAGUS SAMBAR ♡

Serves: 2

1 cup toor dhal (yellow lentils)

3 cups water

6 fresh asparagus spears

2 carrots

1 tablespoon olive oil

1 red onion, finely chopped

1/2 lime

1 tablespoon sambar powder (page 286)

1 teaspoon yellow mustard seeds

1 teaspoon cumin seeds

Wash the toor dhal (yellow lentils) and pressure cook them in 3 cups of water for 10 minutes. Remove from heat and allow pressure to fall naturally. Hand puree the dhal with a wooden spoon and set aside. Wash and cut asparagus into 1-inch pieces (discarding the hard stems). Cut carrots into matchsticks and set vegetables aside. Heat olive oil in a small cast-iron skillet to medium heat; add onion, mustard and cumin seeds and cook until the seeds begin to crackle. Stir seed mixture into the dhal, adding the vegetables at the same time. Cover and let simmer on low heat for 25 minutes. Remove from heat and serve warm.

SPICY BAKED BEANS ♡

Serves: 4

1 cup small lima beans

3 cups water

1 teaspoon brown mustard seeds

1 teaspoon fresh ginger, grated

1 tablespoon fresh garlic, grated

1 teaspoon onion powder

1 tablespoon tamari

1 teaspoon lemon juice

1 tablespoon sesame butter

1/4 cup bean water

Wash beans, place in a pot with water, and bring to a boil. Cover and simmer for 45 minutes on medium-low heat. Remove from stove, strain the beans (retaining 1/4 cup of bean water), and place into a baking dish. Garnish top of beans with ginger, garlic, and onion powder. Mix tamari, lemon juice, and sesame butter with the warm bean water until the mixture is milky smooth, then pour over the beans. Bake the spiced beans for 30 minutes in a 350 degree oven. Serve warm.

SAMBAR POWDER ♡

12 tablespoons coriander seeds

12 tablespoons cumin seeds

1/8 cup chana dhal

2 tablespoons fenugreek seeds

8 tablespoons mustard seeds

8 tablespoons dried red chilis

1/2 teaspoon sea salt

1/2 teaspoon asafetida

Dry roast the coriander and cumin seeds with dhal in a large cast-iron skillet. Add the fenugreek, mustard seeds, and chilis after the dhal begins to turn light brown; continue roasting on very low heat for an additional 5 minutes. Add salt and asafetida at end of roasting. Grind the ingredients together to a fine powder. When cool, store in an air-tight jar.

URAD & OKRA SAMBAR ♡

Serves: 2

Sambar is a South Indian dish of spicy dhal, generally made from urad beans with savory vegetables such as daikon, bitter gourd, snake gourd, ash gourd, and seasoned with delectable spices.

1/2 cup urad dhal (Indian black lentils)

2 1/2 cups water

6 okras

1 small daikon radish

1/2 teaspoon tamarind paste

1/4 cup warm water

4 fresh curry leaves

1 green chili, whole

1/4 teaspoon turmeric powder

2 teaspoons sambar powder (recipe on page 286)

1 teaspoon organic ghee (recipe on pages 150-151)

1 teaspoon brown mustard seeds

1/2 teaspoon rock salt

Wash urad dhal (black lentils) and cook in pressure cooker for 10 minutes. Remove from heat and let the pressure fall naturally. Use a ladle to hand puree urad dhal and set aside. Wash okra and radish, cut into thin rounds, and set aside. Dilute tamarind paste in warm water and pour into the dhal. Stir in curry leaves, chili, turmeric, and sambar powder. Add okra and radish. Cover and simmer for 30 minutes over low heat. Heat ghee in a small cast-iron skillet and roast the mustard seeds for a minute or so over medium heat until they pop. Stir the mixture into the sambar mixture, add salt, and serve hot.

COMFORTING CURRIES & CASSEROLES

SPICY BLACK BEAN BROCCOLI ♥

Serves: 4

2 heads of broccoli

4 cups water

4 tablespoons olive oil

I/4 cup yellow split peas

4 tablespoons urad dhal (Indian black lentils)

3 dried red chilis

I/2 teaspoon mustard seeds

I pinch asafetida

I/2 teaspoon rock salt

Wash the broccoli and cut into thin, long spears. Boil or steam for 5 minutes, strain, and retain a I/2 cup of the broccoli water. In a small skillet, add olive oil and roast the peas, urad dhal (black lentils), and chilis over medium heat until light brown. Add mustard seeds, and when they crackle, add asafetida and salt. Use a mortar and pestle to grind the roasted spices and dhal into a coarse powder. Add broccoli water to the skillet and stir into a thick paste over low heat. Mix paste into the steamed broccoli and serve warm.

WISE EARTH STIR-FRY ♥

Serves: 4

2 cups cabbage, shredded

I cup mung bean sprouts, chopped

I/2 cup broccoli, finely cut

I/2 cup cauliflower, finely cut

I/4 cup red bell peppers, diced

3 tablespoons olive oil

I tablespoon split urad dhal (Indian black lentils)

I teaspoon fresh ginger, grated

I teaspoon brown mustard seeds

I/2 teaspoon cayenne pepper

I/4 teaspoon turmeric powder

I pinch asafetida

I pinch rock salt

Wash vegetables, cut them into fine pieces as indicated, and set aside. Heat the olive oil in a wok or large skillet and brown the urad dhal (black lentils), ginger, and mustard seeds over medium-low heat, before introducing the spice powers. Stir, turn the heat up to medium, and add the vegetables one group at a time, allowing a few minutes between groups in the following order: first add the broccoli and cauliflower, then stir; then add the cabbage and bell peppers. Add a sprinkling of water to prevent sticking. Cover and allow vegetables to cook for 3 minutes or so, before adding the sprouted mung beans. Turn off heat, cover the wok, and let it stand for a few minutes before serving the stir-fry

KARELA KADHI ♥
Serves: 2

Khadi is a classical Vedic dish made from homemade yogurt and seasoned with curry leaves and savory spices. Excellent for the digestive fire, this dish is generally served with crisply cooked vegetables such as karela or bitter gourd.

1/2 cup plain organic yogurt
2 tablespoons chickpea flour
I cup water
I teaspoon mustard oil
1/2 teaspoon ginger, minced
1/2 teaspoon chilis, minced
3 dried curry leaves, crushed
1/4 teaspoon cumin powder
1/4 teaspoon of turmeric powder
4 karela (bitter melons)
2 tablespoons olive oil
1/2 teaspoon sea salt

Blend yogurt, flour, and water into a smooth consistency. Simmer on low heat, stirring constantly to prevent curdling. Heat mustard oil in a skillet and sauté ginger, chilis, curry leaves, cumin, and turmeric for 3 minutes. Stir into yogurt mixture and remove from heat. Cut the karela in half lengthwise, core, and rinse. Slice into 1/4-inch semi-circles. Add olive oil to skillet, heat, and sauté karela on medium heat for 5 minutes. Add salt, uncover, and lightly fry on low heat for 15 minutes until karela pieces are dry and crisp. Pour yogurt mixture over karela and serve warm.

RED PEPPER LOAF
Serves 4: (2 loaves)
2 red bell peppers
2 cups warm water
I teaspoon dried tarragon
1/2 teaspoon cayenne powder
I tablespoon natural yeast

1 teaspoon rock salt
4 cups barley flour
1 teaspoon sunflower oil

Spear the whole peppers with a fork and char over an open flame until the skin turns black. Run cold water over them and peel off the skin. Remove core and seeds and cut into 1/2-inch thick strips. Set aside. Combine water, tarragon, cayenne, yeast and salt. Stir until the yeast dissolves. Add flour gradually along with most of the peepers, setting aside a few pieces for garnishing. Knead into sticky dough and transfer into a large oiled bowl. Cover securely and let rise in a warm place for 40 minutes. Punch down the dough, cover and let rise again for 40 minutes. Divide the dough into 2 equal pieces and put on an oiled baking pan. Brush tops of loaves with oil, garnish with reserved pepper slices, and bake at 425 degrees for 10 minutes. Reduce heat to 350 degrees and bake for 20 minutes more. Remove from oven and allow to sit for 15 minutes. Slice and serve with melted ghee.

CARROT & BEAN AVIYAL ♡
Serves: 4

Aviyal is a appetizing South Indian dish prepared with a variety of seasonal vegetables such as carrots, potatoes, green beans, and ash gourd, then cooked to perfection in a thick gravy made from curd or yogurt, and blended with grated fresh coconut and accented with chilis, coriander, cumin, and other savory spices.

5 carrots
1 plantain
1 pound green beans
1 teaspoon cumin seeds
1/2 cup fresh coconut, grated (if not available, substitute dried coconut)
1 teaspoon coconut oil
1/2 teaspoon turmeric powder
1/2 teaspoon sea salt
1/8 cup water, plus 2 tablespoons
1/2 cup plain organic yogurt
1 tablespoon cilantro, minced, for garnish

Wash vegetables, cut carrots into matchsticks, and cut plantain and green beans into 2-inch pieces. Dry roast the cumin seeds and coconut over medium heat, until golden, and set aside. Heat the coconut oil in large skillet; add vegetables, turmeric, and salt, and sauté on medium-low heat. Add 1/8 cup of water and simmer for 25 minutes. Grind coconut and cumin with 2 tablespoons water to create a paste, then add to cooked vegetables. Stir in yogurt. Pour the aviyal into a serving bowl and garnish with fresh cilantro.

YAM CURRY ♡

Serves: 2

3 medium-size yams

1 tablespoon olive oil

2 onions, diced

2 cloves garlic, finely diced

1 teaspoon ginger, freshly grated

1 tablespoon curry powder (recipe on page 134)

1 teaspoon Wise Earth Garam Masala (see appendix three, "Seasonal Masalas")

1 teaspoon cumin seeds

2 cups water

1/2 teaspoon rock salt

Scrub yams and cut into 1-inch pieces. Heat olive oil in a large skillet and sauté onions, garlic, ginger and spices for a few minutes over medium heat until onions becomes transparent. Add yams and sauté on low heat for 3 minutes before adding water and salt. Stir, cover, and simmer for 35 minutes on medium heat until curry is fairly thick. Serve with basmati brown rice.

NEW POTATO MASALA ♡

Serves: 2

1 pound new potatoes

1 tablespoon olive oil

1 onion, diced

1 teaspoon brown mustard seeds

2 tablespoon fresh cilantro, minced

1/2 tablespoon lemon juice, freshly squeezed

1/2 teaspoon turmeric powder

1/2 teaspoon sea salt

Scrub potatoes and cut into quarters. Add to boiling water and cook on medium heat for 15 minutes until tender. Heat the olive oil in a large skillet and sauté onion and mustard seeds over medium heat for a few minutes until seeds pop. Add cilantro, lemon juice, turmeric, and salt, and stir. Add the boiled potatoes and continue to cook on low heat for about 5 minutes until potatoes are brown.

SAVORY MUSTARD CAULIFLOWER ♡

Serves: 2

1 teaspoon mustard oil

2 cups cauliflower florets

1 teaspoon mustard seeds

3 large mustard leaves, finely cut

4 tablespoons water

Heat mustard oil in a skillet and brown mustard seeds for a few minutes over medium heat until they begin to pop. Cut the cauliflower into small pieces and add to the skillet. Lightly brown the cauliflower before layering mustard leaves over them. Add water, cover, and simmer for 5 minutes or so until cauliflower is tender. Serve warm.

SQUASH KARIKAI ♡

Serves: 2

Karikai is a South Indian dish, traditionally served during holiday festivities. It is a combination of root vegetables such as plantains, butternut squash, taro, and potatoes cooked slowly with grated coconut and spices until it becomes a fairly thick stew of perfection. It is sometimes served as a second course, instead of sambar, in the traditional Tamil dinner.

1 large butternut squash

1 cup boiling water

1/2 teaspoon rock salt

2 tablespoons organic ghee (recipe on pages 150-151)

1 teaspoon urad dhal (Indian black lentils)

1/2 teaspoon ajwain seeds

1/2 teaspoon brown mustard seeds

2 dried red chilis

1/2 teaspoon turmeric powder

1/4 cup fresh coconut, grated (if not available, substitute dried coconut)

Wash, peel, core, and cut squash into 1-inch cubes. In a medium-size saucepan, bring a cup of water to a boil; add squash and salt. Cover and simmer for about 7 minutes. Drain squash, save the cooking water, and set aside. Heat ghee in a medium-size skillet over medium heat and introduce the urad dhal (black lentils), ajwain and mustard seeds, chilis, and turmeric. Lightly roast the mixture until seeds begin to crackle. Add coconut, stir, and sauté for a few minutes. Stir in the boiled squash, along with the reserved cooking water. Cover and cook on low heat for 5 minutes until the broth thickens. Remove from heat and serve warm over cracked wheat or bulgur.

TANGY ROASTED RED PEPPERS ♡

Serves: 2

2 large red bell peppers
1 teaspoon olive oil
1/2 teaspoon black pepper, finely ground
1/2 lime, freshly juiced

Wash peppers and sit each one directly on a medium flame using a pair of tongs to turn them. Turn as needed to roast evenly. Remove from flame and place in a bowl of cold water. Remove the blackened skins by hand and core the pepper to remove the stem and seeds. Be careful not to burn your hands. Slice peppers and serve, sprinkled with olive oil, black pepper, and lime juice.

SAVORY BAKED TOFU ♡

Serves: 4

2 pounds firm tofu
1 tablespoon Wise Earth Garam Masala (see appendix three, "Seasonal Masalas")
1 tablespoon tamari
1 teaspoon fresh ginger, grated
1 teaspoon fresh garlic, finely minced
1 pinch cayenne powder
1 tablespoon olive oil
1 cup hot water

Preheat oven to 375 degrees. Cut tofu into 1-inch chunks and place in a medium-size baking dish. Add garam masala, tamari, ginger, garlic, cayenne, olive oil, and hot water over the tofu. Cover the dish and let the tofu mixture marinate for 30 minutes. Then bake marinated tofu for 30 minutes until the liquid evaporates and the tofu is browned and firm in texture.

CREAMY POTATO SOUFFLÉ ♡

Serves: 4

4 large white potatoes
2 pounds soft tofu
1 teaspoon black pepper, coarsely ground
1 small scallion, minced
1 tablespoon olive oil
1 teaspoon organic ghee (recipe on pages 150-151)
1/2 teaspoon rock salt

Preheat oven to 450 degrees. Oil a large baking dish and set aside. Scrub potatoes and cut into quarters. Boil for 15 minutes. Wash hands and crumble the tofu into a large bowl. Once the potatoes are cooked, peel off the skins, and place potatoes in the bowl with tofu. Add the black pepper, scallion, olive oil, ghee, and salt. Blend ingredients together into a smooth mixture before pouring into the baking dish. Bake for 10 minutes until the top is brown and crusty. Serve hot.

MILLET SUPREME ♥

Serves: 4

3 1/2 cups water

2 cups millet

1/4 cup fresh peas

1 tablespoon sunflower oil

1/4 cup currants

1/4 cup roasted almonds, slivered

1/2 lemon, freshly juiced

1/2 teaspoon turmeric

1/2 teaspoon cumin powder

1/2 teaspoon ajwain seeds

1 teaspoon rock salt

Bring water to a boil in a medium-size saucepan. Thoroughly wash the millet and add to boiling water, along with the peas, turmeric, cumin powder, ajwain seeds, and salt. Cover and simmer on medium heat for 20 minutes. Heat the oil in a small skillet, and add the currants and almonds. Stir for a few minutes until the currants begin to swell. Add the lemon juice. Add mixture to the millet, and continue cooking for 10 minutes more. Serve warm.

SQUASH & SWEET POTATO CASSEROLE ♥

Serves: 4

1 medium butternut squash

2 large sweet potatoes

3 cups water

1/2 cup soy flour

1 tablespoon organic ghee (recipe on pages 150-151)

2 tablespoons fresh cilantro, minced

1 teaspoon fresh basil, minced

1/2 teaspoon cardamom powder

1/2 teaspoon black pepper, ground

1/2 cup soy milk

3 sprigs fresh mint, minced, for garnish

Preheat oven to 500 degrees. Wash and core squash, and cut into quarters. Wash and cut the potatoes into quarters, retaining the skins. Bring water to a boil, add squash and potatoes, and cook for 15 minutes. Strain and retain 1/4 cup of the cooking water. Allow to cool before scooping out the flesh and discarding the skins. Place in a bowl, cover, and set aside. In a large cast-iron skillet, toast the flour for a few minutes over medium heat until it turns light brown. Pour the flour into the bowl of squash and potatoes, and mix well. In a small cast-iron skillet, melt the ghee on low heat and introduce the herbs and spices. Sauté for 30 seconds and stir into the squash mixture. Add reserved cooking water, along with the soy milk and salt. Mix well and pour into an oiled baking dish. Bake the casserole for 10 minutes or so until the top is lightly browned. Garnish with fresh mint and serve hot.

SHAKAHARI SHEPHERD'S PIE
Serves: 6

1 cup spelt groats
4 cups water
2 large sweet potatoes
2 yams
1 large white potato
1/2 cup soy milk
1 tablespoon olive oil
1/4 cup apple cider
1 teaspoon rock salt
2 tablespoons unsalted butter
2 large red onions, coarsely diced
1/2 teaspoon coriander powder
1/2 teaspoon curry powder (recipe on page 134)
1/2 teaspoon cumin powder
1 pinch turmeric powder

Oil and set aside six individual ramekins. Pressure cook spelt groats in 4 cups of water for 45 minutes. Allow pressure to fall naturally before opening the pressure cooker, drain the groats, and retain cooking water. Scrub potatoes and yams and cut into large chunks. Boil in retained cooking water for 20 minutes until soft. Drain and remove skins. In a large mixing bowl, add milk, cider, salt, and butter, then mash potatoes and yams together. Preheat oven to 400 degrees. In a cast-iron skillet, heat olive oil and sauté onions and spices on medium-low heat for a few minutes until onions turn translucent, then stir in the cooked spelt groats. Fill the bowls with the spelt mixture before topping them off with a layer of mashed potatoes. Place in oven and bake for 25 minutes until the edges of potatoes are browned.

RICOTTA & MILLET QUICHE
Serves: 2

Crust:
I Covered Pie Crust, spelt or whole wheat (see Covered Pie Crust recipe on page 304, but do not cover quiche)

Filling:
1/2 cup soft cooked millet
I cup ricotta cheese
1/2 cup soy milk
1/2 teaspoon black pepper
I teaspoon cumin powder
I pinch turmeric powder
2 tablespoons olive oil
1/4 cup water

Preheat oven to 375 degrees. Lightly grease pie pan and place the rolled out pie crust into it and set aside. Wash your hands and ply the millet and cheese into a smooth mixture in a large bowl before adding the milk, spices, olive oil, and water. Pour filling into pie crust, leveling the top. Bake for 30 minutes until the top of quiche turns brown and crusty. Serve warm.

MILLET SUPREME ♡
Serves: 4

3 1/2 cups water
2 cups millet
1/4 cup fresh peas
I tablespoon sunflower oil
1/4 cup currants
1/4 cup roasted almonds, slivered
1/2 lemon, freshly juiced
1/2 teaspoon turmeric
1/2 teaspoon cumin powder
1/2 teaspoon ajwain seeds
I teaspoon rock salt

Bring water to a boil in a medium-size saucepan. Thoroughly wash the millet and add to boiling water, along with the peas, turmeric, cumin powder, ajwain seeds, and salt. Cover and simmer on medium heat for 20 minutes. Heat the oil in a small skillet, and add the currants and almonds. Stir for a few minutes until the currants begin to swell. Add the lemon juice. Add mixture to the millet, and continue cooking for 10 minutes more. Serve warm.

RED CABBAGE & ONION SOUP ♡

Serves: 4

1/2 gallons water

1 small red cabbage, shredded

2 red onions, chopped

1 tablespoon coriander powder

1/2 teaspoon cayenne powder

1 tablespoon dried dill

1 tablespoon dried parsley

2 cloves garlic

1 tablespoon rock salt

1/4 cup cashew butter

1 red onion, thin half-moon slices

Bring water to a boil in a large heavy-bottomed soup pot. Add the shredded cabbage and chopped onions, along with coriander and cayenne powders, dried dill and parsley. Lightly crush the garlic cloves with a hand stone and remove the skin. Add the garlic to the soup mixture. Cover and simmer on medium heat for 35 minutes until onions are practically dissolved. Add cashew butter and stir the soup until it dissolves. Garnish the hot soup with thinly sliced red onions. Remove from heat, cover, and let sit for 5 minutes. Serve hot with a heaping dollop of millet.

MIZUNA & LEMON SALAD ♡

Serves: 4

1 fresh lemon

2 teaspoons rock salt

1 large bunch mizuna leaves

Wash lemon and cut into very thin slices, retaining the skin. Season the lemon slices with salt. Arrange the seasoned lemon slices on top of the mizuna greens, and serve.

NOURISHING BREADS

GARLIC BASIL SCONES

Serves: 6

1 tablespoon sunflower oil

1 tablespoon garlic, minced

2 tablespoons fresh basil, minced

2 green onions, chopped

2 cups barley flour

3/4 cup water
1/2 teaspoon rock salt

Preheat oven to 375 degrees. Heat the sunflower oil in large skillet, and sauté the minced garlic over medium heat until golden brown. Add basil, green onions, flour, water, and salt. Blend into a thick batter. Place plum-size dollops of batter on an oiled baking tray, spacing them 2 inches apart. Bake for 15 minutes until golden brown.

ALMOND SCONES
Serves: 6
1 tablespoon organic ghee (recipe on pages 150-151)
1/4 cup roasted almonds, finely chopped
1/2 teaspoon nutmeg powder
1/2 teaspoon ginger powder
1/2 teaspoon cardamom powder
2 cups spelt flour
3/4 cup water
1/2 teaspoon rock salt

Preheat oven to 375 degrees. Melt ghee in a large skillet over medium heat. Add almonds and spice powders, along with flour, water, and salt. Remove from heat and blend into a thick batter. Place plum-size spoonfuls of batter on an oiled baking tray, spacing them 2 inches apart. Bake for 15 minutes until golden brown.

PUMPKIN CURRANT BREAD ♡ ⓥ
Serves: 6 (1 loaf)
2 cups pumpkin, cooked
1/4 cup currants
1/2 teaspoon cinnamon powder
1/2 teaspoon ginger powder
1/2 teaspoon cardamom powder
1/2 teaspoon mace, ground
1/8 teaspoon cloves, ground
1 cup millet flour
1/4 cup soy milk
1/2 lime, freshly juiced
1/2 teaspoon rock salt

Preheat oven to 400 degrees. Combine all ingredients in a large bowl and mix into a thick batter. Oil a large loaf pan and spoon the batter into it. Bake for 20 minutes until top of loaf is crusty.

BUCKWHEAT GOLDEN BEET SCONES

Serves: 6

1 tablespoon corn oil

1 teaspoon brown mustard seeds

1 small bunch fresh parsley, chopped

1 small bunch fresh chives, chopped

1 large golden beet, peeled and grated

2 cups buckwheat flour

3/4 cup water

1/2 teaspoon rock salt

1/2 teaspoon black pepper, finely ground

Preheat oven to 375 degrees. Heat the corn oil in a large skillet over medium heat. Roast the mustard seeds until they begin to pop. Add parsley and chives, then remove from heat. Mix in the beet, flour, water, salt, and pepper. Blend into a thick batter. Place plum-size spoonfuls of batter on an oiled baking tray, spacing them 2 inches apart. Bake until golden brown and a fork inserted in the center comes out clean.

POTATO DILL SCONES

Serves: 6

2 large potatoes, cooked and mashed

1/2 cup warm soy milk

1 cup soy flour

1 teaspoon coriander powder

1/2 teaspoon black pepper, finely ground

1 small bunch fresh dill, chopped

1 tablespoon corn oil

1 teaspoon cumin seeds

Preheat oven to 375 degrees. Combine mashed potatoes, soy milk, flour, spice powders, and fresh dill in a large bowl; mix into a thick batter. Heat corn oil in a small skillet over medium heat, and roast cumin seeds until golden brown. Blend into the batter. Place plum-size spoonfuls of batter onto an oiled baking tray, spacing them 2 inches apart. Bake for 15 minutes until golden brown.

UNLEAVENED RYE BREAD

Serves: 6 (2 loaves)

1 cup spelt flour

2 cups rye flour

1 teaspoon rock salt

1 tablespoon caraway seeds

2 tablespoons sesame seeds

1 1/2 cups warm water

In a mixing bowl, combine the flours, salt, and seeds. Slowly add just enough water to knead the dough into a ball. Continue to knead dough for 5 minutes. Transfer dough to an oiled bowl, cover with a damp cotton towel, and let sit in a warm place overnight. After dough has risen overnight, preheat oven to 325 degrees. Knead dough again for 5 minutes. Then form into 2 long, oval loaves. Place on a lightly oiled and floured baking sheet. Bake for 75 minutes until golden brown.

OPULENT DESSERTS

CRANBERRY CAKE ♥ ❶

Serves: 6

Topping:

1/2 pound fresh cranberries

1/4 cup water

1 cup grape juice

2 tablespoons maple syrup

Batter:

1 1/2 cups chickpea flour

1/2 teaspoon baking powder

2 tablespoons sunflower oil

2 tablespoons plain organic yogurt

1 tablespoon dried orange peel

3/4 cup water

Preheat oven to 350 degrees. Oil a shallow baking dish and set aside. In a small saucepan, combine all the topping ingredients. Cover and simmer on medium heat for 10 minutes, until the cranberries are tender. In a mixing bowl, sift the flour and baking powder together and then add the sunflower oil, yogurt, and orange peel. Gradually introduce the water and mix into a batter. Pour the batter into the baking dish. Bake for 10 minutes, then pour the cranberry topping over the cake. Continue baking for 20 more minutes. Serve warm.

WALNUT PEAR CAKE

Serves: 4

2 tablespoons organic ghee (recipe on pages 150-151)

1/4 cup unrefined brown sugar

1/2 teaspoon natural vanilla extract

1 teaspoon cinnamon powder

1/2 teaspoon ginger powder

1/2 teaspoon ground nutmeg

1/2 teaspoon rock salt

1/2 cup spelt flour

1/2 cup water

1/2 cup dried pear slices

1/2 cup crushed walnuts

Preheat oven to 350 degrees. Oil and flour a baking pan, then set aside. Combine the ghee, sugar, extract, spice powders, and salt in a bowl. Add a palmful of water and whisk the mixture until smooth. Gradually fold in the flour, adding the remaining water. Mix in the walnuts and dried pear slices. Pour the batter into the prepared pan and bake for 30 minutes at 350 degrees.

EARLY WINTER OATCAKES

Serves: 6

1/2 cup boiling water

1/4 cup raisins

1 1/2 cups rolled oats

1 cup oat flour

1/4 cup sunflower oil

1/2 rock salt

Preheat oven to 375 degrees. Oil and lightly flour a baking sheet. Pour boiling water over raisins. Set aside for 10 minutes. In a mixing bowl, thoroughly mix the oats, flour, oil, and salt together. Strain the raisins, retaining the water, and add to the flour mixture. Gradually pour in the retained water and mix the ingredients into a firm dough. Roll the dough out on a floured surface and cut into small rounds, 2 inches in diameter. Place on the prepared baking sheet. Bake for 12 minutes until the cakes begin to brown. Serve as is, or with a dollop of Almond Cream (recipe on page 259).

CRANBERRY CURRANT COOKIES ♡ ⓦ

Serves: 6

1/2 pound fresh cranberries

1/2 cup currants

1 1/2 cups apple juice

1 1/2 cups soy flour

1/2 teaspoon baking powder

1 teaspoon cardamom powder

1/2 cup rice syrup

3/4 cup warm water

Preheat oven to 400 degrees. Oil and flour a cookie tray. In a small saucepan, combine cranberries, currants, and apple juice. Bring to a boil, reduce heat, and cook for 10 minutes until cranberries are soft. In a mixing bowl, combine and sift the flour and baking powder, then add cardamom powder and rice syrup. Gradually introduce the water and blend mixture into a batter. Stir in the cranberry mixture. Drop the batter by spoonfuls onto the cookie tray. Bake for 10 minutes until cookies are lightly brown. Serve warm.

SHORT CRUST PASTRY SHELL

Serves: 4

2 cups spelt flour*

1/2 teaspoon rock salt

1/2 cup sunflower oil

3 tablespoons unsalted butter

1/4 cup ice water

*Substitute rye, oat, or soy flour for a yeast-free pastry shell.

Combine the flour and salt in a large mixing bowl. Set aside. Blend the sunflower oil and butter thoroughly in a separate bowl, and then cut into the flour mixture. Use your hands to blend the mixture into a flaky consistency. Mix in the ice water a palmful at a time, gathering the dough into a stiff ball. Roll out the dough on a floured surface to form an 8-inch circle. Fit into an oiled baking dish, trimming the edges. Prick bottom and sides of unbaked shell with a fork. Refrigerate for 1 hour. Bake at 425 degrees for 15 minutes until golden brown. (When baking the shell with a filling, follow the baking time set out with the individual pie filling recipes.)

CAROB WALNUT BROWNIES

Serves: 6

1/4 cup unsalted butter

2 tablespoons unrefined brown sugar

2/3 cup soy milk

1/2 teaspoon natural vanilla extract

2/3 cup spelt flour

1 teaspoon baking powder

1/4 cup unsweetened carob powder

1/2 teaspoon rock salt

1/4 cup chopped walnuts

Preheat oven to 350 degrees. Lightly oil and flour a shallow baking pan. In a mixing bowl, blend the butter and sugar together until smooth. Then blend in soy milk and vanilla essence. Sift the flour and baking powder and then gradually fold into butter-sugar mixture. Blend in carob powder, salt, and walnuts. Spoon the batter into the baking pan. Bake for 20 minutes or until a fork inserted comes out clean. Cut into squares when cool.

SPICED PUMPKIN PIE

Serves: 6

Crust:

1 Short Crust Pastry Shell (recipe on page 302)

Filling:

1/2 small pumpkin, cooked and mashed

1/4 cup chickpea flour, lightly browned

1 tablespoon dried orange peel

1/8 cup warm milk

1 teaspoon cinnamon powder

1/2 teaspoon cardamom powder

1/2 teaspoon mace, ground

1/2 teaspoon nutmeg, ground

1/8 cup rice syrup

1 tablespoon corn oil

1/2 teaspoon rock salt

Combine all ingredients in a large mixing bowl, blending the pie filling until it is creamy. Pour filling into an 8-inch Short Crust Pastry Shell (recipe on page 302) and bake at 425 degrees for 15 minutes.

COVERED PIE CRUST (SPELT)
Serves: 4

4 cups spelt pastry flour*
1/4 teaspoon sea salt
1/8 cup chilled sesame oil
1 cup cold water
*Substitute whole wheat flour if spelt is not available.

Mix flour and salt together in a large mixing bowl and ply well. Add sesame oil and water, and thoroughly knead the dough for 4 minutes. Allow to stand at room temperature for 30 minutes or chill for 15 minutes. Divide dough in half and roll 1 part into a circle about 1 1/2 inches larger than the bottom of your pie dish. Lightly oil baking dish and press the rolled dough into it, letting the dough brim a little over the edge of the dish. Fill with prepared filling. If covering the top of the filling with the pie crust, roll out the second piece of dough to cover the pie. Place dough over the filling loosely and press the edges of the upper and lower crusts together with the fingers or with a fork. Poke a few holes in the top of the pie with the fork to allow excess air to escape.

COVERED PIE CRUST (BARLEY FLOUR)
Serves: 4

3 cups barley pastry flour
1/4 teaspoon rock salt
1/8 cup chilled corn oil
1 cup cold water

Mix flour and salt together in a large mixing bowl and ply well. Add corn oil and water, and thoroughly knead the dough for 4 minutes. Allow to stand at room temperature for 30 minutes or chill for 15 minutes. Divide dough in half and roll 1 part into a circle about 1 1/2 inches larger than the bottom of your pie dish. Lightly oil baking dish and press the rolled dough into it, letting the dough brim a little over the edge of the dish. Fill with prepared filling. If covering the top of the filling with the pie crust, roll out the second piece of dough to cover the pie. Place dough over the filling loosely and press the edges of the upper and lower crusts together with fingers or with a fork. Poke a few holes in the top of the pie with a fork to allow excess air to escape.

EARLY WINTER ELIXIRS

ALMOND ROSE ESSENCE TEA ♡
Serves: 2

2 cups almond milk
1/2 cup water

1/2 teaspoon coriander powder

1 teaspoon rose water

1 teaspoon honey

Combine water and milk and bring to a boil. Add spices and simmer over low heat for 5 minutes. Strain, add rose water, sweeten with honey, and serve warm.

SAGE LEMON THYME TEA ♥

Serves: 2

3 cups water

2 tablespoons fresh sage leaves

1 teaspoon fresh lemon thyme

1/2 lemon, freshly juiced

Bring water to a boil, add the sage leaves, and simmer on low heat for 3 minutes. Remove from heat, cover, and let stand for 1 minute. Strain the leaves, add lemon juice to the decoction, and serve warm. Sweeten with 1 teaspoon of honey, if desired.

GINGER HONEY TEA ♥

Serves: 2

3 1/2 cups water

1 tablespoon fresh ginger, grated

1/2 lemon, freshly juiced

1 tablespoon honey

Bring water to a boil. Peel the ginger and finely grate it. Add to water and steep on low heat for 7 minutes. Remove from heat, cover, and let stand for 1 minute before adding the honey and lemon juice. Strain and serve warm.

SORREL LEMON BALM TEA ♥

Serves: 2

3 cups water

2 tablespoons fresh sorrel leaves

1 teaspoon fresh lemon balm leaves

1 teaspoon of orange zest

Bring water to a boil, add the leaves and zest, and simmer on low heat for 3 minutes. Remove from heat, cover, and let stand for 1 minute. Strain the decoction and serve warm. Sweeten with 1 teaspoon of honey, if desired.

LICORICE FENNEL TEA ♡

Serves: 2

2 cups almond milk

1/2 cup water

1/2 teaspoon licorice powder

1/2 teaspoon ginger powder

1 teaspoon fennel seeds

1 teaspoon honey

Combine water and milk and bring to a boil. Add spices and simmer over low heat for 5 minutes. Strain, sweeten with honey, and serve warm.

Part Seven

WINTER

I take The Vow of Ahimsa

To invest in world peace and the protection of all beings

Chapter Eighteen

WINTER AHIMSA PRACTICES FOR REST & REJUVENATION

The bloom of tenderer flowers is past
And lilies droop forlorn,
For winter-time is come at last,
Rich with its ripened corn...
The vines, remembering summer, shiver
In frosty winds, and gain
A fuller life from mere endeavor
To live through all that pain.

—Kalidasa

Rest and reflection are the Living Ahimsa mantras for the late winter season. Winter is the most austere season of the year, and its rhythms invite you to safeguard your inner reservoir of strength and indulge in a well-deserved reprieve from the year's hard work and stressors. Our ancestors wisely conserved their energy and efforts during this time. They understood that Mother Earth was resting and that her stillness generated the necessary rejuvenation of all of her living charges. From the Living Ahimsa perspective, fatigue syndrome, memory loss, and other stress-related conditions are a direct result of our disregard for winter's rhythms and living out of sync with them.

Rest and reprieve are essential to our well-being, and winter's energies provide a critical opportunity for us to fortify our endurance and strength. When we align ourselves with the greater energies of the seasons—winter, in particular—we feed our inner reservoir enough to carry through for the rest of the year. Our tissues are cosseted by the winter energy in the same way that nature's micro-organisms, seeds, and saplings are protected beneath the dried brambles and snows. This blanket of protection provides the necessary cyclical rest for the vital organism. In the northern climates, the undifferentiated aura of the snowy landscape blending into the sky brings a profound sense of harmony, joy and calm to the mind of all creatures; a perfect time to huddle in blissful comfort at the hearth of the home with loved ones. Like the bear that hibernates in its cave, we humans need to acknowledge winter's stoic presence and its profound healing effects on our physical, mental, and spiritual bodies. For this, we must draw our attention closer to home and focus on the well-being of family, tending to the hearth and to the phenomenal opportunity for quantum change that only winter brings.

The sacred space that winter creates is austere and reverent. Its powerful sparseness draws our thoughts into harmony, providing a clean canvas for us to recast our living environment within and without. Indeed, this occurs naturally when we recognize the healing commands of this major season and retreat inward to revive our sacred nourishment and spirit. It is a time to moderate our work schedules and reduce ongoing activities. Observe the replenishing Living Ahimsa winter practices presented in this chapter to refuel the body, mind, senses, and spirit.

Rest and reflection do not mean bringing our lives to a full stop or turning into couch potatoes! Celebrate the winter season through long, brisk walks in her wintry elements, foraging for hidden food treasures underneath her brush. Collect pinecones and evergreen boughs with red berries to decorate and add fragrance to your home. In fact, these are the precious months of the year when we can organically cast off stress and welcome serenity of mind. The still of the season beckons a sense of immutable quiet—a settling time for the body, mind, and spirit to rebalance, recharge, and refocus.

In rural England, where the late winter begins with the new year, blessings of the land accompany the revelry of this cold season of retreat. Bits of cakes are hung on trees and libations of cider are poured onto the Tree of Life to spur its magic. The Chinese people celebrate the onset of late winter with the Feast of the Kitchen God. The smiling, rotund image of Tsao Wang is placed in the home to watch over and safeguard the family. Families congregate in their kitchens to prepare cakes, sweets, and decorated foods as offerings to the Kitchen God. Occasionally molasses is dabbed onto the god's mouth so that only "sweet" words will be transported to the Jade Emperor.

Traditionally, the late winter season is celebrated in the spirit of reawakening Living Ahimsa memory and aspirations. Hindus begin this season by observing silence on the full moon, which falls on the 15th day of the late winter's waxing moon. In the fullness of this winter's moon, the Great Goddess Lalita Maha Tripurasundari, may be seen by her devotees in her full regalia. In this sacred month of *Magha* (January into February), aspirants fast and take a bath in the holy Ganges River. The god Vishnu is worshipped by perambulating the sacred peepal tree. Fasting is practiced by stoic Hindus for the entire fortnight starting at the full moon and ending on the new moon with *Mauni Amavasya*, a day of silence. As you will experience, practicing silence helps you to emulate the resounding spirit of the late winter bringing infinite joy and vitality. The most dramatic seasonal transition occurs at this juncture as the overwhelming silence of winter once again manifests into the delicate sounds of life as the spring awakens.

THE LONGEST NIGHT

The winter solstice marks the beginning of a period of time for profound observances and reverent activities in my culture. Winter is considered a time when the earth, the Great Mother's womb, can be revitalized so it can sustain the memory of sustenance and fertility for the welfare of all her beings.

Lohri is an important occasion (enthusiastically celebrated in North India during mid-January) commemorating the earth's heightened fertility, and rejoicing in the great relief of the end of the coldest month. This is a time when our planet has been at its farthest from the sun and now starts its journey back towards it. Farmers celebrate Lohri by taking a period of rest before the spring harvest.

This season is especially auspicious because it is when Lord Krishna—avatar of dharma and love—manifested himself on earth. Lohri celebrates love and the joy of the family, and in the event of the birth of a newborn or a marriage in the family, it assumes a larger significance. The first Lohri of a new bride or newborn baby is extremely propitious. In Punjab, the bread basket of India, wheat is the main winter crop. Sown in October, the young green fields emerge in the glistening January sun with the promise of an abundant harvest. In the morning on Lohri day, children go from door to door singing traditional songs and expecting their just Lohri rewards—money and sweets made from sesame seeds. As the sun begins to set, huge bonfires are lit near the fields and in the front yards of homes. People circle around the bonfires and offer oblations such as puffed rice and corn into the fire as they chant local invocations in reverence to Agni, god of fire: *Aadar aye dilather jaye* (May we invoke grace and banish poverty). Oblations are hoped to bring blessings to the land and prosperity to the farmers and their families. The day following Lohri is called *Maghi*. In Hindu tradition, this is one of many auspicious days to be charitable and to enjoy a sanctifying bath in the holy rivers.

Each year in South India, *Pongal* is usually celebrated between the 12th and 15th of January to commemorate the harvest of crops and offer thanks to the seasons, the sun, the earth, and the cows. For Hindus, the time of Pongal is extremely auspicious as it marks the sun's entry into the Tropic of Capricorn from the Tropic of Cancer. On this day the sun begins its journey north for a period of six months.

The word *pongal* comes from the Tamil word *ponga*, which literally means "boil," an appropriate name for this festival symbolizing overflowing abundance. Pongal also refers to the name of the special sweet dish cooked on Pongal day. This festival marks the end of the monsoons. It is a harbinger for prodding the spirit to clean out the old and welcome in the new. Seventy-five percent of India's population live in farming villages and understand the value of keeping the earth fertile; not only as a source of food and nourishment, but also to sustain the memory of synchrony between the good earth and human existence. Almost all Hindu festivals are directly linked to Mother Earth and her annual cycle of the seasons and are intended to replenish bountiful memory, fertility, and nourishment.

AWAKENING TO WINTER'S RHYTHMS

To balance the extreme conditions of winter, nature increases our physical, mental, and spiritual digestion. Appetite becomes powerful at this time, and you must feed that inner fire. You may increase the size of your meals and imbibe healthful quantities of nourishing foods that buffer the body and mind against the cold. Freshly baked breads, heavy soups and stews, cooked fruits and root vegetables with ghee or butter and creamy sauces, milk beverages, and wholesome desserts are examples of Living Ahimsa feasts for the winter days. To inspire you into the perfect winter tempo, you'll find scrumptious feasts and simple fasts set out in this section.

Caring for the mind, body, and spirit is imperative if you are to build the foundation of health during this season of deep cold. Body massages with warm, fragrant oils, warm baths, ginger compresses on the lower back, warm clothing, and a cozy environment created in the home are the nurturing demand of this exceptional season.

Particularly nourishing for this time of year are substantial meals prepared from wholesome grains, buckwheat, millet, and wheat. Life-generating pulses (such as mung beans, kidney beans, red lentils, soy beans) and earthy vegetables (like carrots, onions, leeks, turnips, sweet potatoes, yams, winter squashes, and beets) with a dash of greens, a plentiful dollop of creamy butter, cream, ghee, or buttermilk, and dabs of honey, molasses, maple syrup, Sucanat, or turbinado sugar are also nourishing. Live in accord with the rhythms of late winter and you will discover strength, profound stamina, and deepening wisdom for the rest of the year.

THE ENERGY OF LATE WINTER				
PRIMARY ACTIVITY	PREDOMINANT TASTE	PREDOMINANT ELEMENTS	TIME OF YEAR	DOSHIC NATURE
Resting	Bitter	Air and Space	Mid-to-late January through mid-to-late March (Northern Hemisphere)	Vata
			Mid-to-late July though mid-to-late September (Southern Hemisphere)	

Table 18.1

THE PRACTICE: WINTER SOLSTICE MOON FAST

It is best if you can work up to observing 7 fasting days during the winter. The most auspicious time to begin your week-long winter fast would be on the full moon of *Magha*, which occurs at the beginning of March or end of February. This is the most critical time of the year to lay bare the body, mind, and spirit in order to rest, and revitalize your body to its maximum point of fulfillment.

OPTIMUM TIMING:*
Northern Hemisphere:
- 13 days following the full moon at the end of January, counting the full moon day (this brings you into February).
- 12 days following the new moon in February, not counting the new moon day.
- 11 days following the full moon at the end of February, counting the full moon day (this may bring you into March).

Southern Hemisphere:
- 13 days following the full moon at the end of July, counting the full moon day (this brings you into August).
- 12 days following the new moon in August, not counting the new moon day.
- 11 days following the full moon at the end of August, counting the full moon day (this may bring you into September).

*I highly recommend purchasing a Vedic Calendar to calculate the exact timing of the new and full moons for Ekadashi calculations.

Contra-indications: Do not fast during severe illness, menstruation, or while bleeding. The elderly and young children should avoid fasting.

INSTRUCTIONS:
- On the auspicious full moon day that occurs in late February or early March, begin a 7-day Winter Moon Fast. If you need to work up to a 7-day fast, observe as many days as you can. (Refer to instructions in The Practice: Observing a Fast on Ekadashi on pages 70-73.)

This Living Ahimsa lunar observance is practiced to reclaim your state of sacred nourishment and inner balance with cyclical rhythms—to reclaim your grace with nature and thereby heal and nullify personal health and familial challenges. This fortnight of practice is aligned with the waxing and waning tempo of the moon. (If you are unable to complete a full fast, try to observe a modified Semi-Fast, detailed on pages 73-77.)

SILENCE AT WINTER'S NEW MOON—
REVITALIZING COGNITIVE MEMORY

By exploring the profound practice of silence, which I will detail in the following pages, we will cultivate greater memory and awareness. The season of winter, when everything is covered in the undifferentiated serenity of muted coldness, allows us the deepest silence of the year. Winter invites us to delve deeply within to discover the immutable content of the human self—*inner* silence. Our own sense of deep quiet is filled with the sentience of cosmic memory, which, in turn, is nurtured and made effulgent by the vibrations of the cosmic sound. Silence is the transformer of consciousness.

The rishis revealed that human consciousness emerged from the memory of the cosmos—the greater consciousness that is everywhere. Every cell of our being is formed from the essential memories of creation, and every species is further formed from its own set of memories, which are transformed and assimilated from the beginning of time. Memory contains the truth of the universe. It is both the inner guide for each life and a means of exchange with all other beings.

According to Living Ahimsa principles, our memory is nourished and sustained by the vibratory sound of the universe. Indeed, all memory is based in the cosmic sound. The first emanation of creation emerged from *nada,* the inaudible cosmic vibrations known as the primordial sound. Through the transformation of this primordial sound, the entire universe emerged, constantly resolving into other shapes and forms. The *Chandogya Upanishad* reveals cosmic sound as The Word: "The Word makes known heaven, earth, wind, space, the waters, fire, the celestials, humans, animals, grass and trees."

Why have we not retained our entire chain of collective memory from before time began? In short, because as human organisms our memory capacity—what we carry in our physical organism—is limited. The way this phenomenon is explained in the Vedas is that the process of birth and its resulting shock causes us to lose the memories of our extensive past. The purpose of life is to remember who we are and, in so doing, to learn to cultivate the karmas that bring joyful fulfillment of our individual purpose. In essence, we do retain the imprints of all of our lives' memories but only in their essential form. These collective memories, which I refer to as our "cognitive memories," are stored in our buddhi, which is also responsible for storing the precious content of our awareness. This awareness, and the cognitive memories associated with it, is always available to be accessed and recognized.

Let's explore the buddhi. Buddhi is the cognitive instrument that gives us the ability to process our individual awareness, which, in turn, is filtered down from cosmic consciousness. It is the vehicle by which we transform consciousness into expression. It is the most superior block of cosmic memory carried by humans and is located in the frontal part of the brain. When we awaken to the power of our buddhi, we develop that prescient wisdom that makes us intuitive, sensitive, introspective, and sentient beings. Essentially, the buddhi holds the universe's memories within us, and the mind is the vehicle for expressing the memories held within our awareness. When the mind is aligned with the buddhi, we express ourselves consciously. It is said in the *Chandogya Upanishad*, "A person is what his desire is. It is our deepest desire in this life that shapes the life to come. So let us direct our deepest desires to know the self that is born of cosmic silence."

In order to fulfill our individual purpose, we must overcome whatever stands in the way of remembering who we truly are. When our cognitive memories are blocked, we forget who we are. Part of our psyche is also blocked, and we therefore lose our ability to tap into the innate intuitive guidance that keeps us on our life's path. We forget our sacred purpose. The fertility of mind, spirit, and body are entirely dependent on the quality and quantity of our memory. Therefore, it is essential that we reclaim our cognitive memories. The following practice will help you do just that. It will help you explore, develop, and expand your mind's focus on your inner sound. In short, you will recognize that you are the primal source of consciousness.

THE PRACTICE OF SILENCE: MEDITATING ON OM

OPTIMUM TIMING: Mornings from 6:30-7:30 a.m.
- Northern Hemisphere: For two weeks starting at the new moon in March.
- Southern Hemisphere: For two weeks starting at the new moon in September.

Although it may seem paradoxical on the surface to use a sound to achieve inner silence, I assure you it is not! Reflecting on the sacred sound OM is the most direct pathway to quieting the mind, which is the focus of silence. When we pronounce OM, we use the entire spectrum of vocal range from throat to lips, and we recall the most ancient phenomenon: the cosmic sound of consciousness. Contemplation of the Sanskrit sound OM calms the mind and opens the gateway to the vast inner realm of silence and cognitive memory. In Sanskrit the word OM is composed of 3 syllables: A-U-M pronounced AH-OU-MM, representing the 3 states of consciousness in the cosmos. (The buddhi assumes dominance as we enter silence.)

Try to take a day (or several hours) once a month to practice silence. Start the day with 40 minutes of OM meditation. Spend approximately 5 minutes at each of the 4 stages of this meditation, and then 20 minutes enjoying the silence that ensues. As your focus on quieting the mind improves, you may wish to extend the meditation to an hour.

INSTRUCTIONS:
1. Sit in a comfortable posture on the floor or in an upright chair with your feet firmly

planted on the ground. Concentrate on the first syllable of OM, which is AH. The AH aspect of OM refers to the physical body and universe, and the waking state. Say AH for the count of I, then pause for the count of I. Concentrate on the silent pause between the repetitions of AH. Do this for 5 minutes.

2. Now, focus on the second syllable of OM, which is OU. The OU aspect of OM refers to the subtle or astral body, the cosmic mind, and the dream state. Say OU for the count of I, pronounced by puckering your lips into a circle, then take pause for the count of I. Concentrate on the silent pause between the repetitions of OU. Do this for 5 minutes.

3. Next, concentrate on the last syllable of OM, which is MM, pronounced with the lips closed. MM represents a state of sleep. Say MM for the count of I, then take pause for the count of I. Concentrate on the silence between the repetitions of MM. Do this for 5 minutes.

4. Lastly, focus on the whole syllable OM. Say OM for the count of I, then pause for the count of I. Concentrate on the silence between the repetitions of OM. Do this for 5 minutes.

Now that you have attuned to the cosmic sound OM, put away the syllables and audible sounds of the mind. Sit in yourself for 20 minutes or so. Observe your inner silence—your resonant field of awareness, filled with the reverberations of the cosmic OM. When you arise from your practice, continue to harness your sense of quietude for the rest of your day.

THE PRACTICE: WINTER MOON FEAST

OPTIMUM TIMING:
- On winter solstice day.
- During the 4-day long celebration of Pongal occurring in mid-January.
- On the full moon day in the latter part of March.

PREPARATION:
Prepare your Winter Moon Feast for your friends and family from the many lavish recipes provided you in the next chapter of recipes, "Wondrous Winter Repasts." Alternatively, to honor the slim austerity of the pervading season, you may choose to prepare the classical Vedic dish of Pongal (recipe follows). Serve this ancient repast in beautiful, large bowls with a dash of Tila Namak (recipe on page 284), and your guests will surely be filled with warmth, love, and the abundance of simplicity.

First though, take a moment to truly appreciate the Living Ahimsa feast you are about to create by exploring the sacred lessons of the hands in chapter seven. Those teachings will forever change the way you work and commune with food.

Whenever possible prepare your meals and feasts by massaging your hands when you wash grains and legumes. Knead your cosmic energies into the dough. Roll out and pat flatbreads lovingly with your hands. Tear leafy greens with your fingers rather than cutting them with a knife. Nourish yourself, and nurture and heal your family and friends with the creation of a feast made from your own sacred energies.

A BLISSFUL BOWL OF PONGAL:

On the auspicious day of Pongal, the sweet rice dish also called "pongal" is made from a mouth-watering concoction of newly harvested rice, mung beans, jaggery, and fresh milk, all brought to a boil until overflowing from the pot. The pongal is cooked outdoors on an open fire in a new earthenware pot. Fresh turmeric and ginger—herbs symbolic of fertility and vitality—are tied around the neck of the pot. Once the rice is cooked and spilling over into a thick creamy nectar, it is removed from the fire and garnished with raisins and cashew nuts sautéed in ghee. Venerating the sun god, Surya, and the fire god, Agni, the blissful pongal is offered to them on a new banana leaf before it is imbibed by the celebrants.

This harvest festival of Pongal is celebrated over a 4-day period in South India. In Tamil Nadu, celebrants decorate the cows and engage them in lavish processions. Apart from feeding family and guests, pongal is offered as a blessed food to the cows, street dogs, and other animals.

Each day of the Pongal festival has a special significance. On the first day called Bhogi, old clothes and unwanted materials are dispensed with, marking the beginning of a new life. The second day, the actual day of Pongal, is celebrated by boiling fresh milk early in the morning and allowing it to boil over the cooking vessel—a sign of abundance for the coming year. People also prepare savories and sweets and exchange goodwill and gifts within their community for the 4-day long duration of the festivities

To honor this auspicious time of winter and to relish the authentic taste of the season, prepare and hold a blissful bowl of pongal in your hands and feel its warmth radiating through you while savoring the aromatic taste of its nectar. The following are simple recipes for making your own Pongal Feast.

SAVORY PONGAL ♥

Serves: 4

2 1/2 cups water

I cup white rice

1/4 cup split mung beans

1/2 teaspoon turmeric powder

2 tablespoons organic ghee (recipe on pages 150-151)

I teaspoon cumin seeds

I teaspoon peppercorns, coarsely grated

1/2 cup raw cashews, chopped

1/2 teaspoon rock salt (optional)

Bring water to a boil in a large earthenware pot. Add the rice, mung beans, and turmeric powder, and simmer over medium heat for approximately 30 minutes until the rice mixture is cooked to a porridge-like consistency. Cover and remove from heat. Melt the ghee in a small cast-iron skillet, then add the cumin seeds, peppercorns, and cashews. Stir and roast over low heat for approximately 3 minutes until the cumin seeds turn brown. Stir this mixture into the pongal. Add salt and serve piping hot in beautiful bowls.

SWEET PONGAL ♥

Serves: 4

3 1/2 cups water

I cup short-grain brown rice

1/2 cup whole mung beans

I cup whole milk

2 cups jaggery or turbinado sugar

2 tablespoons organic ghee (recipe on pages 150-151)

2 tablespoons cashews, chopped

2 tablespoons raisins

1/2 teaspoon cardamom powder

1/2 teaspoon clove powder

1/2 teaspoon nutmeg, grated

I pinch of saffron threads

Bring water to a boil in a large earthenware pot. Add the rice and mung beans, and simmer over medium heat for approximately 30 minutes before stirring in the milk and sugar. Let the rice mixture cook for an additional 20 minutes over low heat until it becomes a porridge-like consistency. Cover and remove from heat. Melt the ghee in a small cast-iron skillet, then add the cashews, raisins, and spice powders. Stir and roast over low heat for approximately 3 minutes until the raisins swell. Stir this mixture into the pongal and sprinkle the saffron strands on top of it. Serve piping hot in beautiful bowls.

As a reminder, before you serve this or any feast, offer the first bite to the goddess as a token of gratitude. This is also an opportune time to serve your dogs or pets some pongal in their very own bowls. Every dog has his day, and the festivities of pongal are meant to include special care for the animals as well. Animals have a distinct sense of recognizing when they are being truly honored and cared for. I don't mean excitedly pouring mushy attention on an animal, but communicating respect and gratitude. It fascinates me to see how instinctively perfect the animals are. They sniff out your intention well before you are aware of what your intentions are! The street dogs in India who receive pongal blessings and food strut about like little princes on that day, and they conduct themselves with great nobility once they have been garlanded. They know it is their day and seem to avoid any non-decorous behavior and usual skirmishes.

HONORING THE ANIMALS

Following the festival of Dipavali, explored in the Early Winter section of this book, the ceremony of *Govardhana Puja* is observed. This celebration begins on the *Kartika* new moon day, which generally occurs at the end of October or beginning of November. At this time, Hindus observe a five-day period of prayers, offerings, and rituals to honor the animals (specifically the crows, dogs, and oxen) and ending with the care of the animal that is venerated with great passion—the symbol of maternal instinct—the cows.

As a Living Ahimsa practice on every day of the year we should make a point to care for and contribute to the safety and well-being of each and every animal in the world. The heartfelt, conscious ritual activities I am about to propose for the caring of the animals is of absolute necessity today if we are to reclaim our cognitive memory of ahimsa, compassion, and humanity. These observances also demonstrate a living culture of humanity's peaceful coexistence with nature and all of her creatures.

Unfortunately, evidenced by the massive plundering of nature and blatant human disregard for her—and other contributing factors such as modernization and urban living—the numbers of annihilated species, injured or mistreated animals, and homeless animals that crowd the streets are becoming progressively worse every day. At present we live with a treachery of conflicts in this regard. For example, we turn a blind eye to their suffering or are overly attentive to our pets while we contribute to the blatant hurt of other animals by eating them. Through these ancient Vedic practices (which I have unearthed and revived as part of the Wise Earth Ayurveda's Living Ahimsa way of life) we can awaken our cognitive memories from their long slumber and recognize the sanctity of each and every creature. I hope that through this work we will restore our own priceless health as well as that of the animals.

Every Cow Has Its Day

As you know, cows are considered sacred and are treated with great respect in my culture. In fact, all animals are held in great esteem, since we recognize that each life force and species performs an irreplaceable function in the totality of creation. Cows, however, are considered special wards of the goddess Lakshmi—goddess of wealth, well-being, and familial happiness. At this time of year, the goddess is welcomed into the hearts and hearths of the Hindus with rituals involving light, song, prayer, and fresh flowers. Vows of the self are taken so the disciple can remain happy and prosperous throughout the year.

Cows are also identified with the goddess Aditi, mother of the gods. In ancient times cows were considered perfect gifts for the Brahmins—Hinduism's spiritual guardians—and so it came to be understood that killing a cow would be equivalent to killing a Brahmin. Cows represent the giving nature of the Great Mother that sustains life to every Hindu. In Vedic literature, cows are often described as "Mother" since we sustain ourselves by the milk we get from them. By honoring these gentle animals who give more than they take, we honor all creatures. These gentle creatures are venerated as carriers of great maternal value to the earth. The Sanskrit saying: *go-brahmana-hitaya* informs us that the Lord is deeply concerned about the welfare of the cows and the Brahmins, spiritual teachers. On the fourth day of this festival, the cows are honored with flower garlands around their necks and are served delicious vegetarian meals. Having saved the sacred strings worn during the brother-revering celebration of Raksha Bandhana, which I mentioned earlier, celebrants tie them on cows' tails. It is believed that by doing so the cows will help pull them into the celestial sphere after death.

The first day of *Govardhana Puja* and its festivities are relegated to the crows, which are recognized as flying messengers of the ancestors. On this day a special Vedic ceremony is performed: The crows are fed delicious, blessed food they greatly enjoy, before any of the human guests are fed. On the second day of honoring the animals, the dogs are lavished with appropriate attention. Dogs are traditionally recognized as the guardians of both the human habitat as well as the underworld. On this day, bindis of red sacred powder are put on their foreheads, garlands of fresh, fragrant flowers are hung around their necks, and lavish meals are served to them. Although dogs are not vegetarian by nature, on this day they enjoy ritual vegetarian meals of chapati—the favorite food of dogs in India. You can honor all the animals with your kindness and good thoughts at any time, although the time of the *Kartika* new moon is seen as one of the most auspicious times to lavish them with love and good care.

The following is a wonderful practice you may observe to refresh your Living Ahimsa memory of kindness to all living creatures. In general, I recommend you say a prayer for the welfare of all animals, and if permitted, nourish and feed any non-aggressive animals you encounter anywhere. First though, you must inculcate an essential understanding when caring for animals and pets.

In the Vedic culture, it is recommended that dedicated areas and large basins for grooming and bathing pets are set aside. For reasons of propriety, we do not bathe them in the homes or baths we use. In my tradition we recognize that each species carries its own set of memories, concerns, and behaviors. For this reason we do not try to domesticate animals or have them live inside the home since this process inevitably dulls an animal's intrinsic species memories and progressively curbs its natural sense of freedom.

However, we appreciate that domesticated animals serve a purpose in society since they provide companionship, love, a sense of fullness to the human family, and teach children imperative early skills of bonding. We can, however, seek to better understand our pets' primal natures while we gain comfort from their presence in our lives. In so doing, we preserve their integrity. One way of achieving this is to recognize that your pets are part of the animal kingdom, and that anything that we do to hurt animals denigrates them. We must also recognize that animals, like human beings, need a certain amount of privacy and space. Unlike the human, who has the power of speech, the ability to think and plan, and the will to execute programs, animals work largely through instinct—their intrinsic set of memories creates form and function in their own unique ways. Because their instincts are shaped by a fierce and primal need for survival, their intentions can be driven by extremely compelling forces. For example, in my training I have learned that animals, and dogs in particular, are able to extract the nutritive energy from a food, simply by focusing their attention on that food. This is why it is advised that you do not imbibe your meals in the presence of your pets. Feed them at their own appointed time with awareness and a one-pointed sense of attention.

THE PRACTICE: HONORING THE ANIMALS

Renew your bond with your pets in an extraordinary way. Have them join you while chanting a Prayer to the Goddess Mother (following) for their welfare and all animals at large.

OPTIMUM TIMING:
- The *Kartika* new moon occurring in late October or early November.
- At Pongal, the 4-day celebration usually occurring between the 12th and 15th of January.

PREPARATIONS:

Lavish love upon your honored pets by bathing and grooming them, then decorating them with fresh-flower garlands around their necks. Get them new toys, new bowls and collars, and any accessories that will keep them well-groomed and happy.

MANTRA FOR FORGIVENESS:

Prayer to the Goddess Mother, Lalita Maha Tripurasundari
• Facing east, recite 108 repetitions of the following mantra:

Om Krtajnayai Namah
(Pronounced: OOM KRIT-AGH-NYAA-YAI NAH-MAH-HA)

To the Great Goddess Lalita Ambika, who embodies the sun, moon, elements, time and space; the One who knows whatever grievances are committed by Her charges; the One who compensates our transgressions with knowledge when we worship Her.

• After the mantra, speak directly to the goddess asking her forgiveness:

Forgive me for my thoughts and actions that run counter to ahimsa,
the cosmic law of your universe.

Whether by omission or commission, if my thoughts or actions contribute to the
personal or collective misery, violence, anger, or hatred, may I be forgiven.

May I be forgiven for my contribution toward the slaughtering and eating of the
animals. May I recognize the beauty of all creatures, like I do my own pet.

With this mantra, I plead for your benign grace.

May I be free from the travesty of ignorance of my true nature.

May my awareness always be lit by your Light of Knowledge.

• After the prayer, bless your pets with traditional sacred red sindur powder by placing a dab on their foreheads.
• Take them to their favorite park or grassy field for a healthy run; let them show off their newly blessed foreheads and acquired garlands.
• You may also feel inclined to gather homeless animals or visit nearby shelters taking nourishing meals, treats, and blessings for the animals.

Chapter Nineteen

WONDROUS WINTER REPASTS: BREAD, BROTH & BEYOND

Your winter feast is laden with delicious soups and bountiful winter grains, freshly baked breads, accented with winter greens and warming salads. These are the perfect meals for the late winter season—rich and abundant—designed to stimulate your own Inner Medicine healing energies. You'll discover the satisfaction and wholesome nurturance in simply enjoying a large bowl of flavorful soup or the inimitable spirit of Living Ahimsa in kneading, baking, and imbibing the primeval feast that is bread, broth, and beyond.

LATE WINTER MENU PLANNING

The Late Winter Season:
- Northern Hemisphere: Mid-to-late January through mid-to-late March.
- Southern Hemisphere: Mid-to-late August through mid-to-late October.

Vulnerable Time: For Kapha and Vata Types*
- Kapha: Avoid excess cold, unctuous, salty, and fatty foods, and refined sweets.
- Vata: Avoid excess cold, dry, and bitter foods
- * To learn your body type, see appendix one, "Wise Earth Ayurveda Body Types."

LATE WINTER MENU: DO's & DON'T's	
APPROPRIATE FOODS FOR LATE WINTER	FOODS TO AVOID IN LATE WINTER
Sweet, moderately sour, and moderately salty tastes	Pungent, bitter, and astringent tastes
Warm, unctuous, heavy, or substantial foods	Cold, dry, light, fermented, and stale foods

Seasonal grains, earthy root vegetables, cooked or organically canned fruits, beans, organic dairy, good quality and freshly prepared sweets, cakes, porridges, puddings, and breads	Meats, fowl, fish, and eggs

Table 19.1

SAMPLE LATE WINTER MENU

Late Winter Breakfast:
- Kapha: Breakfast is not recommended.
- Pitta and Vata: See appendix three, "Breakfast of Champions," for a wide array of breakfast choices that can be enjoyed throughout the year.

Late Winter Lunch:
- Creamy Butternut Squash Soup (p 328)
- Fresh Baked Seven-Grain Bread (p 336)

Late Winter Dinner:
- Arugula & Currant Salad (p 332)
- Black Bean Tamarind Soup (p 327)
- Stovetop Cornbread (p 338)
- Apple Date Torte (p 342)

Gluten-free recipes are indicated by ♡
Yeast-free recipes are indicated by ⬤

NURTURING SOUPS

MILLET & LENTIL SOUP ♡

Serves: 8

1 1/2 gallons water

1 1/2 cups millet

1 cup brown lentils

4 carrots

4 stalks celery, chopped

3 green onions, chopped

1 teaspoon cumin powder

1 tablespoon dried parsley

1 tablespoon coriander seeds

1 teaspoon mustard seeds

4 cardamom pods

I teaspoon fresh ginger, grated

I 1/2 teaspoons rock salt

I tablespoon organic ghee (recipe on pages 150-151)

1/2 lemon, freshly juiced

I small bunch winter cress, for garnish

Bring water to a boil in a large heavy-bottomed soup pot. Thoroughly wash the millet and lentils and add to the boiling water. Add carrots, celery, green onions, cumin powder, and parsley. Dry roast the coriander and mustard seeds in a cast-iron skillet over medium heat until the mustard seeds begin to pop. Coarsely crush the seeds in a suribachi and add them to the soup along with cardamom pods, grated ginger, and salt. Cover and simmer on medium heat for 45 minutes. Add ghee and lemon juice. Wash and tear the slender-lobed leaves of the winter cress into large pieces and garnish the soup. Remove from heat, cover, and let sit for 10 minutes. Serve warm with a winter bread of your choice.

POTATO & BARLEY SOUP

Serves: 8

2 gallons water

5 large potatoes

3 large carrots

I cup pearled barley

1/2 cup red lentils

I large yellow onion, minced

I tablespoon coriander powder

I tablespoon dried dill

I teaspoon black pepper, finely ground

I 1/2 teaspoons rock salt

I tablespoon sunflower oil

I tablespoon cumin seeds

I small bunch fresh parsley, minced

Bring water to a boil in a large heavy-bottomed soup pot. Scrub the potatoes and carrots well until most of the skins have rubbed off. Cut the potatoes in quarters, and cut the carrots in large chunks, then add both to the boiling water. Wash the barley and lentils then add to the soup broth. Add the onion, coriander, dill, black pepper, and salt. Stir, cover, and simmer on medium heat for I 1/4 hours until the barley becomes plump and soft. Heat the sunflower oil in a small skillet over medium heat and roast the cumin seeds until golden brown. Add the cumin seeds and oil to the soup by stirring the soup with the small skillet (if possible). Add the fresh parsley, cover, and simmer on low heat for 10 minutes more. Serve hot with a winter bread of your choice.

CREAMY CORN & PEPPER SOUP ♡
Serves: 8
1 gallon water
1 pint soy milk
1/2 cup dried corn, coarsely crushed
1 teaspoon rock salt
1/2 teaspoon cayenne powder
1/2 teaspoon black pepper, finely ground
3 dried whole chilis
1/2 cup chickpea flour
1 teaspoon turmeric powder
1 tablespoon soy oil
1 small bunch shepherd's purse, for garnish

Bring water and soy milk to a boil in a large heavy-bottomed soup pot. Add crushed corn, salt, cayenne, black pepper, and whole chilis. Stir and simmer on medium heat for 45 minutes. Dry roast chickpea flour and turmeric in a medium-size skillet over medium heat until golden brown, stirring frequently to avoid burning. Fold the flour mixture into the boiling soup. (If a thinner soup is desired add more water.) Reduce heat to low, stir, cover, and let simmer for 15 minutes more. Lightly sauté the shepherd's purse in soy oil and garnish the soup with it. Serve warm over soft cooked millet or barley.

GOLDEN BEET & CHICKPEA SOUP ♡
Serves: 8
1 1/2 gallons water
6 golden beets, peeled
2 cups chickpeas, soaked overnight
2 yellow onions, minced
4 stalks celery, chopped
2 large carrots, diced
1 teaspoon dried sage
1 tablespoon dried parsley
1/2 teaspoon cayenne powder
1 tablespoon soy oil
1 teaspoon ajwain seeds
1 teaspoon rock salt
1 small bunch celery leaves, chopped, for garnish

Bring water to a boil in a large heavy-bottomed soup pot. Scrub the beets and cut them into bite-size pieces, then add to the boiling water. Strain the chickpeas and add to the water along with the onions, celery, carrots, sage, and parsley. Then add the cayenne powder. Heat the soy oil in a small skillet and roast the ajwain seeds over medium heat until golden brown, then add to soup mixture by stirring the soup water with the small skillet (if possible). Add salt, stir, cover, and simmer on medium heat for 40 minutes until the chickpeas are quite soft. Garnish with celery leaves and serve hot with a winter bread of your choice.

RED CABBAGE & ONION SOUP ♥

Serves: 8

1 1/2 gallons water
2 small red cabbages, shredded
4 red onions, chopped
1 tablespoon coriander powder
1 teaspoon cayenne powder
1 tablespoon dried dill
1 tablespoon dried parsley
3 cloves garlic
1 tablespoon rock salt
1/4 cup cashew butter
1 red onion, thin half-moon slices

Bring the water to a boil in a large heavy-bottomed soup pot. Add the shredded cabbage and chopped onions, along with the coriander, cayenne, dill, and parsley. Lightly crush the garlic cloves with a hand stone and remove the skin. Add to soup mixture. Cover and simmer on medium heat for 35 minutes, until onions are practically dissolved. Add cashew butter, and stir until it dissolves. Garnish the hot soup with the thinly sliced red onion. Remove from heat. Cover and let sit for 5 minutes. Serve hot with a heaping dollop of medium-grain brown rice.

BLACK BEAN TAMARIND SOUP ♥

Serves: 8

1 1/2 gallons water
1 1/2 cups black beans
2 large potatoes, peeled and cubed
2 small carrots, diced
1 teaspoon fresh ginger, grated
1 tablespoon soy oil
1 teaspoon brown mustard seeds
1 teaspoon cumin seeds
1 teaspoon dried oregano

I teaspoon dried sage

I 1/2 teaspoons rock salt

I tablespoon tamarind paste

3 tablespoons warm water

Bring water to a boil in a large heavy-bottomed soup pot. Wash beans and add to the water along with the potatoes, carrots, and grated ginger. Heat soy oil in a small cast-iron skillet and roast the mustard and cumin seeds over medium heat until they begin to pop. Add seeds to the soup water by stirring the pot with the small skillet (if possible). Add oregano, sage, and salt. Cover and simmer on medium heat for 30 minutes. Dilute the tamarind paste in warm water and stir into the soup. Cover and let simmer for 10 minutes more. Serve hot with a heaping dollop of soft-cooked short-grain brown rice.

WINTER YOGURT SOUP

Serves: 8

2 quarts water

I pint soy milk

1/2 cup oat bran

I teaspoon white pepper, finely ground

I teaspoon rock salt

I quart organic yogurt

2 tablespoons sunflower oil

I teaspoon cumin seeds

I teaspoon ajwain seeds

I small bunch celery leaves, for garnish

Bring water and soy milk to a boil in a large heavy-bottomed soup pot. Stir in the oat bran, salt, and pepper and let simmer on medium heat for 5 minutes. Lower the heat and fold in the yogurt, stirring frequently to prevent it from curdling. Heat sunflower oil in a small cast-iron skillet and roast the spice seeds over medium heat until golden brown. Add to the yogurt soup by stirring the soup pot with the small skillet (if possible). Remove from heat. Garnish with celery leaves and serve warm with a winter bread of choice.

BUTTERNUT SQUASH SOUP

Serves: 8

I 1/2 gallons water

I large butternut squash, peeled and cut into I-inch cubes

I cup rolled oats

3 tablespoons fresh cilantro, minced

I tablespoon cumin powder

I teaspoon coriander powder

1/2 teaspoon turmeric powder

1/2 teaspoon black pepper, finely ground

I tablespoon fresh ginger, grated

I lemon, freshly juiced

I tablespoon rock salt

I tablespoon soy oil

2 scallions, chopped

Bring water to a boil in a large heavy-bottomed soup pot. Add the squash, oats, cilantro, spice powders, black pepper, fresh ginger, lemon juice, and salt. Cover and let simmer on medium heat for 35 minutes. Use a flat-bottomed ladle to puree the squash. Heat soy oil in a small skillet and sauté the scallions for about 2 minutes over medium heat, then add to the creamed soup. Cover and simmer for 5 minutes more. Serve hot with a winter bread of your choice and lightly sautéed mustard greens on the side if desired.

WISE EARTH POTATO LEEK SOUP ♥

Serves: 8

1 1/2 gallons water

4 leeks, thinly sliced

2 yellow onions, chopped

4 large potatoes, peeled and quartered

1/2 cup yellow split mung beans

2 tablespoons dried dill

I teaspoon black pepper, finely ground

1 1/2 teaspoons rock salt

I tablespoon organic ghee (recipe on pages 150-151)

1/2 cup fresh roasted sunflower seeds, for garnish

Bring water to a boil in a heavy-bottomed soup pot. Add leeks, onions, potatoes, mung beans, dill, black pepper, and salt. Stir, cover, and simmer over medium heat for 45 minutes until the leeks are almost dissolved and the potatoes crumble. Stir in the ghee. Serve hot garnished with a few roasted sunflower seeds and soft cooked cracked wheat on the side.

ROSEMARY PARSNIP SOUP ♥

Serves: 8

1 1/2 gallons water

6 large parsnips

I teaspoon coriander powder

I teaspoon cumin powder

1 teaspoon black pepper, finely ground

1 1/2 teaspoons rock salt

1 tablespoon dried rosemary

1 tablespoon dried parsley

1 cup chickpea flour

1 tablespoon sunflower oil

3 tablespoons sesame seeds

Bring water to a boil in a large heavy-bottomed soup pot. Scrub parsnips, cut in large chunks, and add to water. Add spice powders, black pepper, salt, rosemary, and parsley. Cover and simmer over medium heat for 25 minutes until the parsnips are tender. Dry roast the flour in a small skillet over medium heat until golden brown, and introduce it into the soup mixture. Heat the sunflower oil in a separate skillet and roast the sesame seeds for about 1 minute over medium heat until golden brown. Add to soup. Cover and let simmer for 5 minutes more. Serve warm with a winter bread of your choice.

DAIKON & TOFU SOUP ♡
Serves: 8

1 1/2 gallons water

4 medium-size daikons

1/2 cup grated carrot

2 tablespoons sesame oil

2 pounds semi-firm tofu

1/2 teaspoon red pepper flakes

1/2 teaspoon black pepper, finely ground

1 1/2 teaspoons rock salt

1 teaspoon fresh ginger, grated

1 lemon, freshly juiced

1 tablespoon unrefined brown sugar

1 small bunch winter cress, for garnish

Bring water to a boil in a large heavy-bottomed soup pot. Scrub daikons and cut on a bias into 1/2-inch thick pieces. Add to the boiling water along with the carrots. Heat the sesame oil in a large cast-iron skillet over medium heat. Cut tofu into 1-inch squares and lightly pan fry for a few minutes, turning the pieces over to lightly brown each side. Add fried tofu to the soup mixture along with pepper flakes, black pepper, salt, ginger, lemon juice, and brown sugar. Stir, cover, and simmer on medium heat for 15 minutes until the daikons are completely translucent. Wash the winter cress, tear into large pieces, and garnish the soup. Remove from heat and serve hot over cooked noodles or with a winter bread of your choice.

GRATIFYING WINTER GRAINS

SOFT LEMON MILLET ♥

Serves: 2

3 1/2 cups boiling water

1 cup millet

4 tablespoons split urad dhal (Indian black lentils)

1/2 teaspoon brown mustard seeds

1/8 teaspoon asafetida

1 pinch rock salt

Lemon slices, for garnish

Bring water to a boil in a medium-size pot. Wash millet and dry roast over medium heat in a large cast-iron skillet until evenly golden, then add to the hot water. In a small skillet dry roast urad dhal and mustard seeds for a few minutes until the seeds start to pop. Add to the grains along with the asafetida and salt, stir well. Simmer on medium-low heat for 45 minutes. Garnish with lemon slices.

CARDAMOM CLOVE SPICED WHEAT

Serves: 2

1/2 cup whole wheat berries

8 whole cloves

4 cardamom pods

2 teaspoons olive oil

1 tablespoon cumin seeds

1 teaspoon rock salt

4 cups boiling water

Fresh parsley, for garnish

Soak wheat berries for 5 hours. Rinse and add to boiling water in a pressure cooker with whole cloves and cardamom pods. Bring to pressure and cook for 35 minutes. Allow pressure to fall naturally. In a small skillet heat the olive oil over medium heat and brown the cumin seeds. Then grind into a fine powder. Allow spiced wheat to cool for 15 minutes before mixing powder into the wheat. Garnish with fresh parsley and serve warm.

SUPPLE CINNAMON RICE ♥

Serves: 2

1 cup short-grain brown rice

5 cups water

1 two-inch cinnamon stick

Wash the rice and add to bottom of pot. Add water and bring to a boil. Cover and simmer on low heat for 60 minutes. The rice should be creamy with a few whole kernels. Serve warm with Tila Namak condiment (recipe on page 284).

SUBLIME WINTER SALADS

WATERCRESS & SCALLION SALAD ♡

Serves: 4

1 large bunch watercress or land cress
1 tablespoon scallions
1 teaspoon fresh ginger, grated
1/2 lemon, freshly juiced
1 teaspoon olive oil
1/2 teaspoon rock salt

Wash watercress and scallions. Tear the cress into bite-size pieces and set aside. Finely chop the scallions, place in a salad bowl, and add grated ginger, lemon juice, oil, and salt. Fold in the watercress and serve.

ARUGULA & CURRANT SALAD ♡

Serves: 6

2 bunches arugula
1 tablespoon olive oil
1 tablespoon cumin seeds
1/4 cup currants
1 teaspoon rice vinegar
1/2 teaspoon orange peel, dried
2 tablespoons warm water
1/2 teaspoon black pepper, finely ground

Wash the arugula, tear into bite-size pieces and set aside. Heat the olive oil in a small skillet and roast the cumin seeds and currants over medium heat until the seeds turn golden brown and the currants are plump. Remove from heat and stir in the rice vinegar, orange peel, water, and black pepper to create the dressing. Pour over the salad and serve immediately.

ENDIVE & BARLEY SALAD

Serves: 6

2 cups pearl barley, cooked
1/2 cup endives, finely cut

1 tablespoon dried basil

1 teaspoon dried rosemary

1 tablespoon walnut oil

1/2 lemon, freshly juiced

1 teaspoon rock salt

Wash the cooked barley with warm water, cover, and set aside. In a large salad bowl, combine the endives and herbs, juice, and salt. Add barley and toss all the ingredients to mix. Serve warm.

SPROUTED MUNG & SESAME SALAD ♡

Serves: 6

1 cup Sprouted Mung Beans (recipe on page 118)

1 head red oak lettuce

1/8 cup hot water

1 tablespoon sesame butter

1 teaspoon tamari

1/2 lemon, freshly juiced

1 tablespoon sesame oil

1 tablespoon sesame seeds

1 teaspoon brown mustard seeds

Wash the mung bean sprouts and lettuce then tear the lettuce into bite-size pieces, place them in a large salad bowl and set aside. Pour hot water into a small bowl and dissolve the sesame butter by whipping it into a smooth base for the dressing. Add the tamari and lemon juice. Pour sesame oil in a small skillet and roast sesame and mustard seeds for 2 minutes over medium heat until they start to pop. Stir the dressing into the skillet then pour the contents over the sprouted mung and lettuce. Toss and serve.

HERBED OAT SALAD

Serves: 6

2 cups cracked oats, cooked

1 tablespoon sunflower oil

2 small shallots, minced

1 teaspoon dried thyme

1 teaspoon dried oregano

1 teaspoon dried rosemary

1 teaspoon dried marjoram

2 tablespoons apple cider vinegar

I teaspoon rock salt
I tablespoon cumin seeds
Handful fresh parsley, minced, for garnish

Wash the cooked oats with warm water to loosen grains, pour into a large salad bowl, cover, and set aside. Heat the sunflower oil in a large skillet over medium heat, sauté the shallots for I minute, then add the cumin seeds. Once the seeds turn golden brown remove from heat and stir in the herbs, vinegar, and salt. Pour the mixture into the oats. Garnish with minced fresh parsley, if available. Toss and serve at once.

CARROT, RADICCHIO & KOMBU SALAD ♡
Serves: 6
4 carrots
2 heads radicchio
I bunch green leaf lettuce
2 strips kombu seaweed
I tablespoon olive oil
4 small shallots, chopped
I teaspoon cumin seeds
I tablespoon rice vinegar

Wash the carrots, cut them into matchsticks, and set them aside in a large bowl. Wash radicchio and lettuce, tear leaves into bite-size pieces, and place into the bowl. Wash and towel dry the kombu strips. Heat olive oil in skillet and fry the kombu for a minute over medium-high heat while turning each piece to brown both sides. Remove from skillet and set the crisp pieces aside to cool. Add shallots and cumin seeds to the hot oil and sauté for a few minutes until the shallots turn translucent in color. Pour mixture into the salad bowl, add vinegar, and toss to mix. Break the kombu strips into tiny pieces and use as a garnish.

GARBANZO & BUCKWHEAT SALAD
Serves: 6
2 cups garbanzo beans, cooked
2 cups buckwheat groats, cooked
I/4 cup fresh parsley, minced
3 licorice mint leaves, minced
I/2 teaspoon cayenne powder
I teaspoon rock salt
I/2 teaspoon black pepper, finely ground

I tablespoon olive oil

I teaspoon ajwain seeds

I ounce raisins

1/2 tablespoon tamari

1/4 cup warm water

In a large salad bowl combine the garbanzo beans and buckwheat groats along with the herbs, spices, salt, and pepper. Heat olive oil in a small skillet and roast the ajwain seeds and raisins over medium heat until the seeds turn golden brown and the raisins are plump. Remove skillet from heat, stir in the tamari and water, and pour the contents over the beans and groats. Toss and serve at once.

WARMING WINTER BREADS

MILLET SQUASH BREAD ♡ Ⓥ

Serves: 6 (2 loaves)

I small butternut squash, peeled and cooked

2 cups millet, cooked

1/2 cup cornmeal, plus additional for garnish

I teaspoon coriander powder

I teaspoon cumin powder

1/2 teaspoon red pepper flakes, finely ground

2 tablespoons corn oil

I teaspoon rock salt

2 cups warm water

Preheat oven to 375 degrees. Combine squash, millet, cornmeal, coriander, cumin, red pepper, corn oil, and salt in a large bowl. Gradually pour in the water and knead until smooth. Divide dough into two equal parts and place in oiled loaf pans. Sprinkle cornmeal on top. Bake for 20 minutes until the top of loaves are brown.

QUINOA OAT BREAD Ⓥ

Serves: 6 (2 loaves)

I cup quinoa

I cup oat bran

I cup rolled oats

I tablespoon natural yeast (optional)

I tablespoon organic ghee (recipe on pages I50-I5I)

I tablespoon unrefined brown sugar

2 cups boiling water

1 tablespoon fresh dill, minced

1 tablespoon fresh parsley, minced

1 teaspoon organic mustard

1 teaspoon rock salt

Preheat oven to 375 degrees. Dry roast the quinoa in a heavy skillet for 5 minutes over medium heat and combine it with the oat bran, rolled oats, yeast (optional), ghee, and brown sugar that has been diluted in the boiling water. Stir, cover, and let sit for 30 minutes Blend in the fresh herbs, mustard, and salt, then knead into sticky dough. If too watery, add oat bran as needed. Divide dough into two equal parts and put in oiled loaf pans. Bake at 375 degrees for 10 minutes, then reduce heat to 325 degrees and bake for 15 minutes more.

ROSE PETAL BREAD

Serves: 6 (2 loaves)

1/4 cup organic dried rose petals

1/4 cup boiling water

1 tablespoon natural yeast

8 drops natural vanilla essence

4 cups barley flour

1 3/4 cups warm water

1/2 teaspoon rock salt

1/4 cup sugarless raspberry jam

Soak the rose petals in boiling water for 10 minutes. Stir in the yeast until it dissolves and then add the vanilla essence. Combine with flour, water, and salt. Knead into sticky dough. Transfer to a large, oiled bowl. Cover securely and let rise in a warm place for 40 minutes. Punch down the dough, divide into two equal pieces, and place in greased loaf pans. Make a deep indentation in the center of each loaf and fill with 2 tablespoons of raspberry jam. Cover and let rise again for 40 minutes. Bake for 10 minutes at 375 degrees. Then reduce heat to 325 degrees and continue baking for 20 more minutes.

SEVEN-GRAIN BREAD

Serves: 8 (3 loaves)

1/2 cup warm water

1 tablespoon natural yeast

2 tablespoons sesame butter

1/2 cup spelt flour

1/2 cup unbleached whole wheat flour

1/2 cup soy flour

1/2 cup millet flour

1/2 cup oat bran

1/2 cup rolled oats

1/2 cup cracked wheat

I tablespoon Sucanat

1/2 teaspoon rock salt

I 1/2 cups warm water

Dissolve the yeast in 1/2 cup warm water and dilute the sesame butter in the yeast solution. In a large bowl combine the flours, bran, rolled oats, cracked wheat, Sucanat, salt, and 1 1/2 cups water. Add the yeast-sesame-butter mixture and knead into a sticky dough. Transfer dough to a large oiled bowl. Cover securely and let rise in a warm place for 40 minutes. Punch down the dough, cover, and let rise again for 40 minutes until it doubles in size. Form dough into 4 loaves and place on oiled baking trays. Bake at 350 degrees for 25 minutes.

RUSSIAN RYE POTATO BREAD

Serves: 8 (3 loaves)

I tablespoon unsalted butter

I tablespoon caraway seeds

2 large potatoes, mashed

1/4 cup yogurt

3 cups rye flour

2 cups warm water

I teaspoon rock salt

Melt butter in a heavy skillet and roast the caraway seeds for 1 minute over medium heat until golden. Combine with the mashed potatoes, yogurt, flour, water, and salt in a large bowl and knead into a sticky dough. Transfer dough to a large oiled bowl, cover securely, and let it sit in a warm place overnight. The dough will turn mildly sour and rise moderately. Divide dough into 4 equal loaves and place in small oiled loaf pans. Bake at 350 degrees for 20 minutes.

CELERY OREGANO BREAD

Serves: 6 (2 loaves)

I tablespoon sunflower oil

I tablespoon celery seeds, plus additional for garnish

I tablespoon natural yeast

I cup warm soy milk

I cup warm water

3 1/2 cups spelt flour
1/4 cup fresh celery leaves, minced
1 tablespoon dried oregano
1 teaspoon rock salt

Heat sunflower oil in heavy skillet over medium heat and roast the celery seeds until golden. Set aside. Dilute yeast in warm soy milk. Combine milk-yeast mixture with water, flour, celery leaves, oregano and salt in a large bowl. Add the celery seed and oil mixture, then knead into a sticky dough. Transfer dough to a large oiled bowl. Cover securely and let rise in a warm place for 40 minutes. Punch down the dough, cover, and let it rise again until it doubles in size. Divide dough into 2 pieces and put into oiled loaf pans. Sprinkle a few celery seeds on top of the dough and bake at 375 degrees for 10 minutes. Then reduce heat to 350 degrees and bake for 20 minutes more.

STOVETOP CORNBREAD ♡ ⓥ
Serves: 8
1 tablespoon corn oil
1 teaspoon brown mustard seeds
1 teaspoon cumin seeds
1 tablespoon organic ghee (recipe on pages 150-151)
2 cups cornmeal
1 cup corn flour
1 cup soy flour
2 1/2 cups warm water
1 cup warm soy milk
1 teaspoon coriander powder
1/2 teaspoon turmeric powder
1/2 teaspoon cayenne powder
1 teaspoon rock salt

Heat the corn oil in a large cast-iron skillet over medium heat and lightly roast the mustard and cumin seeds until the mustard seeds begin to pop. Add ghee. When the ghee melts remove the skillet from heat and set aside. Combine cornmeal, flours, water, soy milk, spice powders, and salt in a large bowl. Pour in the spice seed-ghee mixture and mix into a thick batter. Pour the batter into the unwashed large skillet, cover, and let cook over low heat for 30 minutes until the cornbread is cooked. Carefully cut the cornbread while it is in the skillet and serve warm.

CARROT RICE BREAD ♡ ⓜ

Serves: 8

3 cups short-grain brown rice, cooked

1/2 cup roasted sesame seeds

1/2 cup grated carrots

1 tablespoon sunflower oil

1 large onion, minced

1 small bunch chives, chopped

1 teaspoon rock salt

1/2 teaspoon black pepper, finely ground

1 cup water

Sesame seeds, for garnish

Preheat oven to 375 degrees. Combine rice, sesame seeds, and carrots in a large bowl. Heat the sunflower oil in a skillet over medium heat and sauté onion and chives for a few minutes until the onion turns translucent. Add to the rice mixture along with salt and pepper. Add sufficient water to make a semi-firm batter. Coat 2 loaf pans with oil and half fill each with batter. Sprinkle sesame seeds on top of the batter for garnish. Bake for 25 minutes until the bread is crispy brown on top.

DECADENT DESSERTS

ROSE & ALMOND CUSTARD ♡

Serves: 6

2 tablespoons dried rose hips

2 cups water

1 1/2 cups almond milk

8 drops natural almond essence

1/2 teaspoon cardamom powder

1/4 cup raw almonds, peeled and crushed into paste

1 teaspoon grated fresh lemon peel

2 tablespoons kudzu powder

1/8 cup cold water

3 tablespoons maple syrup

1/4 cup dried organic rose petals

Boil water in a medium-size saucepan and cook rose hips on medium heat for 30 minutes. Strain and reserve the water for tea, discarding the rose hips in your compost. Combine the tea, almond milk, almond essence, cardamom powder, almond paste, and lemon peel in the saucepan. Simmer uncovered on medium heat for 5 minutes. Dilute the kudzu powder in cold water and pour into the tea mixture. Stir frequently until it reaches a smooth, creamy texture and to prevent the kudzu from lumping. Add the maple syrup. Garnish with rose petals. Cover and allow custard to sit for 5 minutes before serving.

SWEET YOGURT SHORTBREAD

Serves: 6

1/2 cup organic ghee (recipe on pages 150-151)

1 cup spelt flour

1 cup barley flour

1/4 cup unrefined brown sugar

1/8 cup plain yogurt

1/2 teaspoon black pepper, finely ground

Preheat oven to 300 degrees. Bring ghee to room temperature and cut it into the flours and sugar in a mixing bowl. Add the yogurt and black pepper. Gather the mixture into a ball. Use your hands to press the ball into an 8-inch circle on a floured surface, about 1/2-inch in thickness. Cut into triangular shapes. Prick with a fork and place on an oiled baking tray. Bake for 35 minutes until the edges turn golden brown.

APPLE ROSE PETAL PIE ♥

Serves: 6

2 pounds cooking apples

1/8 cup chickpea flour

2 tablespoons organic ghee (recipe on pages 150-151)

1/4 cup dried organic rose petals

1/4 cup cold water

2 tablespoons unrefined brown sugar

8 drops natural orange essence

1 tablespoon dried orange peel

1/2 lemon, freshly juiced

1 teaspoon cardamom powder

1/2 teaspoon cinnamon powder

1/2 teaspoon ground cloves

1/2 teaspoon rock salt

1 tablespoon maple syrup

Prepare an 8-inch chilled Short Crust Pastry Shell (recipe on page 302). Place shell into an oiled baking dish. Do not cut off the extra dough hanging over the edge of dish. Set aside extra dough, rolled out and cut into 3-inch wide strips, to decorate the top of the pie.

Preheat the oven to 350 degrees. Wash and core the apples. Slice thinly and set aside in a mixing bowl. Lightly roast the flour in a heavy skillet over medium heat until it turns golden brown. Add roasted flour to the apple slices, fold in the ghee, and blend the mixture together. Soak the rose petals in cold water for 10 minutes. Strain, retain the rose water, and set aside. Into the apple mixture blend the orange essence, orange peel, lemon juice, spice powders, and salt. Pour a palmful of the reserved rose water into the apple mixture, and put aside the remaining rose water for other use. Place the apple filling into the pre-pared pastry shell. Arrange the soaked rose petals on top of the filling, then lay the strips of dough across the dish, creating a lattice effect. Take the extra dough hanging over the edge of the baking dish and curl it up, building a ridge around the edge of the dish and seal-ing the ends of the dough strips into it. Finally, flute the ridge-edge around the dish. Brush dough with maple syrup. Bake pie for 1 hour until the crust is golden brown.

VANILLA BREAD PUDDING
Serves: 6

1 quart soy milk
1 teaspoon vanilla essence
1 teaspoon dried orange peel
1/8 cup currants
1/8 cup unrefined brown sugar
1 vanilla bean, split
4 cups dry whole wheat bread, cubed
1/4 cup chopped walnuts

Preheat oven to 375 degrees. Combine milk, vanilla essence, orange peel, currants, and sugar. Whisk the mixture until it turns foamy. Add the vanilla bean, bread, and walnuts and pour into an oiled baking dish. Bake for 1 hour until the top of the pudding is golden brown. When serving the pudding you may remove the split vanilla bean and discard in your compost.

DRIED FRUIT MEDLEY ♡
Serves: 6

2 cups water
2 tablespoons dried raspberry leaves
1/4 cup dried figs
1/4 cup dried apricots
1/4 cup dried prunes
1/4 cup dried pineapple, unsweetened
1/4 cup dried currants
1 cup rice milk

1/2 teaspoon cardamom powder

1/2 teaspoon ginger powder

1/4 cup chopped pecans, for garnish

Bring water to a boil in a medium-size saucepan and add raspberry leaves. Cover and simmer for 15 minutes. Strain, retain the tea, and discard the leaves in your compost. Chop figs, apricots, prunes, and pineapple into small pieces, and add along with the currants to the tea. Stir in rice milk, cardamom, and ginger. Cover and simmer for 25 minutes on medium heat until the fruits are very tender. Garnish with pecans and serve hot.

APPLE DATE TORTE

Serves: 6

2 cooking apples

1/4 cup dates

1/2 teaspoon cardamom powder

1/2 teaspoon ground nutmeg

1 pinch rock salt

1 cup whole wheat pastry flour

1/2 teaspoon baking powder

2 tablespoons walnut oil

1/8 cup maple syrup

1/8 cup apple sauce

Preheat oven to 350 degrees. Wash and core the apples, thinly slice, and set aside. Remove seeds from dates and cut into thin strips. Combine apples, dates, cardamom, nutmeg, and salt in a mixing bowl and set aside. Sift flour and baking powder into a separate bowl. Add the walnut oil and maple syrup into the flour mixture along with the apple sauce. Mix into a batter and pour into an oiled baking dish. Layer the top of batter with the fruit mixture. Bake for 45 minutes until a fork inserted in center of torte comes out clean. Serve warm.

TANTALIZING TEAS

CLOVE, CARDAMOM & BLACK TEA ♡

Serves: 2

1/2 cup water

2 cups milk

1 teaspoon cloves

2 two-inch cinnamon sticks

1 teaspoon cardamom pods

I teaspoon black tea leaves

I teaspoon honey

Combine water and milk and bring to a boil. Add spices and tea leaves, and simmer over low heat for 5 minutes. Strain, sweeten with honey, and serve warm.

ROSEMARY & SAGE TEA ♥
Serves: 2

3 cups water

2 tablespoons fresh sage leaves

I teaspoon fresh rosemary leaves

1/2 lemon, freshly juiced

Bring water to a boil and add the sage leaves. Simmer on low heat for 3 minutes. Remove from heat, cover, and let stand for I minute. Strain the leaves, add lemon juice to the decoction, and serve warm. Sweeten with I teaspoon of honey, if desired.

GINGER & CINNAMON SPICE TEA ♥
Serves: 2

3 1/2 cups water

I tablespoon fresh ginger, grated

6 whole cloves

1/2 teaspoon cinnamon powder

1/2 teaspoon turmeric powder

Bring water to a boil, peel the ginger and finely grate it. Add to water and steep on low heat for 3 minutes before adding the cloves, cinnamon, and turmeric. Remove from heat, cover, and let stand for I minute before straining. Serve warm.

LICORICE & MINT TEA ♥
Serves: 2

3 cups water

I tablespoon dried licorice root, shredded

5 drops mint essential oil

Bring water to a boil, add the root, and simmer on low heat for 3 minutes. Remove from heat, cover, and let stand for I minute. Strain the decoction, add essential oil, and serve warm. Sweeten with I teaspoon of honey, if desired.

SAFFRON & FENNEL TEA ♡
Serves: 2
1/2 cup water
2 cups milk
1 teaspoon fennel seeds
12 strands saffron

Combine water and milk and bring to a boil. Add fennel seeds and saffron and simmer over low heat for 5 minutes. Strain and serve warm.

WISE EARTH AYURVEDA BODY TYPES

YOUR METABOLIC CONSTITUTION

Each person bears a unique constitution, much like having a metabolic finger-print. As you will learn, the dosha that is dominant in you determines your meta-bolic type. Knowing what type you are provides you with helpful tools for main-taining a healthy life of balance. It also helps in diagnosing disease. Although disease has numerous causes, including genetic, environmental, and karmic fac-tors, irritation of the doshas is always due to ill health. The proportion to which Vata, Pitta, and Kapha exist within you is what makes your constitution different from someone else's.

Your constitution is determined at birth by the states of balance or imbalance of your parents' rhythms during conception, as well as from the particular permuta-tions of the five elements in the sperm and ovum at the time of conception. Once you are born, your constitution remains constant throughout your lifetime, but the condition of your doshas can change according to disharmonious factors in your lifestyle and environment. The practices of sadhana can help bring back the doshas into a state of harmony and certainly can help maintain your health.

There are other clues to help you determine your own or another's constitution. For example, the Pitta type will tend to have straight hair that is reddish in color. Does this mean if you're of African descent you can't be Pitta? Of course not. The Vedic seers who developed Ayurveda were people of color and of course could be dark-skinned and light-skinned. Even if you are dark-skinned and have essen-tially black hair, there may be a reddish tinge to the hair; it can be kinky, but it will get prematurely gray. Pitta skin may have a reddish tone as well, and regardless of the underlying skin color, it will be oily and warm.

Pitta types are more shapely and athletic than Vata or Kapha. Their bodies have the shape of an inverted triangle—with broad shoulders and slim hips. They tend to eat spicy, pungent foods, and sweat a lot. Pitta types can be moderate in weight, and have brown or hazel eyes, or greenish ones like tigers. They may be fiery, vola-tile, or aggressive in temperament. Their physical problems are generally related to the stomach, liver, spleen, and small intestine—hyper-acidity, diarrhea, poor sight, skin rashes, liver, spleen, and blood disorders are some of the common complaints of Pitta types. Their strengths are that of good physical stamina, strong intelligence and mental focus. They also tend to be successful, courageous, and practical in their dealings.

Vata types have hair that is typically thin and dry, and often kinky or frizzy. Their skin has a grayish hue. They tend to be thin and angular because they are formed by the element of wind, like a desert plant. Their eyes are usually brown, narrow, and uneven in shape, and their skin is always dry around the eyes. Likewise, they often have dry, cracked skin. Vata types have trouble putting on weight and often seem mentally distracted. Their physical problems are generally in the lower body—the large intestine and colon—because that's the seat of Vata energy. They tend to develop conditions such as constipation, insomnia, flatulence, arthritis, and osteoporosis. Their strengths are that of a strong and sensitive spirit. They strive for inner freedom and are generally environmentally and spiritually attuned. They have deep faith and are generally flexible and adaptable to life's varying situations.

Kapha types are the most voluptuous, with abundant, wavy hair. They have what I call a "moonlit" complexion, meaning that the hue is very fair regardless of color. Many dark people have translucent skin that looks as if the moon is reflected in it. Their eyelashes are long and curled, and the eyes themselves tend to look like big pools. They have a cool and complacent temperament. They have moist skin that can be oily, but is always cool; their hands and feet are typically cool. The weak spot for Kapha is in the upper body—the lungs, throat, thyroid, and tonsils—and they tend to be susceptible to conditions such as colds, coughs, allergies, tonsillitis, and bronchitis. Their strengths are that of physical and maternal endurance, calmness, and patience. Humility, nurturance, and fortitude are common Kapha virtues.

Once you understand these concepts, you can determine the constitution of the people around you. For example, my assistant is a Vata-Pitta type. Her skin tends to be dry. She has a strong spiritual temperament with a deep spiritual faith. She loves her inner freedom, although she can be impatient. My mother is the rare Kapha-Vata type who is immensely patient and steadfast. My father was a Pitta-Kapha type who had a full head of abundant, wavy locks, with a quick and alert mind. He excelled in meeting life cheerfully regardless of the obstacles he faced.

The table that follows summarizes the characteristics of the nine different body types—Vata, Pitta, and Kapha, and the various combinations of the three doshas.

THE NINE AYURVEDA METABOLIC TYPES

VATA

Element	Air/space
Energy	Cold
Texture	Dry, rough
Temperament	Austere, indecisive
Emotional strength	Spiritually adept
Emotional weakness	Irregularity, fearful
Body structure	Thin, angular, very short or very tall
Complexion	Brownish or grayish

PITTA

Element	Fire/water
Energy	Hot
Texture	Oily, soft
Temperament	Fiery, vibrant
Emotional strength	Materially adept, visionary
Emotional weakness	Indulgent, aggressive
Body structure	Athletic, well-shaped
Complexion	Yellowish or reddish

KAPHA

Element	Water/earth
Energy	Cool
Texture	Smooth, dense
Temperament	Methodical, slow
Emotional strength	Maternal, nurturing
Emotional weakness	Attachment, greediness
Body structure	Heavy, compact
Complexion	Pale, clear

VATA-PITTA

Element	Dominant—air/space, subordinate—fire/water
Energy	Cool
Texture	Sometimes dry, sometimes oily
Temperament	Sometimes indecisive and sometimes fiery
Emotional strength	Spiritually inclined, goal-oriented
Emotional weakness	Irregular, fearful, and sometimes aggressive
Body structure	Thin, tall, or lanky
Complexion	Brownish or yellowish

PITTA-VATA

Element	Dominant—fire/water, subordinate—air/space
Energy	Warm
Texture	Oily, sometimes dry
Temperament	Cheerful, sometimes aggressive
Emotional strength	Materially adept, goal-oriented
Emotional weakness	Ambitious, intolerant
Body structure	Moderate to thin, well-shaped
Complexion	Yellowish or tan

KAPHA-VATA

Element	Dominant—water/earth, subordinate—air/space
Energy	Cold
Texture	Smooth, dense, sometimes dry and rough
Temperament	Extremes: sometimes methodical, sometimes indecisive
Emotional strength	Nurturing, spiritually inclined
Emotional weakness	Unmotivated, attached
Body structure	Moderate to heavy (easily gains and loses weight)
Complexion	Pale, sometimes dark

VATA-KAPHA

Element	Dominant—air/space, subordinate—water/earth
Energy	Cold
Texture	Dry, sometimes smooth
Temperament	Extreme tendencies, mercurial, irregular
Emotional strength	Spiritually adept, maternal
Emotional weakness	Isolated, fearful
Body structure	Thin to moderate (easily gains and loses weight)
Complexion	Dark, sometimes pale

PITTA-KAPHA

Element	Dominant—fire/water, subordinate—water/earth
Energy	Warm
Texture	Soft, moist
Temperament	Decisive, patient
Emotional strength	Well-balanced, materially adept, vital
Emotional weakness	Possessive, indulgent
Body structure	Well-shaped, moderate to heavy
Complexion	Reddish, sometimes pale

KAPHA-PITTA	
Element	Dominant—water/earth, subordinate—fire/water
Energy	Cool, sometimes warm
Texture	Smooth, dense, moist
Temperament	Slow but methodical
Emotional strength	Excellent stamina, tenacious
Emotional weakness	Stubborn, lethargic
Body structure	Solid, curvaceous, and heavy
Complexion	Pale, sometimes reddish

UNDERSTANDING THE DOSHAS

Before we address the best way to care for your individual metabolic type, let us explore the doshas in depth. Knowing which dosha is dominant in your body helps you understand your physical rhythms. All Ayurveda diagnosis begins with the doshas. The doshas are a classic example of energy and matter in dynamic accord. The literal Sanskrit meaning of the word *dosha* is "fault" or "impurity," since doshas become visible usually when they are in a state of imbalance. The existence of doshas suggests that the human body is vulnerable to disease; in a state of balance or health we cannot detect the doshas. In a state of imbalance or disequilibrium, however, the doshas become visible as mucus, bile, wind, and all other bodily discharges. If we ignore these early signs of disorder, imbalances can quickly become full-blown diseases.

The three doshas coexist to varying degrees in all living organisms, and each is formed by a union of two elements in dynamic balance. Air and space, both ethereal elements, form the dosha Vata. In the Vata dosha, air expresses its kinetic power of mobility, which is Vata's physio-psychological nature. Dryness is an attribute of motion and when excessive, it introduces irregularity and change-ability into the body and mind. The element of fire forms the dosha known as Pitta. In the Pitta dosha, fire expresses its transformational power, Pitta's physio-psychological nature. Heat is an attribute of transformation, and when in full force it produces irritability and impatience of the body and mind. In the Kapha dosha, water expresses a stabilizing force. Heaviness is an attribute of stability, Kapha's physio-psychological nature. Excessive heaviness introduces lethargy into the body and mind.

Each dosha also has a primary function in the body. Vata is the moving force, Pitta is the force of assimilation, and Kapha is the force of stability. Together they are an impressive example of seemingly adversarial forces in potential harmony. Vata is the most dominant dosha in the body since air, its main element, is much more pervasive in the world than fire and water. Vata tends to go out of balance much more quickly than Pitta and Kapha. Vata governs bodily movement, the nervous system, and the life force. Without Vata's mobility in the body, Pitta and Kapha would be rendered lame. It is most influenced by the rajas principle.

Pitta governs enzymatic and hormonal activities and is responsible for digestion, pigmentation, body temperature, hunger, thirst, and sight. Further, Pitta acts as a balancing force for Vata and Kapha. Pitta is most influenced by the sattva principle.

Kapha governs the body's structure and stability. It lubricates joints, provides moisture to the skin, heals wounds, and regulates Vata and Pitta. Kapha is most influenced by the principle of tamas.

Vata, Pitta, and Kapha pervade the entire body, but their primary domains are in the lower, middle, and upper body, respectively. Kapha rules the head, neck, thorax, chest, upper stomach, fat tissues, lymph glands, and joints. Pitta pervades the chest, umbilical area, lower stomach, small intestines, sweat and sebaceous glands, and blood. Vata dominates the lower body, pelvic region, colon, bladder, urinary tract, thighs, legs, arms, bones, and nervous system.

Apart from its main site, each dosha has four secondary sites located in different areas of the body. These five sites are considered to be each dosha's center of operation, which include the various support systems through which the entire body functions.

The doshas interact continuously with the external elements to replenish their energy within the body. Each dosha's five sites have a specific responsibility toward the maintenance of the organism. Doshas also exist in the more subtle aspects of the body and universe, such as the life force and the mind. Thus they are energetically much more influential in the maintenance of our overall health than their mere physiological expressions would suggest. In fact, as they manifest within the physical body, they need to be continually cleansed out of the body in order to maintain harmonious internal rhythms.

Each dosha's seat is associated with organs where its energy and function are most manifested. The primary seat of Vata, for example, is the large intestine. The air of the colon also affects the kidneys, bladder, bones, thighs, ears, and nervous system. Vata's four remaining seats are the skin, lungs, throat, and stomach.

The stomach is Pitta's main seat in the body. The fire of the stomach affects the small intestine, duodenum, gall bladder, liver, spleen, pancreas, and sebaceous glands. Other seats for Pitta are the blood, heart, eyes, and skin.

Kapha's main seat is also the stomach; the water of the stomach affects the lymph glands and fat tissues. Other sites for Kapha are the heart, tongue, joints, and head. The water of the head also affects the nose, throat, and sinuses.

Since each dosha is formed from two elements, it bears the qualities of both. Vata types, for example, influenced by the reigning elements of air and space, tend to be somewhat ungrounded. Pitta types are generally fast, fluid, and fiery, patterned as they are after fire and water. And those in whom Kapha is dominant tend to be slow and methodical, since they are heavily affected by the characteristics of their main elements, water and earth. Every moment of every day, we are able to see the doshas in action through the elemental qualities we find in ourselves and the environment.

ELEMENTAL SOURCES OF THE METABOLIC TYPES

Vata	Air/Space
Pitta	Fire/Water
Kapha	Water/Earth

QUALITIES OF THE METABOLIC TYPES

VATA (like wind)	PITTA (like fire)	KAPHA (like water)
Astringent	Dense	Cool
Bitter	Fetid	Heavy
Cold	Fluid	Intense
Dry	Hot	Oily
Erratic	Light	Salty
Light	Oily	Smooth
Mobile	Pungent	Sour
Pungent	Salty	Stable
Rough	Sour	Sweet

NURTURING YOUR METABOLIC TYPE

The Ayurveda principle of "like increases like" helps us nourish our individual rhythms and achieve balance in our lives. According to this principle, we are nurtured by the elements and inclinations other than those innate to our metabolic type. Just as an individual who has a predominant quality of air in her nature has to work on building more stability, one who is extremely fiery needs to develop more moderation in his activities. You should avoid the intake of things that are like your own qualities—qualities that you already have—and increase the intake of things that are unlike your constitutional attributes. The chart on the following page lists the properties that nurture each metabolic type.

NURTURING PROPERTIES FOR YOUR METABOLIC TYPE

VATA: NURTURED BY FIRE, WATER & EARTH

Consistent

Heavy

Hot

Moist

Salty

Smooth

Sour

Sweet

PITTA: NURTURED BY WATER, AIR, SPACE & EARTH

Aromatic

Astringent

Bitter

Calm

Cool

Substantial

Sweet

KAPHA: NURTURED BY FIRE, AIR & SPACE

Astringent

Bitter

Dry

Light

Pungent

Stimulating

Warm

NURTURING YOUR PERSONAL RHYTHMS

These balancing principles are to be applied especially during your most vulnerable seasons. Each dosha is increased in its own seasons. These are times of increased opportunity to gain a deeper understanding of our inner rhythms. The Vata seasons are rainy season/early fall and autumn. The Pitta seasons are spring and summer. The Kapha seasons are early and late winter. Follow the recommendations that follow for activities most appropriate for your metabolic type as determined in the previous chart. And keep in mind that depending on your imbalances and seasonal demands, you may be able to engage from time to time in nourishing regimens other than those for your own prakriti.

NOURISHING REGIMENS FOR YOUR METABOLIC TYPE

FOR VATA TYPES: NOURISHING QUICK & IRREGULAR RHYTHMS

Balancing Principle: Stability
- Maintain a steady routine around eating and sleeping habits.
- Choose only the activities that create ease and allow yourself adequate time to complete them.
- Take ample rest.
- Eat wholesome, fresh, warm, moist, and nourishing foods.
- Avoid bitter, cold, fermented, stale, and raw foods.
- Buffer yourself against cold, damp, and wet environments.
- Make an effort to embrace warmth, love, healthy rituals, and routines.

FOR PITTA TYPES: NOURISHING FAST & DECISIVE RHYTHMS

Balancing Principle: Moderation
- Rise with the sun and go to bed by 10 p.m.
- Plan activities ahead to avoid time pressure.
- Ease yourself out of all stressful activities and maintain only those projects that create ease.
- Eat wholesome, moderately cool or warm, substantial, and calming foods.
- Avoid hot, spicy, oily, salty, fermented, and stale foods, as well as the use of stimulants.
- Shield yourself against hot, humid, and stressful environments.
- Make an attempt to embrace serenity and calmness.

FOR KAPHA TYPES: NOURISHING SLOW & METHODICAL RHYTHMS

Balancing Principle: Stimulation
- Engage in stimulating physical exercise every day.
- Open yourself to new and invigorating experiences.
- Rise with the sun every day.
- Eat wholesome, light, warm, pungent, and stimulating foods.
- Avoid cold, oily, rich, and excessively sour or salty foods.
- Buffer yourself against cold, damp, and wet environments.
- Unburden yourself of all old loads and lighten your heart.

THE SIX SEASONS OF
THE VEDIC CALENDAR

As I mentioned in chapter six, "Living in Harmony with the Seasons," a solar year in the Hindu Calendar has 365 days and 12 months, (a leap year has 366 days) similar to the Western Calendar. But the Vedic solar year is divided into six seasons of two months each: spring, summer, rainy season/early fall, autumn, early winter, and late winter. One solar month consists of the number of days taken by the sun to move from one sign of the zodiac, or rashi, to another, and each rashi is identified with its corresponding Gregorian zodiac sign. In this system of measuring time, Hindu months will straddle two months of the Western Calendar. According to the Hindu Calendar the year begins with the month of *Chaitra* (March-April) when the sun enters the zodiac sign of Aries on the day after the spring equinox.

THE SIX SEASONS OF THE VEDIC CALENDAR			
VEDIC SEASON	SANSKRIT NAME OF SEASON	OCCURS DURING THE MONTHS OF	SANSKRIT NAMES OF MONTHS
Spring	Vasanta	March April	Chaitra Vaishakha
Summer	Grishma	May June	Jyeshta Ashadha
Rainy Season/ Early Fall	Varsha	July August	Shravana Bhadrapada
Autumn	Sharada	September October	Ashvini Kartika
Early Winter	Hemanta	November December	Margashirsha Pausha
Late Winter	Shishira	January February	Magha Phalguna

THE TWELVE ZODIAC SIGNS

GREGORIAN ZODIAC SIGN	VEDIC ZODIAC SIGN	OCCURS DURING THE MONTHS OF
Aries	Mesha	March-April
Taurus	Vrishabha	April-May
Gemini	Mithuna	May-June
Cancer	Karkata	June-July
Leo	Simha	July-August
Virgo	Kanya	August-September
Libra	Tula	September-October
Scorpio	Vrischika	October-November
Sagittarius	Dhanur	November-December
Capricorn	Makara	December-January
Aquarius	Kumbha	January-February
Pisces	Mina	February-March

VEDIC FESTIVALS & OBSERVANCES

The following summary of Vedic festivals and observances lists only those that are mentioned throughout the pages of this book.

SPRING–VASANTA

Northern Hemisphere: Mid-to-late-March through mid-to-late-May		Southern Hemisphere: Mid-to-late September through mid-to-late November	
THE BIRTH OF LAKSHMI	**GANGUARA**	**RAMA NAVAMI**	**VASANTA PANCHAMI**
Occurs: on the first day of spring, the 3rd day of the waxing moon following the new moon occurring at the end of March. The Birth of Lakshmi is a day to celebrate joy, prosperity, and wellness, as Lakshmi is the goddess of family bliss and prosperity. In Vedic astronomy, the world was created on this day and the computation of time began from sunrise on this day many epochs ago. (See page III.)	Occurs: on the first day of spring, the 3rd day of the waxing moon following the new moon occurring at the end of March. Ganguara is a woman's festival celebrating the fresh spring moon. Young and elder women alike venerate Goddess Gauri who bestows marital happiness and familial bliss. (See page III.)	Occurs: on the 9th lunar day of the month that generally falls in April (*Vaishakha* in the Vedic Calendar). Rama Navami celebrates the birth of Lord Rama, god of dharma-righteous action, and also marks the completion of the annual cycle of the 6 seasons. (See page 105.)	Occurs: on the 5th day of the waxing moon of *Magha* (February-March). Vasanta Panchami celebrates Saraswati, goddess of wisdom, art, and learning. Mirth, gaiety, sweetness, and fragrance are the essences of this day. Yellow clothing is worn and saffron rice is prepared representing the golden hue of maturity and spirituality. (See pages 105-106.)

SUMMER–GRISHMA

Northern Hemisphere: Mid-to-late May through mid-to-late July	Southern Hemisphere: Mid-to-late November through mid-to-late January

SNANAM YATRA	GANGA DUSSHERA
Occurs: on the first full moon of summer. Snanam Yatra is an auspicious bathing festival celebrated by millions of Hindus in Crissag through the recitation of Vedic mantras. 108 pots of consecrated water are poured on the forms of the deities that preside over this occasion. After the bath the deities are dressed in ceremonial cloth and are retired in seclusion for 15 days. (See page 146.)	Occurs: on the 10th day of the first waxing moon of summer, generally occurring around mid-May. Ganga Dusshera is celebrated during this auspicious time of the summer when millions of Hindu people take early morning dips in the sacred Ganges River. They do so to wash away despair, tiredness, negative emotions . and experiences, disease, and misfortune. (See pages 147-148.)

RAINY SEASON—VARSHA

Northern Hemisphere:
Mid-to-late July through
mid-to-late September

Southern Hemisphere:
Mid-to-late January through
mid-to-late March

GURU PURNIMA	NARALI PURNIMA	THE BIRTH OF GANESHA	RAKSHA BANDHANA
Occurs: on the full moon day in July. Guru Purnima is a festival in which the guru or enlightened Vedic spiritual teacher is venerated with an outpouring of love, devotion, and gratitude. This tradition dates back to ancient times with the introduction of the first guru—Veda Vyasa. (See pages 189, 194.)	Occurs: on the first full moon falling in August which coincides with Raksha Bandhana and marks the end of the monsoons. Narali Purnima is a festival in which coconuts are offered by the fishermen in Maharastra to the sea-god Varuna and to show gratitude to him for the benevolent rains. In my tradition the coconut fruit, which is used prolifically in Hindu ceremonies, is symbolic of the cosmic womb that produces prosperity, nourishment, and fertility. (See page 190.)	Occurs: on the fourth day of the waxing moon in August, generally lasting for 10 days. The Birth of Ganesha celebrates the beloved elephant-headed deity—with his curving trunk, potbelly, and huge ears—beloved by millions of people around the world. Known for his massive power to remove obstacles from his disciples' paths, Ganesha is venerated at the onset of virtually every activity in Hindu life. In India, villagers mark this occasion by immersing clay figurines of Ganesha in the rivers and streams. (See page 190.)	Occurs: on the first full moon falling in August. Raksha Bandhana is a ceremony for strengthening family bonds, a time when men and boys renew their traditional vows to safeguard their sisters. Young girls and women tie an amulet around the right wrists of their brothers as a token of affection and protection against negative forces. (See pages 190, 320.)

AUTUMN–SHARADA

Northern Hemisphere: Mid-to-late September through mid-to-late November	Southern Hemisphere: Mid-to-late March through mid-to-late May

JANMASHTAMI	PITRI PAKSHA	NAVARATRI
Occurs: on the 8th day of the waning moon at the end of August or beginning of September.	Occurs: during the waning moon of *Ashvini* that falls in September and October.	Occurs: on the first lunar day of the waxing moon in *Ashvini* that falls in September and October.
Janmashtami is a festival commemorating the birth of Lord Krishna. Krishna and his consort, Radha, symbolize the eternal and divine lovers. On this day images of both deities are bathed and adorned with fineries after early morning ablutions. (See page 224.)	Pitri Paksha is an observance honoring the spirit of the dead and departed ancestors. It helps to revive within us the memory of our people, and to nourish the spirits of our ancestors. The practice involves 2 weeks of reciting special prayers as well as making offerings of grain, water, and milk to appease the ancestors. (See pages 230-232, 235.)	Navaratri, celebrated in India twice a year, honors Goddess Durga, the 10-armed celestial warrior. According to Vedic lore, Goddess Durga rides a lion, plays the rattle drum, and defeats evil to protect her people. Sacred grass, flowers, leaves, lamps, incenses, and grains from the autumnal harvest are offered in gratitude to the goddess for her protection. Barley is sprouted in clay pots and its sheath worn on caps and behind the ears, symbols of the final day of Navaratri. (See pages 108, 224, 237-238.)

EARLY WINTER—HEMANTA

Northern Hemisphere:
Mid-to-late November through
mid-to-late January

Southern Hemisphere:
Mid-to-late May through
mid-to-late July

DIPAVALI

Occurs: on the last day of the waning moon in *Kartika* (October-November).

Dipavali is a lavish 5-day long celebration of light. Throughout India, millions of lights are lit on cotton wicks and placed in tiny clay bowls filled with ghee or oil. The festival commemorates the victory of God Rama over Ravana, the malevolent king, symbolizing the triumph of universal and ethical principle over evil. (See pages 270, 272-273, 278.)

LATE WINTER—SHISHIRA

Northern Hemisphere: Mid-to-late January through mid-to-late March	Southern Hemisphere: Mid-to-late July through mid-to-late September

MAUNI AMAVASYA	LOHRI	PONGAL
Occurs: on the new moon that falls on the 15th day of the late winter's waxing moon. Mauni Amavasya is an observance of silence that begins the late winter season. In the fullness of this winter's moon, the Great Goddess, Lalita Maha Tripurasundari, may be seen by her devotees in her full regalia. In this sacred month of *Magha* (February into March), aspirants fast and bathe in the holy Ganges River. The god Vishnu is worshipped by perambulating the sacred peepal tree. Fasting is practiced by stoic Hindus for the entire fortnight starting at the full moon and ending on the new moon with Mauni Amavasya, a day of silence. (See page 310.)	Occurs: in North India in mid-January. Lohri commemorates the winter solstice, when the earth's fertility is heightened, and heralds the end of the coldest month of the year. Farmers celebrate Lohri by carving out a period of rest before the spring's harvest begins. Lohri celebrates love and joy of the family, and in the event of the birth of a newborn or a marriage in the family, it assumes a larger significance; the first Lohri of a new bride or a newborn baby is considered extremely propitious. (See page 311.)	Occurs: on the solar calendar generally between the 12th and 15th of January. Pongal is an extremely auspicious celebration for Hindus as it marks the sun's entry into the Tropic of Capricorn from the Tropic of Cancer. Each year in South India, Pongal is celebrated in January to commemorate the harvest of winter crops and offer thanksgiving to the seasons, sun, earth and the cows. (See page 311, 316-317.)

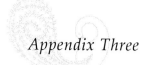

BREAKFAST OF CHAMPIONS

THE WHOLESOME GRAIN BREAKFAST

For Pitta and Vata types, breakfast is the most important meal of the day. A peaceful and nourishing meal goes a long way to fortify your strength and stamina for the day's activities. Kapha types must be careful to not invigorate the appetite too early in the day, and generally fare well without breakfast, or with only an invigorating cup of tea or very light fare in the mornings. A vegetarian breakfast is the easiest meal to prepare, and in my opinion, the best for one's overall well-being.

Following are some delicious breakfast recipes. The more complicated repasts may be used on celebratory occasions. Imagine how wonderful you'll feel by starting your day with a wholesome breakfast of whole grains, such as sweet rice, millet, amaranth, oats (steel cut or rolled), wheat, spelt, and kamut (cracked). They are even better if you add dried fruits such as raisins, currants, dates, or fresh apples and peaches to your whole grain porridge. Spice them up with cardamom, cinnamon, clove, and ginger powders and sweeten with Sucanat or maple syrup for a satisfying and uplifting breakfast.

In the Vedic tradition, grains and beans are freshly ground into variable textures for daily use. The timeless hand grinders are still the best grinding tools because you are using your hands when you work with them. The grinding processes are simple, and once you incorporate them into your daily cooking routines you'll find it difficult to revert to cooking with lifeless flour. On occasion, especially if you're short on time, you can take your breakfast with you to work: Pack a whole-grain muffin, or toast daubed with ghee, yogurt, or a small jar of nut butter and some fruit in your breakfast pack.

STRAWBERRY CREAM OF WHEAT

Season: Spring

Serves: 2

1 1/2 cups milk

1/2 cup Cream of Wheat

1 cup strawberries, sliced

1/2 teaspoon ginger powder

A few drops vanilla extract

1 tablespoon slivered almonds, toasted

2 tablespoons honey

Bring milk to a boil and add Cream of Wheat while stirring over medium heat. Add straw-berries, spices, and vanilla extract. Leave uncovered and cook for 5 minutes or so, while stirring occasionally. Remove from heat; serve warm with toasted almonds and honey as desired. (Be careful not to cook the honey.)

CREAMY SESAME COUSCOUS

Seasons: Spring & Summer

Serves: 2

2 cups water

1 cup couscous

1 cup raisins

1/2 cup sesame seeds, roasted

1 tablespoon organic ghee (recipe on pages 150-151)

Bring water to a boil in a medium-size saucepan, stir in couscous, cover and let stand for 5 minutes. Remove from heat, then add the roasted sesame seeds and ghee. Serve warm.

BUTTERMILK PANCAKES ♡

Season: Summer & Early Fall

Serves: 4

1 cup buttermilk

1/2 cup water

2 tablespoons sunflower oil

1 1/2 cups brown rice flour

1/2 cup maple syrup

Pour the buttermilk into a large mixing bowl, and whip buttermilk and water together. Mix in oil and brown rice flour. Stir and blend well until the batter is smooth and fluid in consis-tency. Lightly oil a pancake skillet, or a tava, (a flat cast-iron or stainless-steel skillet used for making chapatis). On medium heat, pour about a quarter cup of batter onto the skillet and use the back of a ladle to spread the batter in clockwise circles as thinly as possible on the skillet. (If batter is too wet add a little more brown rice flour.) Once one side is cooked after a minute or so, use a spatula to flip it over. Cook the other side for just about a min-ute. Serve hot with maple syrup, if desired.

COCONUT FRUIT PLATE ♡
Season: Summer
Serves: 2
4 peaches, quartered
2 tangerines, peeled and separated
I banana, sliced
2 tablespoons raisins
I/2 cup coconut, shredded
I/2 cup flaxseeds
IO strands of saffron
I/2 lime, freshly juiced

In a large bowl, combine all fruits, add the seeds, saffron, and lime juice, and mix together. Serve with a dollop of plain organic yogurt, if desired.

ALMOND & DATE CREAM OF WHEAT
Seasons: Spring & Summer
Serves: 2
I cup milk
I/2 cup water
I/2 cup Cream of Wheat
3/4 cup dates or figs, chopped
I/2 teaspoon cardamom powder
I/2 teaspoon cinnamon powder
I tablespoon slivered almonds, toasted
3 tablespoons honey

Bring milk and water to a boil; add Cream of Wheat while stirring over medium heat. Then add fruit and spices. Leave uncovered and cook for 5 minutes or so, while stirring occasionally. Remove from heat; serve warm with toasted almonds and honey as desired. (Be careful not to cook the honey.)

APPLE MUESLI
Season: Early Fall & Autumn
Serves: 2
I I/2 cups apple juice
I cup rolled oats
2 tablespoons raisins
2 tablespoons dried apple, finely cut
5 dates, chopped

I/2 teaspoon cinnamon powder

I/2 teaspoon coriander powder

I/2 teaspoon clove powder

I pinch of nutmeg

Combine all the ingredients in a small saucepan. Gently warm over medium heat and serve.

BLUEBERRY SPELT MUFFINS
Seasons: Early Fall & Autumn
Serves: 12

3 cups spelt flour

I I/2 teaspoons baking powder

I/2 teaspoon rock salt

I I/2 cups soy milk

I/4 cup maple syrup

2 tablespoons walnut oil

I cup fresh blueberries

Preheat oven to 400 degrees. Combine flour, baking powder, and salt in a bowl. In a separate large mixing bowl, combine soy milk, maple syrup, and walnut oil, and let stand for 3 minutes. Add the flour mixture and blend the ingredients with your clean hands. Fold in blueberries and spoon into lightly oiled muffin tins. Bake for 25 minutes until golden brown, or until a toothpick inserted in the center of a muffin comes out clean. Cool on a rack, remove muffins from tins, and serve warm, or store in an airtight container in a cool, dry place.

BUCKWHEAT CARROT MUFFINS
Seasons: Autumn & Early Winter
Serves: 12

2 cups buckwheat flour

I/2 cup oat bran

I teaspoon ginger powder

I teaspoon cinnamon powder

I/2 teaspoon cardamom powder

2 teaspoons baking powder

2 cups shredded carrots

I/2 cup turbinado brown sugar

I tablespoon organic ghee (recipe on pages 150-151)

2 cups warm water

I/2 cup currants

I/4 cup chopped walnuts

Preheat the oven to 350 degrees. Combine the flour, bran, spices, and baking powder in a bowl. In a large mixing bowl, combine the carrots, brown sugar, and ghee, and stir together until smooth. Make a hole in the center of the dough and pour in the warm water. Fold in the shredded carrot-sugar-ghee mixture and mix thoroughly. Then stir in the currants and walnuts. Divide the mixture into 12 equal parts and place in lightly oiled muffin tins. Bake for 20 minutes, or until a toothpick inserted in the center of a muffin comes out clean. Cool on a rack, remove muffins from the tin and serve warm, or store in an airtight container in a cool, dry place.

DECADENT OATMEAL
Seasons: Early Winter, Late Winter & Spring
Serves: 2
2 cups water
1 cup rolled oats
2 tablespoons raisins or chopped dates
1/4 teaspoon clove powder
1/2 teaspoon cinnamon powder
1/2 teaspoon orange zest
1/4 cup milk
2 teaspoons maple syrup

Bring water to a boil in a covered saucepan over high heat. Stir in rolled oats, raisins, spices, and zest. Reduce heat, cover, and simmer for 15 minutes, stirring occasionally. Serve garnished with milk, maple syrup, and flaxseed oil.

CREAMY CROCKPOT OATS
Season: Late Winter
Serves: 2
2 cups milk
1 cup water
1/4 cup turbinado brown sugar
1 teaspoon organic ghee (recipe on pages 150-151)
1/4 teaspoon rock salt
1 cup steel cut oats
1/2 cup fresh apple, diced
1/2 cup raisins
1/2 cup flaxseeds

Lightly oil the inside of a crockpot. Place all ingredients in it and mix well. Cover and let simmer on low heat for approximately 2 to 3 hours. Stir and serve while piping hot.

THE ULTIMATE GRANOLA
Season: All Year
Serves: 8
1/2 cup apple juice concentrate
1/2 cup maple syrup
2 tablespoons warm water
1 teaspoon almond extract
8 cups rolled oats
1 cup chopped almonds
2 tablespoons organic ghee (recipe on pages 150-151)
1 cup raisins, currants, or chopped dates

Combine apple juice concentrate, maple syrup, water, and almond extract in a mixing bowl and mix well. Combine oats and almonds in a large roasting pan, spread the syrupy mixture over it, then coat with the ghee. Bake in a 350 degree oven for 25 minutes, or until golden brown, stirring occasionally. Remove from oven, sprinkle the dried fruits on top, cover, and allow to cool before storing in airtight containers in a dry place.

DOSA–VEDIC PANCAKES ♥
Season: All Year
Serves: 4
Dosa is traditional to South India and is made from freshly ground urad dhal (black lentils) and basmati rice. The dhal and rice are soaked in water and ground separately and then combined. The dosa batter is allowed to ferment for one day before use. The grains recommended for the following recipe revert to earlier times when ancient cultures used only processed grains sparsely. Whole grains that are freshly ground produce the most nutritious and wholesome results.

1 cup basmati white rice
3/8 cup urad dhal (Indian black lentils)
1 pinch of rock salt
1 tablespoon sunflower oil

Soak rice and dhal in water separately for 8 hours. Drain and grind together. Place in a bowl, cover with a cotton cloth, and store in a warm place for 8 hours. Add enough water and a pinch of salt to make a pancake batter consistency. Lightly oil griddle and pour batter about 1/8" thick. Cook each side thoroughly for about 3 minutes until lightly browned, just like you would a pancake. Serve with the appropriate chutney for the season (see recipes on pages 370-372).

IDLI–BASMATI RICE & URAD DHAL ♡

Season: All Year

Serves: 4

The king of the fresh grain and bean foods is idli. It is a 3" dome-shaped steamed patty made from slightly fermented ground rice and dhal batter. Idli is the traditional breakfast food of South India and is served with Sambar, a highly spiced dhal and vegetable mixture, or chutney. (See recipe for Urad & Okra sambar on page 287.)

I cup urad dhal (Indian black lentils)
2 cups brown basmati rice*
1/4 teaspoon rock salt
I tablespoon organic ghee (optional)
*Occasionally white basmati rice may be used

Wash dhal and rice separately; using a small amount of water, grind each separately to a fine consistency. Combine the two batters, cover with a cotton cloth, and let sit for 8 hours to mildly ferment. Add salt and ghee immediately before steaming. Use an idli steamer available from Indian grocery stores. Resembling an egg poaching pan, the idli steamer has perforations for the steam to escape through. Lightly oil the idli holders and place 2 tablespoons of batter in each indention. Place in a large pot of boiling water, with the level of the water below the bottom of the idli holders. Keep the water boiling rapidly. Cover and steam for 20 minutes. Scoop the idlis out with a rounded soup spoon. Serve hot with a seasonal fruit chutney of your choice. (See chutney recipes on pages 370-372.)

WISE EARTH TOFU SCRAMBLE ♡

Season: All Year

Serves: 2

I tablespoon olive oil or ghee
I handful of green onions, chopped
I handful of fresh peas
1/4 teaspoon coriander powder
1/2 teaspoon cumin powder
1/2 teaspoon turmeric powder
I pound medium-firm tofu
I teaspoon fresh Italian parsley, minced
I pinch of black pepper
1/2 teaspoon rock salt

Heat olive oil or ghee in a frying pan over medium heat and sauté the green onions and peas for about 3 minutes. Stir in the spice powders. Use your hands to crumble the tofu in a bowl. Fold it into the spice mixture, along with the parsley, black pepper, and salt. Cover, lower heat to low, and cook for about 7 minutes until the tofu begins to brown slightly. Stir occasionally. Serve rolled in chapatis, or on Seven-Grain Bread (page 336) toast.

BREAKFAST CHUTNEYS

Chutneys are an essential accent to food and digestion in my tradition. Made fresh for daily use, their flavors range from savory, spicy, tart and sour, to the exquisitely rich and sweet—each created in harmony with the seasonal requirements. The secret to making great chutney depends on the choice of spices, fruits, and the time you allow them to marinate and meld. You may make your chutneys every 2 weeks and use a dollop of it over your breakfast grains to add verve and inspiration to your day. Following is a chutney recipe for each season—fit for the most auspicious breakfast occasion. I hope you will be inspired to create your own combinations of seasonal fruits in your chutneys as you become adept at chutney making.

SPRING STRAWBERRY & MINT CHUTNEY ♥

Season: Spring
Serves: 8
2 cups fresh strawberries
10 mint leaves, minced
1/2 teaspoon black pepper
1/2 teaspoon fresh ginger, minced
1 tablespoon organic ghee (recipe on pages 150-151)
2 tablespoons honey

Semi-puree strawberries in a small saucepan; add minced mint leaves, black pepper, and ginger. Warm the mixture over low heat for 10 minutes. Add ghee, remove from heat, and allow to cool. Stir in the honey before placing the chutney in a glass jar. Store at a cool temperature.

SUMMER CHERRY & TANGERINE CHUTNEY ♥

Season: Summer
Serves: 8
1 cup fresh cherries, seeded
1/4 cup tangerine pulp
8 mint leaves, fresh

I/2 teaspoon cinnamon powder

I/2 teaspoon cardamom powder

I/2 teaspoon black pepper

I/2 teaspoon rock salt

I tablespoon organic ghee (recipe on pages 150-151)

I tablespoon maple syrup

Semi-puree cherries in a small saucepan; add tangerine pulp, mint leaves, cinnamon, cardamom, and black pepper. Warm the mixture over low heat for 10 minutes, then add ghee and maple syrup. Remove from heat and allow to cool. Place in a glass jar and store at a cool temperature.

EARLY FALL DATE & COCONUT CHUTNEY ♥

Season: Early Fall

Serves: 8

I tablespoon organic ghee (recipe on pages 150-151)

I/4 cup dates, finely cut

I/2 cup dried coconut, shredded

2 tablespoons raisins

I teaspoon fresh ginger, minced

I tablespoon fresh cilantro, minced

IO strands saffron

3 tablespoons almond meal

I/2 cup water

Melt the ghee over medium heat in a heavy cast-iron skillet, and add the dates, coconut, raisins, ginger, and cilantro. Sauté over low heat for 5 minutes. Add saffron and almond meal along with the water. Stir, cover, and cook for an additional 5 minutes over low heat. Remove from heat, allow to cool, and place in a glass jar. Store at a cool temperature.

AUTUMN CURRANT & PLUM CHUTNEY ♥

Season: Autumn

Serves: 8

2 pounds ripe plums, pitted

2 tablespoons organic ghee (recipe on pages 150-151)

I/2 teaspoon minced ginger

I teaspoon grated orange zest

I/2 cup currants

I/4 teaspoon ground mace

1/4 teaspoon ground cinnamon
1/4 teaspoon ground coriander
1/8 teaspoon ground cloves
1/2 cup grape juice
1/2 cup Sucanat

Wash plums and cut into quarters. In a stainless-steel saucepan, melt the ghee over low heat and add the ginger and orange zest. Raise the heat to medium, stir in the plums, currants, spices, juice, and Sucanat, and bring mixture to a boil. Reduce the heat and continue to cook the chutney for 20 minutes until it becomes a thick jam. Remove from heat, allow to cool, and place in a glass jar. Store at a cool temperature.

EARLY WINTER GINGER CHUTNEY ♡
Season: Early Winter
Serves: 8
4 tablespoons umeboshi, or rice vinegar
1/2 cup fresh ginger, grated
1 teaspoon rock salt
1 pinch turbinado brown sugar

Warm vinegar; mix in ginger, salt, and sugar. Place in a glass jar and store in cool temperature.

WINTER FIG & CURRANT CHUTNEY ♡
Season: Winter
Serves 8
2 tablespoons walnut oil
1/2 cup dried figs, finely chopped
1/2 cup dried apricots, finely chopped
1/2 cup currants
1/2 teaspoon cayenne powder
1/2 teaspoon turmeric
1 teaspoon rice vinegar
1/2 cup water
1 pinch of rock salt

Heat the walnut oil in a cast-iron skillet over low heat, and add the fruits along with the spices. Simmer on low heat for 5 minutes, then stir in the vinegar, water, and salt. Cover and simmer for about 3 more minutes until the ingredients soak up the liquid. Place in a glass jar and store at a cool temperature.

SEASONAL MASALAS

Every state in India has a variation of the masala. A variety of seasonal spices can be used to create your own divinely nourishing, stimulating masalas: cumin, coriander, fennel, roasted coconut, saffron, turmeric, poppy seeds, and neem leaves. All types may use any combination of the above mentioned spices. The addition of peppercorns, nutmeg, ginger, sesame seeds, mace, cassia leaves, and mustard seeds may be used interchangeably for creating a variety of flavors. I recommend making a batch of masala fresh every fortnight.

NORTH INDIAN GARAM MASALA ♥

1/2 cup cumin seeds
1/4 cup cardamom pods
1/4 cup coriander seeds
1/8 cup whole cloves
I teaspoon nutmeg, finely grated
4 cinnamon sticks

Dry roast the seeds and cinnamon in a heavy cast-iron skillet for 2 minutes. Pound the roasted cinnamon sticks and cardamom pods with a mallet on a grinding stone into small bits. Add the sticks and seeds together. Use a hand spice grinder or a suribachi to grind to a fine powder then add the nutmeg. Store the masala in an airtight jar in a cool place.

SOUTH INDIAN GARAM MASALA ♥

I cup cumin seeds
1/2 teaspoon ajwain seeds
1/4 cup coriander seeds
4 black cardamom pods

Dry roast the seeds and pods, then grind each individually using a hand grinder or suribachi. Grind to a fine powder and add the nutmeg. Store the masala in an airtight jar in a cool place.

WISE EARTH GARAM MASALA ♥

I tablespoon coriander seeds
I tablespoon cumin seeds
1/2 teaspoon fennel seeds
I teaspoon black peppercorns
5 cloves

Grind all the seeds and spices using a hand grinder or mortar and pestle into a fine a powder. Store in an airtight glass jar.

SPRING MASALA ♡
1 teaspoon cumin seeds
2 tablespoons coriander seeds
1 tablespoon yellow mustard seeds
1 teaspoon cardamom seeds
1 teaspoon black peppercorns

Grind all the seeds and peppercorns in a hand grinder or mortar and pestle to a fine a powder. Store in an airtight glass jar.

SUMMER MASALA ♡
2 tablespoons coriander seeds
1 tablespoon poppy seeds
1 teaspoon cardamom seeds
1 tablespoon fennel seeds
10 saffron strands

Grind the saffron strands along with the fennel seeds. Do not roast them.

EARLY FALL MASALA ♡
2 tablespoons celery seeds
1 tablespoon black mustard seeds
1 tablespoon white peppercorns
1 teaspoon ginger powder
1/2 teaspoon nutmeg, freshly grated

Roast and grind the spice seeds before adding the ginger powder and grated nutmeg.

AUTUMN MASALA ♡
1/2 cup sesame seeds
1 teaspoon cayenne powder, freshly ground
1 teaspoon rock salt

Roast and grind the sesame seeds before adding the cayenne and salt.

EARLY WINTER MASALA ♡

2 tablespoons cumin seeds

2 tablespoons caraway seeds

1 teaspoon yellow mustard seeds

1 teaspoon turmeric powder

1 teaspoon garlic powder

Roast and grind the seeds before adding the spice powders.

LATE WINTER MASALA ♡

2 cloves garlic

1 2-inch piece of fresh ginger root

3 dried red chilis

2 tablespoons coriander seeds

1 teaspoon turmeric

Peel the garlic and ginger, roast the coriander seeds, and grind all the ingredients together on a grinding stone. Use half of a palmful of water to meld the ground ingredients. Add turmeric powder toward the end of the grinding.

WISE EARTH AYURVEDA CULINARY SPICES

Ajwain seed: Bishop's weed; relative of the caraway and cumin seeds. It resembles the minute celery seeds. Ajwain has the flavor of the thyme herb. It is to be used mostly by Vata and Kapha types.

Amchoor: A powder made from sun-dried slices of mango. It has a pungent flavor and is generally used like pomegranate seeds or lime juice in North Indian cuisine. It is to be used mostly by Vata types.

Ancho chili: The pod of the poblano chili is sun-dried to a dark brown color. It is used in the fried spice seasonings of curries and dhals. All chilis are good for Kapha types and occasionally for Vata types.

Asafetida: Also known as *hing* or *hingu*. It is a highly pungent dried gum resin, obtained from the ferula plant. It is deep brown in color and is used in Ayurveda medicine as well as in South Indian cuisine. It is used in Ayurveda pharmacology for breast-feeding mothers to cleanse and increase milk. This resin is used sparingly in foods for Vata and Kapha types.

Basil: Tulsi. There are two varieties of basil in India, one has purple-brownish leaves and the other has green leaves. Both are used for worshipping Lord Krishna and Rama throughout India. Both the flowers and leaves of this divine herb are used profusely in religious ceremonies. The camphor basil known as *karpura* is used for Indian cooking. This herb is to be used mostly by Vata and Kapha types.

Bay leaves: Sweet Laurel. This leaf resembles the cassia leaf used in the cuisine of Bengal and the eastern regions of India. Bay leaves are highly aromatic and pungent and are to be used sparingly. This leaf is for Vata and Kapha use only.

Black cumin: *Shahi jeera* or royal cumin; also called *kala jeera*. Black cumin grows abundantly as a wild annual of the Himalayas. The seed is black, slender, and is closely related to the common cumin seed. This cumin is used mostly in the Kashmir, Punjab, and Uttar Pradesh regions of India. This glorious seed may be used by all three doshas.

Black salt: *Kala namak.* This is a dark crimson-grey salt, strong and pungent in flavor. It is high in trace minerals and iron, and is used almost exclusively in India. This salt is to be used mostly by Vata types and occasionally by Kapha types.

Camphor: *Kacha karpura.* This is an edible crystalline compound obtained by distilling the fragrant leaves of the Indian and Chinese evergreen. This raw and natural camphor is used in very tiny pieces to flavor milk beverages, puddings, and sweets in the eastern regions of India. This crystal is also used in Ayurveda medicine in Kapha remedies.

Caraway: This aromatic seed grows on the wild *carum carvi* plant in the foothills of the Himalayas. In India, it is used predominantly in the Kashmir region. This seed is best for Vata and Kapha use, but may be used occasionally by Pitta.

Cardamom: Ela. Green pods and large black pods. The cardamom plant is native to South India. The dark brown seeds are encased in small green pods or large black pods. The green pods are high in volatile oils, and have a flavor that resembles eucalyptus. The seeds of the green pods are mostly used in beverages and sweets. Cardamom has been used for centuries in Ayurveda medicine. This seed is best for Vata and Kapha types, but may be used occasionally by Pitta due to its aromatic flavor.

Cassia leaves: *Tejpatta.* Native to Sri Lanka and South India. These 7-inch long leaves are olive green and are sun-dried. They are pungent in nature and are used as a fried herb seasoning in India's eastern regional cooking. It may be used by Vata and Kapha types.

Cayenne pepper: *Puissi lal mirch.* These are red hot chilis which are sun-dried and ground into a highly potent powder. India exports great quantities of cayenne abroad. Cayenne is used in Ayurveda medicine to reduce phlegm and inflammation in the Kapha dosha.

Charoli seed: *Chironji.* These are large seeds with an almond flavor. They are toasted and used frequently in place of almonds in many Indian desserts. These are best for Vata types and as an occasional spice for Kapha.

Chilis: There are hundreds of varieties of red and green chilis from various *Capsicum* plants. The heat and intense taste are mostly held in the seeds. The smaller the chili, the hotter it is. The large bell-shaped peppers are less pungent. Chilis have been used even before the Vedic period in India. They are a vital mainstay of the Vedic kitchen. India has a great many Kapha and Vata people, and thus the use of so many heating and stimulating spices by the culture.

Colocasia leaf: *Arbi patta;* elephant ears. These plant leaves are blanched and used to wrap various stuffing. They are excellent for all three doshas.

Cinnamon: *Twak* or *dalchini.* Cinnamon is the dried bark of the *Cinnamomum aromaticum,* or cassia tree. It is native to South India. Both the bark and the cassia leaves are used extensively in South Indian cooking. The cassia cinnamon is more pungent with a thicker quill than the thinner bark found in the United States. Cinnamon is another essential ingredient in many Ayurveda remedies. It is good for Kapha and Vata types, due to its heating energy. Pitta may use occasionally.

Cloves: *Lasuna* or *laung.* Cloves are the small pointed dried buds of the evergreen tree. They contain the antiseptic, volatile clove oil and are used in small amounts as a ground spice in masala. Cloves are used extensively in Ayurveda pharmacology. They are good for Vata and Kapha types.

Coriander leaves: *Har dhania;* cilantro. This fragrant and cooling herb is grown profusely in South America, India, and in most tropical climates. It is used predominantly in the Gujarat, Punjab, Rajasthan, and Maharashtra regions of India. The cooling energy of cilantro is used to reduce high Pitta conditions, and the cilantro juice is used to neutralize the poisons of snakebites and insect stings. The seeds of the plant are also widely used in Ayurveda pharmacology. Good for all three doshas.

Coriander seeds: *Dhania.* This round, light seed is used extensively in Vedic cooking. They are slowly roasted, powdered, cracked, and crushed into a variety of masalas. They are sweet and cooling in nature and are the mainstay spice for Pitta types. Coriander is good for all three doshas.

Cumin: *Jeera* or *safed jeera.* This golden aromatic seed is a relative of caraway. It is an ancient spice and is used in cooking throughout India. They are dry roasted and ground into powder or coarsely crushed for vegetables and dhals, or used as an accent in kichadi, which is part of a cleansing diet in Ayurveda. Like coriander seeds, the energy of cumin is suitable for all three doshas.

Curry leaves: *Neem, meetha neem* or *kadhi patta.* Curry leaves are highly fragrant with a touch of citrus to their scent. They are a tiny version of the lemon leaf. The curry leaf has been used since Vedic times and grown profusely throughout India. Due to its extensive use as a masala in the *kari* dishes of South India, most Indian sauces became known as curry. They are a main ingredient in curry powder, even though many masalas are made without them. Fresh neem juice is extremely bitter and is administered to diabetics and to persons with high Pitta conditions. It is also used for reducing weight. The neem leaf has a multitude of uses. The twigs were used as toothbrushes to prevent tooth and gum decay. They were also planted in companion gardens as a natural pesticide.

Curry powder: Curry powder is a truly exotic blend of some of India's finest spices. It can be mixed to be mild or hair-raisingly hot. The most well-known curry powder comes from Madras. Although in Guyana, the elders made the most superb curry masala I have ever tasted. Generally, a curry masala is made from fresh curry leaves (or dried), cumin seeds, mustard seeds, fenugreek seeds, black peppercorns, chilis, coriander, and turmeric. It is best for Kapha types, occasional used for Vata, and rarely used for Pitta types.

Daru: *Anardana*; wild pomegranate seeds. These are grown in the foothills of the Himalayas. The daru fruit is not the edible kind; only the seeds are used. The seed is dried, roasted, and ground or used whole to lend a sour taste to vegetables, soups, and dhals. This is an especially suitable spice for Vata types. Daru has also been used in Ayurveda medicine as far back as the Vedic period.

Fennel seed: *Saunf.* The fennel plant is similar to the dill plant. Both the delicate fennel leaves as well as the seeds are used in cooking. The bulk and the stalks are also used for their post-digestive qualities. The seed is similar to cumin and close in taste to the anise seed. Fennel is delicate and fragrant. The roasted seeds are ground in masalas or used as a breath refresher after meals and as a digestion aid. Fennel seeds are excellent for the Pitta constitution and have been used in Ayurveda pharmacology for many thousands of years. It is an excellent seed for all three doshas.

Fenugreek leaf: *Methi sak.* This leaf has a strong and unusual scent. It is densely bitter and pungent in taste. Its energy, when added to vegetables and dhals, is very pervasive. It is a good stimulant for Kapha types, but too pungent for Pitta and too bitter for Vata. These leaves are used either fresh or sun-dried.

Fenugreek seeds: *Methi.* This seed is considered more a small bean than a seed. It has a golden yellow color and an odd shape. It is generally dried and moderately roasted before use. Like the leaves, the fenugreek seed is also bitter. The seeds are used mainly in pickles, dhals, and masalas. The fenugreek seed is also used in Ayurveda pharmacology for hair replenishing. The seeds are soaked overnight and mashed by hand into a paste. This paste is massaged into the scalp and is left on the hair for 30 to 45 minutes, then rinsed off. The hair gleams, left with subtle oils. It is good for Kapha types, although Vata may use occasionally. All types may use externally.

Ginger root: *Sunthi.* This rhizome has been used in both Ayurveda and Chinese medicine for over five thousand years. It is native to Asia, and is widely used throughout Indian cuisine. Ginger has heating, cleansing, toning, and stimulating properties. It is used for thousands of health purposes such as digestive problems, muscular pain, constipation, and so on. There are hundreds of varieties of ginger from the small green type to the delicate shell-pink ginger available in the spring in India. Many fresh chutneys and condiments are made with ginger. It is also used in various curries, dhals, and vegetables. It is best for Vata and Kapha types, although Pitta may use occasionally. All types may use it externally.

Green mango: *Kacha aam.* The young green mango is peeled and grated and used in many dhals, chutneys, and vegetable dishes in India. It is an excellent mango for pickling. It may be used in moderation for all three doshas.

Horseradish root: This root is used moderately in areas such as Bengal and Orissa for cooling. It is best for Kapha types and occasional use for Vata types.

Lotus seeds: *Makhana.* Several varieties of lotus and water lilies exist in India. In the summer, the lotus stems, leaves, and pods are harvested along with water chestnuts and the fruits of the water bamboo. The lotus seeds are removed from the pods, peeled, and dried. They are roasted in hot beach sand until they pop and become light and fluffy. This is a great delicacy in India. The dried seeds are pressure-cooked with rice in Japan and are also used in soups. These seeds are good for Vata and Pitta types and occasional use for Kapha.

Lotus roots: *Bhain, kamal.* These roots are native to the Kashmir region of India and also to China and Japan. The lotus flower is the most auspicious flower in the Hindu culture due to its symbolism of purity in yoga. They are white, blue, and pink. The stamens of the flowers are used for tea by the yogis. The roots resemble the heart. When cross cut their open chambers resemble a chakra. They are used as a vegetable in North Indian cuisine. The dried root is an important medicine in Ayurveda pharmacology, used for Pitta and Vata conditions.

Mace: *Javitri;* a fibrous covering of the nutmeg fruit which comes from the nutmeg tree. It is dried, roasted, and ground into a masala with other spices or used to flavor sauces. The fibers of mace do not dissolve and are thus removed before the sauce is served. Mace is good for Vata and Kapha types, and occasional use for Pitta (infused in milk).

Mint leaves: *Pudina.* Mint leaves are widely used in India. There are several varieties that grow worldwide. They are great in rice, dhals, and vegetable dishes, and are especially superb in mint chutneys. Most mints can be used by all three doshas.

Nigella seeds: *Kalonji.* This is a tear-shaped black seed which has the misnomer of a black onion seed. It is aromatic and peppery and is used in masalas and pickles in India. It is good for Vata and Kapha types and occasional use for Pitta.

Nutmeg: *Jatiphala, jaiphal.* This sleep-inducing nut is found in the center of the fruit of the evergreen tree. The nut should be grated fresh for use. It is used in many milk beverages and in masalas in Indian cuisine. Nutmeg is excellent to induce sleep and relaxation for Vata types. It may also be used by Kapha types.

Paprika: *Deghi mirch.* These are a mild variety of chili grown in the Kashmir region. They are used for their mild pungency and red and orange colors in food. They are good for Vata and Kapha types, and may be used occasionally by Pitta.

Peppercorns: *Marica, kali mirch, safed mirch.* Grown in profusion along the world's oldest spice shores, the Malabar Coast, and throughout the southwest regions of India; there are notably three colors of black, white, and green. Although there are a variety of colors grown throughout the world, the peppercorn is used in a great variety of foods. It is the dried fruit or berry of a vine. They are harvested unripened and then sun-dried. They are ground, crushed, or used whole. Great for digestive stimulation, this is one of the three heating spices used in the ancient Ayurveda formula called *trikatu.* The other two ingredients are ginger and pippali.

Poppy seeds: *Khas khas, pusta.* These are the off-white, tiny seeds of the poppy plant. They are used ground, wet-ground, or whole in many vegetable dishes. They have high oil content like most seeds and lend a nutty flavor to foods. Both the off-white and blue poppy seeds are available in the US. They may be used by all three doshas.

Rock salt: *Sendha namak.* A salt mined from the underground dry sea beds in its crystalline form. It is recommended in Ayurveda for use with cooking foods. It has the highest mineral content of any salt.

Saffron: *Kesar.* The stigmas of the saffron crocus have been cultivated in Asia Minor, India, China, and the Mediterranean. The deep carmine strands are a very expensive and sattvic accent to food. It is used in many milky desserts to add a perfumed sweetness and with basmati rice in Indian cuisine. The best saffron strands are available from Kashmir and Spain. It is excellent for Pitta types, but may be used by all types.

Sesame seeds: *Til.* These seeds are tiny, tear-shaped, and come in black and ivory colors. They grow in the pods of the sesame plant. They are fragrant and rich in oil and protein. They are washed and roasted, ground or used whole in dhal, rice, and milk. Sesame seeds are used profusely in religious ceremonies. The black seeds are generally used in ceremonies for the deceased and are thus not used for cooking in India. The sesame oil is used extensively in Ayurveda massage therapies. These seeds are good for Vata types.

Tamarind: *Imli.* The tamarind tree is native to India. The pulpy, podded tamarind fruit is used for its sour and fruity taste, and for its somewhat cooling effect in the hot weather. It is used throughout India in dhals, vegetables, and rice. It is also used to make confections. It is excellent for Vata types and occasional use for Pitta.

Turmeric: *Haldi.* Native to Southeast Asia and South India; like ginger, the rhizomes may be used dried or fresh. The roots are boiled, then sun-dried for several weeks. It is then ground and used in masalas, curries, dhals, rice, vegetables, and desserts in India. Although it is bitter, it is considered in Ayurveda to be good for all three doshas.

Varak: Varak is the exquisite soft filigree foils of gold and silver that are slivered and used to adorn foods from ancient times in India. The custom is derived from the Ayurveda use of *bhasma* with precious metals, pearl, and the conch shell. The sheets are made from the pure metal dust molded in between two parchment sheets and hammered until the dust sets into a foil. The gold varak may be used by Vata and Kapha types and the silver by Pitta.

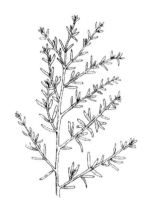

WISE EARTH AYURVEDA CULINARY ESSENCES

Essences are called *ruh* in India. Essences are extracted from herbs, spices, fruits, flowers, root, bark, wood, and the leaves of the trees. Essences are used in foods to help the body remember the cosmic nature of our beings. Scents and fragrant tastes are both important therapies in Ayurveda. The aromatic oils and essences invoke the peaceful sattvic nature of the human.

Essences have been used even before the Vedic period. They are water distilled and extracted without the use of chemicals or alcohols. The most popular essences used in Vedic cooking are from the rose petals, the vetiver's roots, the flowers of the screw pine, and from sandalwood. They are used in the sweet brews, beverages, puddings, and desserts of India. Essences and essential oils are added to food only after the food has been removed from the fire.

Khus essence: *Khas khas.* Khus essence is extracted from the roots of the vetiver grass grown throughout the typical world. The roots are used for making hand fans. The essence of the khus grass is sweet and cooling. The khus oil has a strong, deep aroma of the forest. This essence is good for all three doshas.

Sandalwood essence: *Ruh chandan.* The wood is known as *chandan* and the oil as *chandan tel.* Sandalwood is native to India and grows in Tamil Nadu and Mysore. This is the most exquisite wood and has been used to carve deities and build temples. The chandan paste is used in Hindu ceremonies and worn on the forehead as a constant inducement of our calmer nature. It is a cooling paste, powder, oil, or essence. Sandalwood is used in Ayurveda pharmacology and aromatherapy. It is also used in small amounts in Vedic cooking. The oil is mixed in syrup as a revitalizer. Sandalwood paste can be made by using a piece of sandalwood and rubbing it on a flat stone. Add a few drops of water to allow a paste to form. This essence is excellent for all three doshas.

Screw pine essence: *Ruh kewra.* This essence comes from screw pine trees. This pine grows mostly in South India. The screw pine bears beautiful perfumed flowers and sweet fruits. This essence is good for Vata and Kapha types and for occasional use by Pitta.

Rose essence: *Ruh gulab.* The ruh essence is extracted from the petals of the rose. The rose water or *kewra* is extracted through a process of infusion and distillation. The rose oil, essence, and water is used throughout India to accent sweet beverages. The rose essence and oil are used in Ayurveda aromatherapy. This essence is excellent for both Vata and Pitta types.

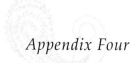

Appendix Four

VEDIC RESOURCES

**Wise Earth Ayurveda Education
Program Leaders**
Nina Molin, MD
P.O. Box 82
Lenox, MA 01240
Telephone: 413-822-0852
E-mail: ninamolin@ananda-health.com

Sarita Linda Rocco
734 Penn Avenue
West Reading, PA 19611
Telephone: 610-376-2881
E-mail: yogainlet@verizon.net

**Wise Earth Ayurveda
Education Coordinator, US**
Yogamaya Doe Wails
102 S 6th Avenue
West Reading, PA 19611
Telephone: 610-750-3572
E-mail: yogamaya@wisearth.org

Wise Earth School of Ayurveda, Ltd.
P.O. Box 160
Candler, NC 28715
Telephone: 828-258-9999
E-mail: inquiry@wisearth.org
Website: www.wisearth.org

Mother Om Mission
Executive Office
4255 Seton Avenue
Yonkers, NY 10466
Telephone: 347-804-8661
E-mail: mom@wisearth.org
Website: www.motherom.org

Mother Om Media
Sales & Marketing
P.O. Box 2094
Sinking Spring, PA 19608
E-mail: sales@motherommedia.com
Website: www.motherommedia.com

Mother Om Media
Public Relations
P.O. Box 277
New York, NY 10014
Telephone: 646-982-7595
E-mail: press@motherommedia.com
Website: www.motherommedia.com

Living Ahimsa Foundation
(My Peace Vow)
c/o Wise Earth School
P.O. Box 160
Candler, NC 28715
Website: www.MyPeaceVow.com

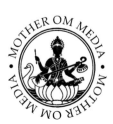

WISE EARTH AYURVEDA
UNITED STATES INSTRUCTORS

Joa Agnello-Traista
Center for Health and Harmony
P.O. Box 106
(264 Harvey Road)
Worthington, MA 01098
Telephone: 413-238-5336
E-mail: joasong@surfglobal.net

Jane Allen
P.O. Box 1116
Cornelius, NC 28031
Telephone: 704-973-0962
E-mail: janeallen@mindspring.com

Chris Arcucci
Divine Play Holistic Health
P.O. Box 2175
Mammoth Lakes, CA 93546
Telephone: 760-934-9343
E-mail: chris@divineplay.us

Margo Bachman
The Heart of Wellness
P.O. Box 4352
Santa Fe, NM 87502
Telephone: 505-670-4506
E-mail: info@heartofwellness.com

Latika Polly Breen
Blisslight Yoga
21430 Blakely Shores Drive
Cornelius, NC 28031
Telephone: 704-280-0805
          704-439-3195
E-mail: mbnamaste@aol.com

Karen Ling Chestnut
204 Crighton Circle
Fort Washington, MD 20744
Telephone: 240-351-3335
E-mail: klccye@yahoo.com

Sangita Hilary Clark
379 Baltic Street
Brooklyn, NY 11201
Telephone: 347-228-4634
E-mail: hdreamerc@aol.com

Blanca Colón-Simon
1546 Citrus Avenue
Chico, CA 95926
Telephone: 530-893-4792
E-mail: blancuz@pacbell.net
blancacolonsimon@gmail.com

Bhavani-Rebekah Crisp
104 Standish Drive
Chapel Hill, NC 27517
Telephone: 928-282-6060
E-mail: iiiiam1@hotmail.com

Brooke Dillane
900 Pinecrest Avenue, SE
Grand Rapids, MI 49506
Telephone: 616-855-2517
E-mail: beehive@dillane.net

Natalie Donnellon
4381 Barchester Drive
Bloomfield Hills, MI 48302
Telephone: 248-417-2628
E-mail: natalied3@mac.com

Cada Driscoll
88 Oak Hill Road
Barrington, NH 03825
Telephone: 603-285-5450
E-mail: Cmdriscoll3@plymouth.edu

Rebecca Egbert
362A Chase Way
Bozeman, MT 59715
Telephone: 406-581-1157
E-mail: rebecca@greenmidwife.com

Debra Farmer
6395 US HWY 53
Eau Claire, WI 54701
Telephone: 715-832-4436

Gretchen Fellon
300 Wall Street Unit 703
Saint Paul, MN 55101
Telephone: 651-228-7796
E-mail: sweetiepea78@hotmail.com

Carrie Finnegan
1788 Treasure Lake Section 15 Lot 198
Dubois, PA 15801
Telephone: 903-390-8526
E-mail: finnegancarrie@yahoo.com

Ilene Fischman
5 Crossgate Lane
Robesonia, PA 19551
Telephone: 610-693-6880
E-mail: fsh5sb@verizon.net

Margo Gebraski
2138 Countryside Circle
Naperville, IL 60565
Telephone: 630-609-8215
E-mail: mgebraski@yahoo.com

Ganga Suzanne Goldston
Ancient Roots Yoga & Ayurveda
1823 Kempton Avenue
Charleston, SC 29412
Telephone: 843-343-6848
E-mail: gangamagoddess@aol.com

Meredith Hart
P.O. Box 108
Plainfield, VT 05667
Telephone: 802-324-4434
E-mail: riversgraceyoga@me.com

Frank Heller
Acupuncture Ayurveda Chiropractic
    Clinic, Ltd.
550 40th Avenue NE
Columbia Heights, MN 55421
Telephone: 612-871-7190
E-mail: frankhellerdc@gmail.com

Karen Moore Holliday
1414 Drift Road
Westport, MA 02790
Telephone: 508-636-7361
E-mail: girijasings@yahoo.com

Lila Linnea Lindberg Jepsen
Great Grains Conversations for Health
1658 Dauphin Avenue
Wyomissing, PA 19610
Telephone: 610-372-7248
E-mail: linnealj@verizon.net

Rosemary Didi Jordan
40 East 9th St. #10J
New York, NY 10003
Telephone: 310-795-7782
E-mail: rosemarydidijordan@gmail.com

Ellen Joseph
P.O. Box 35
Embudo, NM 87531
Telephone: 505-579-4540
E-mail: raquel19482003@yahoo.com

Kathryn Julyan
The Veda Project
2114 South Wall Street
Spokane, WA 99203
Telephone: 509-710-9123
E-mail: thevedaproject@gmail.com

Lolo Khan
P.O. Box 99846
Emeryville, CA 94662
Telephone: 415-717-6319
E-mail: lkveda@yahoo.com

Leanne Korb
10 Leicester Way
Pawtucket, RI 02860
Telephone: 401-726-1521
E-mail: lkorb4@aol.com

Judith Daya Kubish
921 West Glendale Avenue
Glendale, WI 53209-6513
Telephone: 414-221-9293
E-mail: judithkubish@mcleodusa.net

Barbara Loomis
1621 SE Elliott Avenue
Portland, OR 97214
Telephone: 503-341-0663
E-mail: barbara@nurturance.net

Linda Mandolos
289 Maple Grove Road
Mohnton, PA 19540
Telephone: 610-777-5768
E-mail: friendlyflo@aol.com

Lindsey Mann
238 Second Avenue
Decatur, GA 30030
Telephone: 770-335-7292
          706-338-4835
E-mail: lindseyemann@gmail.com
ashtangayogaatlanta@gmail.com

Laura Martin-Eagle
Moon Jewel Healing
2 East 7th Street
Lawrence, KS 66044
Telephone: 785-550-8931
E-mail: bemovedstudio@yahoo.com

Cat Matlock
West Asheville Yoga
602 Haywood Road
Asheville, NC 28806
Telephone: 828-350-1167
E-mail: info@westashevilleyoga.com

Ambika Theresa McGhee
Lotus Center for Health & Healing
1369 Glenwood Avenue
Atlanta, GA 30316
Telephone: 404-561-8873
E-mail: tessmcghee@yahoo.com

Kathryn Shankari McKann
152 Hidden Trails Road
Port Townsend, WA 98368
Telephone: 360-379-9209
E-mail: unmutable@wildmail.com

Devi Elizabeth McKenty
265 Coleman Road
Middletown, CT 06457
Telephone: 860-670-4880
E-mail: queeneliz@snet.net

Marcia Meredith RN, NP
Surya Ayurveda Wellness Center
1552 Osceola Avenue
Saint Paul, MN 55105
Telephone: 651-503-0471
E-mail: Marcia@suryaayurveda.com

Nina Molin, MD
Ananda Health Center for
   Integrative Medicine
P.O. Box 82
Lenox, MA 01240
Telephone: 413-822-0852
E-mail: ninamolin@ananda-health.com

Kimberly Mulvaney
1904 Spring Garden Street #44
Philadelphia, PA 19130
Telephone: 484-716-5190
E-mail:
kimberly_mulvaney@yahoo.com

Monica Novak
4064 N Lincoln Box 104
Chicago, IL 60618
Telephone: 312-929-9007
E-mail: Monicanovak17@gmail.com

Sandra Paradis
617 Union Ave Unit 1-11
Brielle, NJ 08730
Telephone: 732-528-5860
E-mail: Sandi-d@verizon.net

Nitya Jess Oppenheimer
Healing With Plants
143 Eagle Street #4
Albany, NY 12202
Telephone: 518-495-5085
E-mail: healingwithplants@gmail.com

Ailene Sunari Radcliffe
Ayurveda Center for Natural
   Healthcare
665 Emory Valley Road, Suite A
P.O. Box 6408
Oak Ridge, TN 37831
Telephone: 865-406-1143
             865-482-0981
E-mail: tennessee226@comcast.net

Medha Shilpa Rao
1304 West Marlboro Drive
Chandler, AZ 85224
Telephone: 480-963-5683
E-mail: shilpakka@cox.net

Mary Vaishnavi Roberson, PhD
Ayurveda Center for Natural
   Healthcare
665 Emory Valley Road, Suite A
P.O. Box 6408
Oak Ridge, TN 37831
Telephone: 865-482-0981
E-mail: ayurvedacentertn@bellsouth.net

Sarita Linda Rocco
   & Dhira Michael Rocco
Yoga Inlet
734 Penn Avenue
West Reading, PA 19611
Telephone: 610-376-2881
E-mail: yogainlet@verizon.net

Todd Roderick
238 Second Avenue
Decatur, GA 30030
Telephone: 770-335-7292
            706-338-4835
E-mail: lindseyemann@gmail.com
ashtangayogaatlanta@gmail.com

Marci Rhodes
3927 Maravic Place
Sarasota, FL 34231
Telephone: 941-363-0783
E-mail: yogaonthekey@comcast.net

Shasvati Ellen Rosenkrantz
Yoga Inlet
734 Penn Avenue
West Reading, PA 19611
Telephone: 610-223-2466
E-mail: shaswati@dejazzd.net

Linda Rowe
The Mindful Way
52 Main Street, 2nd Floor
Houlton, ME 04730
Telephone: 207-551-4055
E-mail: mindfulway@mfx.net

Bridget Shields
c/o Pratima Ayurvedic Skincare
    Clinic & Spa
110 Greene Street, Suite 701
New York NY 10012
Telephone: 646-373-1336
E-mail: info@bridgetshields.com

Mary Ann Shultz
1290 Union
Platteville, WI 53818
Telephone: 608-348-2604
E-mail: mashultz4@hotmail.com

Marianne Steenvoorden, RYT
Heaven on Earth Yoga
8818 Golfview Drive
Orland Park, IL 60462
Telephone: 708-349-1874
E-mail: msteen4den@sbcglobal.net

Susan Stibler
44 Oak Hill Road
Barrington, NH 03825
Telephone: 603-664-2423
E-mail: susans@metrocast.net

Mary Ann Shultz
1290 Union
Platteville, WI 53818
Telephone: 608-348-2604
E-mail: Mashultz4@hotmail.com

Chelynn Tetreault, LMT
Little Lotus
240 John Ford Road
Ashfield, MA 01330
Telephone: 617-939-7657
E-mail: chelynnt@hotmail.com

Floriana Tullio
6658 Youree Drive, #180
P.O. Box 151
Shreveport, LA 71105
Telephone: 718-744-4256
E-mail: flori12@hotmail.com

Cary Dharani Twomey
Haymarket Pilates & Yoga Center
311 North Eighth Street, #210
Lincoln, NE 68508
Telephone: 402-477-5101
Email: carytwomey@aol.com

Joan Warwick
1112 Third Street, Suite 2
Neptune Beach, FL 32266
Telephone: 904-349-0529
E-mail: joanwarwick@bellsouth.net

Mary Beth Weber, DC
Center for Kriya Studies
3102 Chesterfield Avenue
Charleston, WV 25304
Telephone: 304-346-6688
E-mail: mbmango@hotmail.com

Deb Young
209 Wales Way
Blandon, PA 19510
Telephone: 484-797-0075
E-mail: dyoung0511@msn.com

Joy Young
125 Keough Road
Collierville, TN 38017
Telephone: 901-861-4885
E-mail: radiantwealth81@yahoo.com

Kalyani Evy Zavolas
1500 Hudson Street, Apt 4T
Hoboken, NJ 07030
Telephone: 551-998-2346
E-mail: evykalyani@gmail.com

WISE EARTH AYURVEDA INTERNATIONAL INSTRUCTORS

Australia

Wise Earth Ayurveda Program Leader
Priti Kotecha
Lotus Yoga Centre
457 Brookfield Road
Kenmore Hills
Brisbane, QLD 4069
Australia
Telephone: +61-07-3374-1495
E-mail: lotusyogacentre@gmail.com

Katie Manitsas
Jivamukti Yoga, Sydney
76 Wilford Street
Newtown, NSW 2042
Australia
Telephone: +61-02-9517-3280
E-mail: katiemanitsas@hotmail.com

Mary Woolley
Ananda Veda
15 Madison Drive
Adamstown Heights, NSW 2289
Australia
Mobile: +61-04-00-494166
Telephone: +61-02-49-575727
E-mail: mary@anandaveda.com.au

Brazil

Wise Earth Ayurveda Program Leader
Dr. Ana Maria Araújo Rodrigues
Avenida Afonso Peña 4273 / 7ñ
Belo Horizonte, Minas Gerais
CEP 30130-008
Brazil
Telephone: +55-31-3227-9855
+55-31-3264-3152
E-mail: dra.ana.clinicadasaude@gmail.com

Canada

Wise Earth Ayurveda
Program Leader
Jennifer Lynn Gillis
Mangalam Mandiram
109-2133 Dundas Street
Vancouver, BC V5L1J7
Canada
Telephone: 778-893-1859
E-mail:
mangalam.mandiram@gmail.com

Dana Lerman, ND
Doctor of Naturopathic Medicine
Pure Intent Healing Arts Center
64 Oxford Street
Toronto, ON M5T1P2
Canada
Telephone: 416-466-3237
E-mail: dana@pureintent.ca

Parvati-Angela Lytle
405-151 Robinson Street
Oakville, ON L6J7N3
Canada
Telephone: 289-838-8716
E-mail: parvati@lilayoga.com

Tanya Nash
383 Ravenhill Avenue
Ottawa, Ontario
K2A 0J5 Canada
Telephone: +1-613-325-9642
E-mail: tanya@omammamoon.com

Glynnis Osher
405 West 5th Avenue
Vancouver, BC V5Y 1J9
Canada
Telephone: 917-239-5594 (US)
         604-876-3994 (Canada)
E-mail: info@themysticmasala.com

France

Margarita Prokunina
68 Rue de la Vierge
01710 Thoiry, France
Telephone: +33-606-49-90-14
E-mail: mprokunina@gmail.com

India

Durga Amy Kowalski
Sivananda Yoga Vedanta
    Dhanwantari Ashram
P.O. Neyyar Dam, Trivandrum
Kerala 695 572, India
E-mail: sivadurga108@yahoo.com

United Kingdom & Ireland

Patrizia Faggi
Blooming Lotus Wellness
6 Blithfield Street
Kensington
W8 6RH
London, UK
Cellular: +0207-598-428-395
Telephone: +0207-937-4916
E-mail: info@bloominglotuswellness.com

Rosemarie Sellers
Nutrition & Well Being Center
    for Women
Mill Farm, Bitterley
Ludlow, Shropshire SY8 3HF, UK
Telephone: +01-584-891144
Cellular: +07-738-392307
E-mail: rosemarie@loka.org.uk

Cliodhna Mulhern
Flowstone
Lisardhalla Lodge
127 Ardmore Road
Derry-Londonderry
BT47 3TD, N Ireland
Telephone: +00-44-0-792-932-8513
E-mail: cliodhna@flowstone.org.uk

For updates on the Wise Earth Ayurveda Directory of Instructors, go to www.wisearth.org.

Kindly Note: *We do not recommend or endorse merchants, vendors, and suppliers: Instead, we recommend that you conduct an online search for suppliers in your country for ceremonial ingredients and utensils, as well as Vedic prayer beads and calendars mentioned in this book. However, at the time of printing this edition of* Living Ahimsa Diet, *we are aware of the following vendor:*

Himalayan Academy eStore
Kauai's Hindu Monastery
107 Kaholalele Road
Kapaa, HI 96746
Telephone: 1-808-822-3012
E-mail: contact@hindu.org
        www.minimela.com
- Free Online Vedic Calendar
- Vedic Art of Gods and Goddesses
- Prayers Beads (Malas)
- Puja Kits

INDEX

ABOUT THE AUTHOR

Having served more than a quarter century as a Vedic monk, belonging to India's prestigious Veda Vyasa lineage, Maya Tiwari (Mother Maya) has been praised by the Parliament of the World's Religions for her outstanding work in creating peace, inner harmony, and wellness in the world. Mother Maya's time-tested ability to inspire and create change in human behavior and understanding is a matter of flawless record from the past 27 years of her devout work in the United States and around the world. She founded the Wise Earth School of Ayurveda, Mother Om Mission, and the Living Ahimsa Foundation, and received the prestigious Dhanvantari International Award in 2011 for her pioneering work in Ayurveda education.

She is the embodiment of unwavering peace, and a spiritual pioneer who serves humanity through her award-winning work awakening the spirit of ahimsa, harmony, in every person whose life she touches. In her extraordinary service to humanity, Mother has helped nourish, nurture, and heal thousands of individuals and families, affecting hundreds of communities. She works from the trenches of the inner cities to the halls of the privileged, transcending cultural and social barriers. Her revolutionary work in spiritual healing education has served scores of at-risk communities in Guyana, India, and the United States.

Mother Maya has been tirelessly guiding and educating humanity with her charitable holistic work through hundreds of venues around the world. For more than two decades, Mother has been addressing large audiences and training thousands of volunteer instructors to help serve hundreds of communities. In her work through Wise Earth School and Mother Om Mission, she pioneered the Inner Medicine health and spirituality programs based in Ayurveda; as well as the Living Ahimsa work that is deeply based in the principle of inner harmony, honoring the sanctity of all beings, all species, nature and her sacred resources.

In 2010, Mother made the stunning decision to renounce her monastic title and spiritual moniker—Her Holiness, Sri Swami Mayatitananda—and, as she puts it, "walk a simpler and more accessible life in service of the populations in need." Mother's universal path to inner harmony and non-hurting brings with it a renewed sense of joy, freedom, and stability for all—reconciling the myriad conflicts in our everyday lives, and bringing about a lasting sense of harmony. Author of many best-selling books on health, wellness, and spirituality, her potent spirit of ahimsa touches the hearts of people across the world. Her books include: *Living Ahimsa Diet: Nourishing Love & Life, Women's Power to Heal through Inner Medicine; The Path of Practice: A Woman's Book of Ayurvedic Healing; Ayurveda: A Life of Balance; and Ayurveda Secrets of Healing.*

Mother Maya's Keynote Presentation at the 2009 Parliament of the World's Religions, alongside the Dalai Lama and other great men and women of faith, had a dramatic impact on the consciousness of each of its participants. She eloquently addressed the theme of global reconciliation through the lens of her Living Ahimsa work: "By cultivating personal awareness of ahimsa we can find a common language that needs no words—a communion centered in the heart of oneness. If each one of us makes a commitment to inner harmony, we will surely succeed in achieving the ultimate goal of our human destiny—that of a spiritual freedom that unites us. Ultimately, it is the work of awareness within the individual person that will change the world for the better."

For information on Mother Maya's itinerary and Living Ahimsa World Tour visit:
www.mothermaya.com ~ www.facebook.com/MayaTiwari
www.MyPeaceVow.com

Living Ahimsa Diet: Nourishing Love & Life and other Mother Om Media titles can be purchased through the following distributors:

US:
Ingram
Amazon.com
Baker & Taylor
Barnes & Noble
NACSCORP
Espresso Book Machine

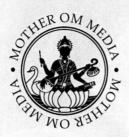

MOTHER OM MEDIA

More than a series of revolutionary books on
Ahimsa, Health, Harmony, Love, Life & Nourishment

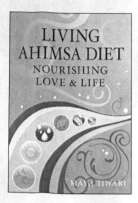 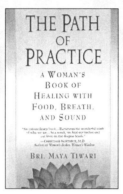 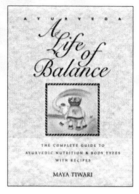 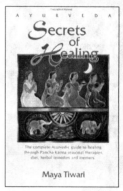

Mother Maya (Maya Tiwari) is an extraordinary spiritual teacher who healed herself from ovarian cancer at the age of 23, and went on to become an expert in Ayurveda education and a world spiritual leader as Her Holiness, Swami Mayatitananda, before renouncing her monastic title to "walk a simpler and more accessible life in service of the populations in need."

Also available from Mother Om Media:

Women's Power to Heal through Inner Medicine
Love! A Daily Oracle for Healing

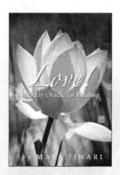 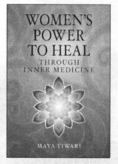

Be the First to Learn More!

New and upcoming titles from Maya Tiwari
Living Ahimsa Workshops schedule
Connect with Wise Earth Ayurveda community at large

motherommedia.com • ahimsalife.com • mothermaya.com • facebook.com/MayaTiwari

Breinigsville, PA USA
08 March 2011
257155BV00005B/1/P

9 780979 327926